Nutrition in Institutions

D1493036

Nutrition in Institutions

Maria Cross
and
Barbara MacDonald

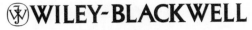

WILEY-BLACKWELL

A John Wiley & Sons, Ltd., Publication

This edition first published 2009
© 2009 Maria Cross and Barbara MacDonald

Blackwell Publishing was acquired by John Wiley & Sons in February 2007. Blackwell's publishing programme has been merged with Wiley's global Scientific, Technical, and Medical business to form Wiley-Blackwell.

Registered office
John Wiley & Sons Ltd, The Atrium, Southern Gate, Chichester, West Sussex, PO19 8SQ, United Kingdom

Editorial offices
9600 Garsington Road, Oxford, OX4 2DQ, United Kingdom
2121 State Avenue, Ames, Iowa 50014-8300, USA

For details of our global editorial offices, for customer services and for information about how to apply for permission to reuse the copyright material in this book please see our website at www.wiley.com/wiley-blackwell.

Library of Congress Cataloging-in-Publication Data

Cross, Maria.
Nutrition in institutions / Maria Cross and Barbara MacDonald. – 1st ed.
    p. cm.
  Includes bibliographical references and index.
  ISBN 978–1-4051–2125-5 (pbk. : alk. paper) 1. Public institutions–Food service.
    2. Public institutions–Food service–Great Britain. 3. Nutrition. 4. Nutrition–Great Britain.
    I. MacDonald, Barbara. II. Title.

  TX946.C76 2009
  363.8′2—dc22

                                                                    2008022793

A catalogue record for this book is available from the British Library.

Set in 10/12.5 pt Sabon by Newgen Imaging Systems Pvt. Ltd, Chennai, India
Printed in Singapore by Utopia Press Pte Ltd

1   2009

Contents

Part 2   Hospitals   103

Barbara MacDonald

Part 3   Care homes for the elderly   217
Barbara MacDonald

Part 4   Prisons   275
Maria Cross

Part 5   Armed forces   361

Maria Cross

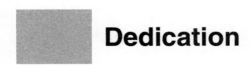 # Dedication

Barbara MacDonald would like to dedicate Part 3 – Care Homes for the Elderly – to Norman Lewis Perryman 1928–2006.

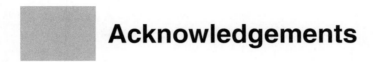

Acknowledgements

Maria Cross and Barbara MacDonald would like to thank Peter Cross and William MacDonald for their constant support in the writing of this book. Special thanks go to Peter Cross for providing all the technical drawings. The authors would also like to express their appreciation to all the individuals and organisations, too numerous to mention, who kindly provided so much invaluable information.

Introduction

'All public sector bodies, especially those that serve the most vulnerable in our society (for example, children and especially looked-after children, the sick, the elderly, the disadvantaged), have a duty to provide appetising, healthy and nutritious meals, consistent with expert advice. Appetising, healthy food can lead to faster patient recovery times, less malnutrition, better educational attainment, less disruptive behaviour, higher productivity and less food waste'. (DH, 2005a)

Large-scale institutional feeding has its roots in the workhouse, and although the workhouse no longer exists, many people still rely on institutions for their food, with hundreds of millions of meals being served annually.

Fortunately, the quality of institutional food has improved since the austerity of workhouse provision was last inflicted on its unfortunate recipients, but in many cases there is still some way to go in terms of quality and service. There is much variation among different types of institution, and within the establishments of each institution, with the result that provision is far from equitable. All five institutions described in this book have experienced peaks and troughs along the road to dietary adequacy, with some making more progress than the others. There have been times in the past when there was remarkably more dedication to better provision than there is now, and after centuries of providing food in institutions, the art of doing so has still not been uniformly perfected.

Institutions have a moral obligation to feed those in their care as well as possible, regardless of their perceived value to society. This obligation requires a non-judgemental ethos which does not bestow greater entitlement on one group over another. In the long term, ensuring good food for all is to everyone's advantage. Children are better behaved and better able to learn; prisoners – who in the vast majority of cases will return to society – are calmer and less aggressive; the military perform better. The sick are more likely to recover faster, and therefore reduce the burden on the NHS and the elderly more likely to enjoy their final years.

Regardless of the policy ideology behind food provision, the fact is that people eat primarily because they are hungry and because they enjoy eating, not because they want to stave off heart disease, or be better behaved. Within each institution, food means something different to those who eat it. Food can be symbolic of authority and control; it can make people feel powerless, and naturally inclined to rebel against it. Choices may be restricted, and the freedom to not only choose but grow and then cook one's own food (for many a normal human activity) is removed. In prison, food can be a trigger for aggressive behaviour, but also provide comfort, as it can to members of the armed forces in combat situations. In hospitals and care homes food can provide something to look forward to, perhaps to break the monotony of the day. Some institutions provide an opportunity for communal dining, which itself can be a positive experience, especially for those children who are used to eating their evening meal alone at home.

Whatever its symbolism, feeding people in institutions is always a complex logistical exercise in which those responsible have to cater for large numbers of people within strict budgetary controls. Meals have to be produced in large quantities at pre-determined times. These meals have to be maintained at certain temperatures for extended periods, whilst both meeting health and safety standards and maintaining an appealing appearance. Religious and lifestyle dietary requirements must be accommodated and minimum choices made available; nutritional standards (where applicable) have to be met, and inspections passed. The more criteria that must be met, the greater the risk of failing to meet them. Thus, for millions of people, their health, healing, strength, behaviour, concentration and learning are often at the mercy of caterers, food suppliers and institutional staff, all of whom operate on different agendas.

It is not surprising therefore that complaints about food in institutions are a long-standing tradition, because whichever institution one may find oneself in, there are bound to be times (frequently, in prisons) when a certain amount of resentment towards that institution is felt and criticising the food provided is a form of dissent.

It is not just those who have to eat what's provided who are now finding fault with the service. Never before has food in institutions attracted so much media and public attention or provoked so much debate. It started with schools (the 'Jamie Oliver effect') and the shock of seeing on television just what was being served up to the nation's children. There has been a groundswell of criticism of food served in hospitals and care homes, but to a lesser extent and largely dominated by issues relating to malnutrition.

The Department of Health in its 2004 annual report admits that budgetary constraints and other issues mean that '*the nutritional value of food is often pushed to the bottom of the checklist during the tendering process*' (DH, 2005a). To be fair, the nutritional value of food is also to be found, quite frequently, at the bottom of the checklist of the people who actually eat it. We have seen that across institutions people do not always make healthy choices – in fact most of the time they would rather eat familiar, preferred foods. New Labour has repeated the mantra of choice many times, but there remains the question of whether or not choice is always a good thing. This is especially relevant to children who have, until recently, been free to choose all the processed food they could manage at school. The current backlash against 'nanny state' government interference overlooks the fact that children constitute a population group much neglected by nanny in recent years. In other institutions, other ethical dilemmas arise. Is it immoral to provide 'unhealthy' food in hospitals, and allow fast food purveyors to ply their wares to the sick? Conversely, should the elderly be force-fed healthy food, when all they want in their final years is good, tasty food that is familiar, fresh and plentiful? Does entitlement to healthy food mean an obligation to eat it?

Simply providing 'healthy' options may not improve the diet of consumers if they are always able to choose 'unhealthy' options. In reality, choice is frequently more about giving food manufacturers the freedom to concoct and sell food of appalling nutritional quality but considerable consumer attraction. Processed food is cheap, so appeals to both manufacturers and procurers. Education is frequently proposed as a means of persuading people to make the right (i.e., healthy) choices. This book shows that education alone has little influence on what people choose to eat. We eat for different reasons, and determinants of choice can be complex and have little to do with health and nutrition. Awareness of healthy eating does not necessarily lead to healthy eating in practice. This is particularly true of children who are surprisingly enlightened on the value of healthy food, but have little interest in applying their knowledge.

The public sector in England (including the NHS, central government, local authorities, the education system, prisons and the armed forces) spends nearly £2 billion annually on food and catering services (DH, 2005b). Not only are there variations in quality of provision, there are also wide variations in expenditure between public sector bodies, as evidenced by Table I.1.

More spending should not, however, be taken as an indication of better food. Our research has found that the armed forces are more likely than any other

Table I.1 Public sector food expenditure, 2004–05.

Food procurer	Daily food cost per individual (£)	Annual food cost (£ million)	Meals per day
Primary schools	0.40–0.65 (range) (lunch only)	234 (approx)	1
Secondary schools	0.5–0.64 (range) (lunch only)	126 (approx)	1
Hospitals[a]	2.50 (average)	300	3
Prison service	1.87 (average)	43	3
MoD	2.00–2.20 (range)	135 (including delivery costs)	3

[a] Figures not available for care homes.

Source: NAO (2006a).

institution to provide good quality food, even though they do not have the greatest expenditure. Even within the same institution, variations in expenditure and quality are evident.

It is crucial that available funds are wisely invested, and best value viewed in a broad context. Historically, government policy on food procurement has been formulated on the principle of value for money, and the Department of Health has admitted that its definition of value for money is narrow and short-term (DH, 2005a). It does not take into account the financial burden of chronic disease, even though the DH acknowledges that cancer, heart disease and stroke, the major causes of death in England, are all diet related and estimates that the cost to the NHS of treating the effects of poor diet is around £4 billion per year (DH, 2005b).

Environmental and sustainability issues have also, in the last few years, emerged as priorities on the public sector food procurement agenda. According to the NAO:

'The particular challenge faced by public sector food procurers today is to reduce the costs of catering, while making progress towards Government objectives on increasing sustainability and nutritional quality'.   (NAO, 2006b)

It is generally acknowledged that the provision of food for large numbers of people is bound to impact on the environment. Much of what is procured for institutions within the UK is sourced from outside (2005a). Table I.2 shows the percentage of UK-produced food supplied by public sector procurers. In 2003 the Public Sector Food Procurement Initiative (PSFPI) was launched, under the auspices of the Department for Environment, Food and Rural Affairs (DEFRA) to help deliver *'a world-class sustainable farming and food sector that contributes to a better environment and healthier and prosperous communities'.* The PSFPI aims to encourage a broader approach to the procurement of food consumed in public institutions and canteens by advocating: higher standards of production; increased tenders from small and local producers; increased consumption of healthy food; reduced adverse environmental impacts and increased capacity of small and local suppliers to meet the demand. This is a formidable remit, not least because food buyers must adhere to free trade regulations and not restrict purchases to specific locations or suppliers (DEFRA, 2006).

Efficient procurement should not be interpreted as buying the cheapest available, a policy which in the past has proven to be disastrous. In its broadest sense, best

Table I.2 Percentage of UK produce purchased by public sector procurers.

	NHS Supply Chain	Ministry of Defence	HM Prison Service
UK-produced food as a percentage of all food supplied	40	43	67

Source: PSFPI (2008).

value not only encompasses good nutrition and food safety at the best price, but also takes into consideration local producers, communities and the natural environment. To this end the government launched, in March 2006, a website – the National Opportunities Portal (http://www.supply2.gov.uk) – with the aim of making local suppliers aware of forthcoming public sector tenders and supply opportunities. *In Smarter food procurement in the public sector*, the NAO (2006b) concluded that:

> 'There is significant scope for increasing efficiency simply through raising the professionalism of public sector food procurement, and by the public sector's pursuing a more joined up approach, and that such measures need have no negative effect on the quality of food served. Indeed, increasing efficiency can have a positive impact on sustainability and nutrition, by enabling organisations to use cost savings in some areas to help to finance improvements in others; for example, savings resulting from better checks on goods delivered could be used to improve the quality of ingredients purchased, or improved nutritional quality could lead to reduced hospital stays and so improve the overall efficiency of NHS trusts'.

The drive for more sustainable procurement is the latest development in an ongoing process of improvement and follows efforts across all institutions to impose standards on the nutritional quality of food provided. Those standards, however, are not necessarily met, even when they are statutory. Standards do not have to be statutory to be effective, as the armed forces have demonstrated. The reason for this is clear: if standards do not have a robust, effective system of audit and monitoring in place, they become ineffectual and therefore meaningless. For that reason, it is difficult to be optimistic about new Food Standards Agency (2007) guidelines on the provision of food in UK institutions – *Guidance on food served to adults in major institutions*. These guidelines are little more than a reiteration of existing government guidelines on healthy eating in general and reference nutrient intakes for adults aged 19–74 years. No advice is offered on enforcement and the guidelines are not institution-specific.

In drawing up guidelines for the provision of food in institutions there is little to add which has not already been said in the past. Writing for the *American Journal of Public Health*, in 1955, the chief nutritionist for the State Board of Health in Indianapolis laid out the objectives of a new institutional feeding programme (Dunham, 1955). These were to:

- standardise the food service
- establish uniformity in distribution of food
- provide sufficient amounts of the right kinds of food to meet the nutrition needs of the patients and employees of these institutions
- initiate an economical food purchasing programme (Dunham, 1955).

Today, some establishments have indeed adopted some or all of these objectives; many have not. Institutions would perhaps gain from observing each other's catering practices and adopting those methods which have proven most effective in attaining such objectives. From our research it has become clear that there are certain approaches which work well in practice. These are outlined in Table I.4 and include:

- Centralisation of management: The armed forces are the only institution to have a fully centralised management system and as a result the service is stream-lined, efficient and cost-effective. Central management means that the institution has full control over every aspect of food procurement and provision.
- In-house catering: Central management does not preclude a certain degree of independence within the establishments of each institution. There is, in some establishments, a small but growing trend towards bringing the catering service back in-house, after having previously out-sourced contracts to private, commercial companies. Doing so gives establishments more control and say over how the service is operated. They can also, where appropriate, employ those in their care in the kitchens.

  In-house catering can also be more economical: in the long term it is cheaper to buy in raw ingredients and pay someone to cook them than leave the whole service to an outside organisation. The problem with outsourcing the catering contract is that the institution in question is unaware of routine, volume-based discounts and rebates that the caterers may be receiving but not passing on (NAO, 2006b). The National Audit Office estimates that the largest UK catering firms may be earning up to around £95 million in discounts and rebates from suppliers, just through their contracts with public sector clients (NAO, 2006b). Prices of commonly purchased items have indeed been found to be consistently higher in those organisations which contracted out the catering service, compared with those who retained in-house services – see Table I.3.

- Stringent, well monitored standards: It is not essential for standards to be statutory – what matters is that they are mandatory within each institution and are strictly monitored. There needs to be a robust framework of audit and monitoring in place, with well-defined responsibilities for all concerned

Table I.3 Organisations that outsourced their catering paid more per item.

	Milk (1 pint whole milk) (pence)	Bread (800 g wholemeal) (pence)	Specified brand of cola (330 ml can) (pence)
In-house (average)	25.3	64.8	22.3
Contracted-out (average)	33.6	84.1	27.7

Source: NAO (2006b).

with procurement and provision. Ideally, standards should be subject to both internal and external monitoring, and those who actually eat the food provided should be allowed an opportunity to regularly express their views and make suggestions.

- Well-trained, well-valued catering staff: All too frequently, catering staff, especially those who are not employed in-house, are poorly paid and poorly trained. Despite poor pay and conditions, it often falls to caterers to acquire sound nutritional knowledge and encourage their customers to make healthy choices. It is hardly surprising when they fail to do so. Catering should be viewed, and valued, as an integral part of the overall service offered by the institution, and not as an essential if bothersome 'add-on'.

- Ability to provide quality food within the available budget: Those who rely on institutions for their food should, as a basic human right, be able to obtain at least five portions of fruit and vegetables a day. This is very often not the case, especially for those who are totally dependent on the institution in question for all their meals and snacks.

In those institutions where the recipients pay for their food (schools and armed forces) one of the greatest challenges currently facing the catering services is customer loyalty. The higher the take-up, the greater the income. Customers are at liberty to take their custom elsewhere if they do not like what's on offer. Therefore, prices must be competitive enough to keep customers on-site. One way to offer more competitive prices is to adopt more efficient sourcing of food products. In *Smarter food procurement in the public sector,* the NAO (2006b) describes case histories from schools, hospitals and the armed forces[1] and highlights the considerable variations in the costs of basic commodities purchased across the public sector. For example, a pint of milk ranged from 17 to 44 pence. Food procurement is common to many public bodies, so there is clearly potential for food procurers to come together to increase their purchasing power by aggregating demand and making joint purchases.

At the moment, the quality of food provided in institutions varies among institutions and frequently between the establishments of those institutions, because each takes a different approach. Table I.4 serves to highlight the different practices (as well as levels of commitment) of each institution.

I.1 Conclusion

All people in all institutions have the right to good and adequate food, but so far the service remains inequitable. In 2003 the media made much of a report published by the Soil Association which claimed that more money was spent per person on lunch in prisons than in schools (Soil Association, 2003). The result was public outrage, but this outrage was misplaced, not least because adults have greater dietary requirements than children. It is not so much wrong and outrageous

Table I.4. Comparison of provision of nutrition in institutions.

	Schools	Hospitals	Care homes	Prisons	Armed forces	Comments
Centralisation of management						
Centralised purchasing system	x	x	x	x	✓	Hospitals: may purchase via NHS contracts or through local negotiation Prisons: purchasing is not central, but central and regional contracts are in place
Same budget across all establishments	x	x	x	x	✓	
In-house catering						
In-house option available	✓x	✓x	✓	✓	✓	Schools & hospitals: option available only where the establishment is equipped with a kitchen
Opportunity for those in care of institution to prepare their own food	x	x	✓x	✓x	✓x	Care homes: depends on health status of resident and/or attitude of proprietor Prisons: inmates can prepare own food only in exceptional cases Armed forces: recipients do not have to eat in messes so can prepare their own food elsewhere.
Stringent, well-monitored standards						
Nutritional standards in place	✓	✓	✓	✓	✓	Schools: standards only in place since 2006/07
Are those standards statutory?	✓	✓	✓x	x	x	Care homes: not enforceable but are taken into account when assessing regulations Prisons & armed forces: standards are mandatory but not statutory
Are standards met?	✓	✓x	✓x	✓x	✓	Schools: only one inspection since introduction of new standards Hospitals: different surveys provide different results Care homes: seems to be dependent on staffing levels Prisons: most standards met but many are still not
Comprehensive manual available to caterers	✓	✓	✓	✓	✓	

Criterion	Schools	Hospitals	Care homes	Prisons	Notes
Effective, standardised monitoring system in place	✓	x	✓	✓	Schools: only since 2006/07 Hospitals: standards are self-assessed by Trusts Care homes: Doubts exist regarding unqualified inspectors
Standard procedure in place to monitor recipient's views	x	✓x	✓x	✓	Hospitals and care homes: limited questioning
Well-trained and valued catering staff					
Possibility for caterers to obtain qualifications	✓	✓	✓x	✓	Schools: only since new standards were introduced Prisons: only if in-house catering, where prisoners are employed, is provided
Members of institutions able to work in kitchens	n/a	n/a	n/a	✓	Prisons: only if in-house catering is provided
Ability to provide quality food within budget					
Sufficient quantities/calories provided	✓	✓x	✓x	✓	Hospitals & care homes: only if patient/resident is able to eat the food available Prisons: calorific value can be excessive, except in Scotland where it may be inadequate
At least 5 portions of fruit and vegetables daily	n/a	✓x	x	✓	Schools: choice of fruit and vegetables available at lunch Hospitals and care homes: if sample menus are followed
Choice of meals available	✓	✓	✓	✓	Care homes: often depends on attitudes of staff
Water freely available	✓	✓x	✓x	✓	Prisons: water available at mealtimes and at cell door if prisoner is allowed to have a flask
Religious or lifestyle requirements catered for	✓x	✓	✓	✓	Schools: it is up to the individual school but they are 'encouraged' to do so Hospitals: protected mealtimes in place.
Suitable timing of meals	✓	✓x	✓x	✓	Care homes: concerns that evening meal may be provided very early with snack not provided later Prisons: evening meal often supplied very early but small snack usually available for later.
Are efforts made to promote healthy eating	✓	✓	✓x	✓	Care homes: debatable whether relevant Prisons: depends on the establishment

that people in prisons should be adequately and humanely fed, but wrong and outrageous that those in other institutions – especially hospitals and care homes – are so often inadequately fed, and with so little humanity. The armed forces were quick to understand the provision of food as being crucial to the smooth running of the military machine and constitute the only institution to consistently value the link between diet and health and performance. Others are catching up fast, having previously been more focussed on the link between diet and financial gain. School food has recently been revolutionised and the Government should be congratulated on the bold changes it has instigated. The Prison Service has also made considerable and laudable progress in recent years in its efforts to improve the provision of food across the prison estate. But it is clear that those who are most vulnerable, and unable to stand up for themselves (quite literally), or riot on rooftops, are those most likely to receive the poorest quality food service. The most vulnerable have not so far found a campaigner to champion their cause, as Jamie Oliver did for schools. If all institutions aspired to the standards set by the armed forces, and applied the same level of organisation and commitment, the provision of nutrition would be more universally commendable.

Note

1   Prisons are covered in a separate report – NAO: *Serving Time: Prisoner Diet and Exercise*, (2006a).

References

DEFRA (2006) Unlocking opportunities: Lifting the lid on public sector food procurement. www.defra.gov.uk/farm/policy/sustain/procurement/index.htm (accessed 8 February 2008).

Department of Health (2005a) On the state of the public health: Annual report of the Chief Medical Officer 2004.

Department of Health (2005b) *Choosing a Better Diet: A Food and Health Action Plan.* London: HMSO.

Dunham, M.A. (1955) Institutional feeding – a challenge. *American Journal of Public Health*, 45:869–873.

Food Standards Agency (2007) *Guidance on Food Served to Adults in Major Institutions.* October 2007. FSA.

National Audit Office (NAO) (2006a) *Serving Time: Prisoner diet and exercise.* Report by the Comptroller and Auditor General. HC 939 Session 2005–2006. 9 March 2006. London: The Stationery Office.

National Audit Office (NAO) (2006b) *Smarter food procurement in the public sector.* Report by the Comptroller and Auditor General. HC 963-1 Session 2005–2006. 30 March 2006. London: The Stationery Office.

Public Sector Food Procurement Initiative (2008) *Proportion of domestically produced food used by Government departments and also supplied to hospitals and prisons under contracts negotiated by NHS Supply Chain and HM Prison Service.* www.defra.gov.uk (accessed February 2008).

Soil Association (2003) Food for Life: healthy, local, organic school meals. www.foodforlife.org.uk (accessed February 2008).

1 Schools

Maria Cross

1.1 Introduction

'The young need protection and it is proper that the state should take deliberate steps to give them opportunity ... Feeding is not enough, it must be good feeding. The food must be chosen in the light of knowledge of what a growing child needs for building a sound body. And when the food is well chosen, it must be well cooked. This is a task that calls for the highest degree of scientific catering; it mustn't be left to chance'. (Woolton, 1945)

The school dinner has carried a tarnished image throughout its history and remains a much-reviled feature of school life. The now infamous turkey twizzler has become a metaphor for the more parlous aspects of the school canteen. Yet anyone whose school days were lived out during the 1970s or earlier will easily recall the equally maligned daily dispensation of mashed potatoes, gravy, lumpy custard, and so on. Most would also recall that there was little or no choice, but that there was always a hot meal, consisting, in the main, of meat or fish, vegetables and potatoes which was followed by a traditional pudding.

The pre-1980s school meal may have been generally unloved, but there was little wastage. This may be because the post-war culture of easy disposablity had not at that stage fully emerged, but also because pupils had little or no recourse to alternative food sources. Some schools did run a tuck shop, but the now ubiquitous vending machine was still to enter school food culture. Children did not as a rule carry much money about them and perhaps would have regarded spending precious financial resources on food as profligate, especially as food was already provided at no additional personal cost.

The nature of the school meal, and the means by which it is provided, have undergone regular transformations ever since its nationwide introduction in 1906. In the post-war years it was a central and vital part of the welfare state, viewed as it was then as a medium to combat poverty, inequality and malnutrition. But in 1980 it was revolutionised on a massive scale by the new Conservative government and the changes introduced by the 1980 Education Act. Whereas pre-1980 grumblings about school meals were focussed on their gastronomic and quantitative shortcomings, post-1980 grievances have been, in the main, concerned with the nutritional quality and health implications of what is served up. It may be a human weakness to reflect on the past with an unrealistic conviction of its superiority, but few need to be persuaded of the rapid decline of school food post 1980. That year saw the transformation of the school meal from a means of providing essential nutrition to children to a privatised, commercial operation driven by market forces. The changes in the service were also widely regarded as part of an attempt to dismantle the welfare state overall.

Not only has the nature of school meals changed beyond recognition, so has the way they are produced and provided. Whereas children in the past were merely 'given' their meal, or 'fed', they are now consumers making choices in a commercially driven society. As a result, they are targeted by market forces which have to compete for each child's loyalty. Having this freedom to choose preferred foods, and having the money to do so, is extremely popular and appealing to children, especially those making the switch from primary to secondary school (Brannen & Storey, 1998).

The school lunch may only provide children with five out of twenty-one potential meals per week but for many children it is the main meal of the day, and often the only hot meal they receive. School meals make an important contribution to the diet and nutrition of school children, providing between one-quarter and one-third of the daily intake of energy, fat, fibre, iron, calcium, vitamin C and folate in 11 to 18-year-old children (Gregory et al., 2000). Primary school children consume one-fifth to one-third of their daily food intake at lunchtime (Gregory et al., 2000). People in lower socioeconomic groups tend to eat less fruit and fewer vegetables and fibre-rich foods (Acheson, 1998). Their diets tends to provide cheap, high-energy foods from dairy products, meats, sugar and cereals, with little intake of vegetables, fruits and wholegrains (James et al., 1997). A study published in 1983 found that children from lower income families ate larger school meals and obtained a larger proportion of their daily nutrient intake from school meals than children from higher income families (Nelson & Paul, 1983). In 2000, one in three children in Britain was found to be living in poverty, that is, their household income was less than 50% of average earnings (Nelson, 2000). The school environment therefore provides what is potentially an excellent opportunity to give a child, especially a child living in poverty, a healthy and nutritious meal.

For all children, the school is also an ideal setting to adopt healthy eating practices and learn about food – its provenance and how it affects health. The Government itself declared, in its 2004 White Paper *Choosing health: making healthy choices easier* that *'people's patterns of behaviour are often set early in life and influence their health throughout their lives. Infancy, childhood and young adulthood are critical stages in the development of habits that will affect people's health in later years'* (DH, 2004).

Unfortunately, however, making healthy choices does not appear to be something that concerns children a great deal. Surveys consistently show that children are perfectly aware of what constitutes a healthy meal – and what doesn't – but when given the choice will nearly always select an unhealthy option. Critics of Government policy claim that children should have restricted choice when it comes to school food.

Government initiatives to improve the quality of food in schools have, until recently, concentrated largely on voluntary self-regulation of the food industry and those who provide school meals, and decentralisation of responsibility of provision. Non-governmental organisations have persistently called for legislation, claiming that the food industry, whose whole raison d'être is to make a profit, can never effectively self-regulate. The main priority of school meal provision must, they claim, be the health of the child. Nutritional standards were abolished in 1980 and then replaced in 2001 by statutory standards, which were not effectively monitored and proved to be pointless. Alarm at the continued worsening of the quality of school food, and deteriorating health status of children of school age in the United Kingdom led to the introduction of new, compulsory standards from 2006 with monitoring by Ofsted. We can all only hope that these will go some way towards reversing the worrying trends which have come to dominate children's dietary choices.

1.2   The health of UK schoolchildren

'... A child of school age, habitually underfed at home, and unable in consequence to receive to purpose the instruction on which the State insists, presents one of the most difficult problems which modern civilisation is called upon to solve'.   (Booth, 1970)

Children fed a monotonous diet of poor quality, predominantly processed food do not thrive.   (School Meals Review Panel (SMRP), 2005)

There is little doubt that health and diet are inextricably linked, and that health in childhood is paramount if healthy adulthood and longevity are to be attained. Whereas surviving beyond childhood and its perils was once a goal in itself, the focus today has shifted from the dangers of infectious diseases to those of chronic diseases, which are largely determined by diet and nutrition (World Health Organization, 2003). Despite this knowledge, never before in our history have we, or our children, eaten such highly processed food, high in saturated fat, trans fatty acids, added sugar and salt. It is these highly processed foods which are thought to be responsible, to a large degree, for the demise of children's health. Chronic diseases, such as type 2 diabetes, once seen almost exclusively in adults, are now manifesting in children (Ebbeling et al., 2002). This is a global concern; the burden of diseases such as diabetes, cancer, cardiovascular disease and obesity is increasing rapidly in both developed and developing countries, appearing earlier in life than ever, and affecting all socioeconomic groups. It has been projected that, by 2020, chronic diseases will account for almost three-quarters of deaths worldwide (WHO, 2003). They have been traced from foetal to adult life and in adulthood are a reflection of lifetime exposures (WHO, 2003). A high calorie intake in childhood, for example, may be related to an increased risk of cancer in later life (WHO, 2003) and childhood obesity is associated with later development of heart disease and other chronic diseases (Cole *et al.*, 2000; Ebbeling *et al.*, 2002).

Obesity, a major cause of chronic disease, reduces life expectancy by 9 years, on average (NAO, 2001). The prevalence of obesity in children appears to be increasing, affecting a wide age range, most ethnic groups and every socioeconomic group (Ebbeling *et al.*, 2002). The proportion of obese girls aged 2 to 15 increased from 12.0% in 1995 to 18.1% in 2005. The proportion of obese boys aged 2 to 15 increased from 10.9% in 1995 to 18.0% in 2005 (IC, 2006). The National Audit Office has predicted that by 2010 one in four adults will be obese.

Levels of obesity have been shown to increase with age. In 2005 the Government established the National Child Measurement Programme which weighs and measures children in reception year (aged 4–6 years) and year 6 (10–11 years). Figures 1.1 and 1.2 show the prevalence of overweight and obese children in England for 2006–2007. In reception year, almost one in four children were

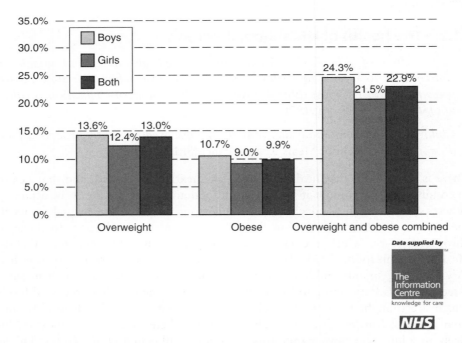

Figure 1.1 Prevalence of obese and overweight children in reception year, by sex. England, 2006/07. (DH *et al.*, 2008. Copyright 2008. Reused with the permission of The Information Centre. All rights reserved.)

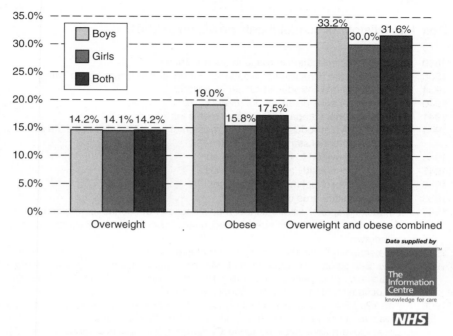

Figure 1.2 Prevalence of obese and overweight children in year 6, by sex. England, 2006/07. (DH *et al.*, 2008. Copyright 2008. Reused with the permission of The Information Centre. All rights reserved.)

classified as either obese or overweight; in year 6 the rate was nearly one in three. Prevalence rates for obesity are greater in year 6 than in reception year. The rate of overweight children is only slightly higher in year 6 than in reception year (DH *et al.*, 2008).

Of particular concern is the recent increase in central overweight and obesity in children, indicated by increased waist circumference (McCarthy & Ellis, 2003). Increased waist circumference is a risk factor for diabetes type 2, heart disease and metabolic disorders. This new trend is especially worrying for children of South Asian origin who are at greater risk of developing type 2 diabetes and coronary heart disease (McKeigue *et al.*, 1991).

In its 2004 White Paper *Choosing health: making healthy choices easier* (DH, 2004) the Government states that halting the growth in childhood obesity is its prime objective. It set a national target to halt the year-on-year increase in obesity among children under the age of 11 by 2010, as part of its strategy to tackle obesity in the population as a whole. In 2007, the Government postponed that target to 2020 in light of further evidence of the worsening of the obesity crisis. It was clear that such a target was plainly over ambitious.

Box 1.1   History of school meals provision to 2001.

1880	Compulsory education introduced across Britain
1906	The Education (Provision of Meals) Act introduced in England and Wales
1934	Free school milk introduced for needy children
1940	Government subsidised school meals by 70%
1941	First nutritional standards for school meals introduced
1944	Education Act introduced statutory provision of school meals in all state schools
	Further nutritional standards introduced
1946	Free milk provided to all schoolchildren
1947	Government subsidy increased to 100%
1950	Charge for a school meal standardised
1955	Nutritional standards updated
1967	Financial responsibility for school meals passed from central control to LEA
1968	Free school milk discontinued in secondary schools. 100% government grant withdrawn
1971	Free school milk limited to 5- to 7-year-olds only
1980	New Education Act introduced. LEAs no longer obliged to provide school meals, except to pupils entitled to a free meal. Fixed pricing removed, as was the obligation to meet any nutritional standards
1988	The 1986 Social Security Act introduced. This restricted eligibility for free school meals to pupils whose parents received Income Support only
	Local Government Act introduced Compulsory Competitive Tendering (CCT). This obliged all LEAs to put school meals services out to tender
1992	The School Meals Campaign launched, calling for the reinstatement of nutritional standards for school meals. The Expert Working Group on Nutritional Guidelines for School Meals established by the Caroline Walker Trust
1999	Under Fair Funding, the school meals budget delegated to schools (compulsory for secondary schools, optional for primary and special schools)
2000	CCT replaced by Best Value
2001	National Nutritional Standards for school meals implemented in England

1.3   A history of school meal provision to 2001

The history of the provision of meals in schools, as outlined in Box 1.1, begins in 1906, although independent efforts to nourish schoolchildren, in various cities and counties, were being made well before then. During the nineteenth century, charities such as the Destitute Children's Dinner Society provided meals for children considered 'necessitous'. By the end of the 1860s, the charity had set up 58 dining rooms in London (Sharp, 1992). Many children were, in the nineteenth century, very necessitous: a survey of the poor of London between 1889 and 1903 found that about a quarter of the population did not have enough money to live on. Similarly, a survey in York reported that almost half of the wage-earning population could not afford enough food to maintain health (Gillard, 2003). In 1879 Manchester became the first city to provide free school meals for the very needy (McMahon & Marsh, 1999).

The 1870 Education Act resulted in many more children from poor homes attending school for the first time. Compulsory education began in the whole of Britain in 1880, and this brought to light the extent of the problem of underfed children, so malnourished that they were unable to learn. It was left to each school to make provisions for its most needy children; school meals were provided by voluntary workers, including teachers (Sharp, 1992).

The nutritional status of schoolchildren was not made a public or government concern until 1904, when a parliamentary committee reported the poor condition of men recruited to fight in the Boer War. As many as 50% of the recruits were found to be undernourished, small and sickly. Concern about the fighting fitness of the military led to the 1906 Education (Provision of Meals) Act which was introduced in England and Wales. (In Scotland, the Education (Provision of Meals) Act came into force in 1908, along similar lines.) This Act gave all local education authorities (LEAs) for elementary education the power to provide meals to children, either free or at a reduced cost, in order to allow those who were *'unable by reason of lack of food to take full advantage of the education provided for them'*. This provision was not however compulsory; LEAs were under no obligation to provide meals if they thought it unnecessary. The Act was not broadly welcomed, amid fears that the provision of school meals might encourage parents to abandon their parental responsibilities (Gustafsson, 2002). It was also feared that such provision might destroy family life (Welshman, 1997). As a result, some LEAs were quick to introduce school meals whereas others took no action (Brannen & Storey, 1998). Among LEAs which did provide school meals, the selection criteria of children and the provision of meals varied. Rural areas, most notably, were unlikely to provide any food (Brannen & Storey, 1998). Free meals were only given to those children considered by medical experts to be suffering from malnutrition (Gustafsson, 2002). LEAs were however able to provide school meals to children not deemed needy, as long as they charged at least the cost price. These meals were often better than those provided for the needy children, and were also served in a separate eating place (Sharp, 1992).

It wasn't just the need to produce fit, fighting men which brought about the introduction of school meals, or *feeding,* as it was then known. The provision of food in schools was regarded as a medical intervention: there was at that time a strong drive to produce a disciplined workforce capable of intense industrial production, and it was recognised that this was not possible without adequate nourishment.

By 1914 around 160 000 children were receiving a school meal (Sharp, 1992). After a government grant covering 50% of expenditure was introduced in that year, that figure rose swiftly to half a million during the First World War. These meals were prepared and served at what were termed 'feeding centres' in the style of soup kitchens (Fisher, 1987). However, in the post-war depression years the government reduced the total expenditure of LEAs for school meals and this resulted in the number of children taking meals falling to 150 000 in 1922–23. In 1934 the government imposed further restrictions on free or reduced cost meals: children had to be both poor and malnourished to qualify (Sharp, 1992). During this whole period grammar schools continued to provide middle-class children with a nutritious meal, paid for by their parents (Gustafsson, 2002).

Also in 1934 the provision of free milk at school was introduced for needy children under a Milk in Schools scheme. Other children were able to buy it if they wished. Milk had in fact been available since 1921 at a cost of 1d for a third of a pint (Welshman, 1997). By the late 1930s there were increasing demands for more free milk to be made available; by March 1939, 55.6% of schoolchildren were receiving free or subsidised milk (Welshman, 1997).

Despite the efforts made after the introduction of the 1906 Education Act, malnutrition and ill-health among children were still not uncommon in the 1930s (Welshman, 1997). A *Political and Economic Planning* report on poverty pub-lished in 1937 concluded that '*the development of nutrition policy ought to take precedence over all other claims for the expansion of health services*' (Le Gros Clark, 1942). The beginning of the twentieth century was considered the 'golden age' of nutrition and nutritional experts were enthusiastic about putting knowledge into practice.

1.3.1   Winning the war

During the Second World War, changes in policy meant that school meals had to be provided for all schoolchildren if requested, at a cost almost equivalent to the cost of the food, or free for cases of hardship (Sharp, 1992). By 1940 the govern-ment grant to LEAs was increased to 70% of expenditure and a main midday meal was provided for all children whose parents wanted them (Sharp, 1992). Despite the difficult conditions of the war years, the school meal service was transformed into a public service for all schoolchildren (Fisher, 1987). Foods were chosen for their nutritive value and supplies controlled and purchased centrally.

The first, albeit rudimentary, nutritional standards for school meals were introduced in 1941, as specified in Government Circular 1571 (Board of Education 1941). The school meal had to provide 1000 kilocalories and contain 20–25 grams of 'first class' protein and 30 grams of total fat (Sharp, 1992). The circular specified quantities of fat and protein because the foods they were found in were rationed at that time and likely to be deficient in the home diet (Passmore & Harris, 2004). The circular also emphasised the importance of providing meals that were both highly nutritious and attractive to children (Passmore & Harris, 2004). There was a massive drive to increase the uptake of school meals, and to this aim the government grant to LEAs was raised to a maximum of 95% and the school meals service was given priority in the supply of rationed and other food stuffs, as well as equipment (Sharp, 1992). The term 'school feeding centre' had been replaced by 'school canteen' and uptake increased by 50% (Sharp, 1992).

The Education Act (1944) was a milestone in the history of the school meal. It meant that the provision of school meals in all state schools became enshrined in statutory law, as a significant feature of the welfare state. All LEAs had a duty to provide school meals '*suitable in all respects as the main meal of the day*'. These meals were based on specific guidelines drawn up by nutrition experts on the precise nutrient requirements of a child, with each meal designed to provide one-third of a child's daily allowance of nutrients and energy, according to scientific knowledge at that time. The meal, the price of which was fixed, basically consisted of meat, two vegetables and a pudding. The Act stated that:

- All pupils attending a state school were entitled to a midday school meal on every school day.
- The meals were to be free to those pupils whose parents were either unemployed or on low incomes. The price of the meal could not exceed the cost of the food.
- For other pupils, the parents were to pay.
- Each local authority was to report to the Ministry of Education on the quantities of ingredients used.

Despite the demands of the Second World War, the government was keenly aware of the importance of adequate nutrition for children, particularly in view of the mass employment of women at that time. A Ministry of Education circular, in 1945, described the school meal as having '*a vital place in national policy for the nutrition and well-being of children*' (Sharp, 1992). In that year, around half the children in state schools were eating a midday meal; evidence of malnutrition was no longer a requisite for free meal entitlement. The effects of wartime policy, under the Ministry of Food, became evident. Official records show that the height and weight of children increased, they grew faster and had better dental health (Fisher, 1987). There were extended benefits, including improved social behaviour (Fisher, 1987). The school meal – no longer just about feeding the necessitous – became a vital part of school life and was valued as a *quick, cheap and easy way of improving and protecting the health of children and of nations* (Fisher, 1987).

1.3.2   The post-war years

In 1946, free milk, which since 1934 had been given to needy children only, was provided to all schoolchildren, with each child entitled to one third of a pint of milk a day. This practice was discontinued in secondary schools in 1968 as a cost-cutting measure. Primary schools were not affected until 1971, when free school milk was limited to pupils aged from five to seven years only, and all pupils in special schools. It was however still available to other pupils provided they paid for it (Sharp, 1992).

By 1947 the government was meeting 100% of the net cost of school meals and in 1950 the charge for a school meal was standardised, a policy which stayed in place for the following thirty years (Sharp, 1992). The post-war years saw further improvements in the school meal, not least the policy that every school should have its own kitchen, even though this was not always workable (Fisher, 1987).

Nutritional standards for school meals were updated in 1955. Each meal was to contain 650–1000 kcal, depending on the age of the child, with 20 grams of 'first class' (animal) protein and 25–30 g of fat (Sharp, 1992). These changes were stipulated in Government Circular 290, appendices to which listed the amounts of foods such as meat, milk and vegetables to be provided and included the recommendation that 'fruit of some kind should be served at least once a week' (Passmore & Harris, 2004).

In 1965, guidelines were updated to include the recommendation that fresh meat should be served on three days a week, with other animal proteins provided on the remaining days (Sharp, 1992). The school meal was to provide a third of the daily nutritional requirements as laid down by the Department of Health. The school meals service reached its peak in 1966, when 70% of children in state schools were eating a school meal. But there was change in the air which was to set in motion a reversal of priorities and a decline in the post-war enthusiasm for a nation of adequately nourished children. The Wilson administration of the 1960s was keen to reduce government subsidies and in 1967 financial responsibility for school meals passed from central control to each LEA. Giving the LEA greater discretion over pricing policy resulted in successive increases in the charge for the school meal. Although Margaret Thatcher's new Conservative administration of 1979 has been widely blamed for the dismantling of the school meal service, the seeds of its demise were sown much earlier.

In 1968 the 100% government grant for school meals was withdrawn and the 1970s saw a decline in the numbers of children taking a school meal, as costs rose. In 1975 some changes were made to nutritional standards: minimum quantities of fat in a school meal were no longer specified, though it was recommended that food be fried in vegetable oil rather than animal fats. There was also no longer a standard for animal protein. Milk and cheese were to be encouraged, as a source of calcium, and margarine fortified with vitamin D was to be used in catering.

It was during the 1970s that concerns over the excesses of children's diets were first expressed. Children were starting to reject the standard 'school dinner' in favour of more enticing, if less nutritious, options that had become available to them. The 1970s saw the birth of a new consumer culture which offered children more choice. The way food was prepared and served also underwent transformations: the school kitchen was increasingly replaced by cook-freeze and cook-chill centres and canteen-style dining rooms and snack bars were gaining popularity.

1.3.3 The end of an era

The arrival of the newly elected Conservative government, in 1979, ushered in massive changes to the school meal service. The new government was committed to reducing public expenditure, and the 1980 Education Act was to have a profound effect on the school meals service and consequently children's dietary habits, as the service underwent deregulation. The Act oversaw the removal of the duty of

LEAs to provide school meals, through the repeal of the 1944 Act, except to those pupils entitled to free meals (i.e. whose parents received supplementary benefit or family income supplement). Nutritional standards and fixed prices were abolished. Entitlement to free school milk in primary schools was also removed. Similarly, the Education (Scotland) Act 1980 deregulated school meals and also removed nutritional standards.

The reasons for these sweeping changes were, the government stated, both financial and innovative (Sharp, 1992). School meals were identified as an area within education where cost-cutting could bring substantial savings and the cash cafeteria was considered more efficient and offered more consumer choice.

The delegation of full responsibility for the provision of school meals meant that each LEA was able to set the cost of meals provided in what was now a discretionary local service. The 1986 Social Security Act, which came into force in 1988, brought further changes which were to undermine free school meal provision. The right to free meals was limited to children whose parents received Income Support; children whose parents received Family Credit were no longer eligible, though they did receive a notional amount of cash which was paid as part of Family Credit. As a result, the number of children who could claim free meals was reduced by over 400 000 (White *et al.*, 1992).

Further neoliberal transformations were to come in 1988, when the Local Government Act introduced compulsory competitive tendering (CCT) for all catering services in the public sector. This completed the transformation of the provision of school meals from a health service into a commercially competitive operation, obliging LEAs to put school meal services out to tender with the private sector. Contracts had to be offered to the catering company offering the cheapest price – even the LEA's own in-house service, known as the Direct Service Organisation (DSO) had to win the tender if it was to continue to operate. It was unlawful for local authorities to engage in what might be considered 'anti-competitive behaviour' (Davies, 2005). With no nutritional standards in place and no fixed pricing, the LEA could provide whatever it wanted at whatever cost. It also meant that it could divert funds to other priorities in education. One of the effects of the Local Government Act was a sharp rise in the price of a school meal. After the introduction of the 1980 Act, the national charge for a school meal was ranged from 35p to 55p. Within a year of the introduction of CCT prices across England ranged from 35p to £1, with an average cost of 65p. As a result, there was a marked drop in numbers of children eating a school meal in many LEAs. CCT was widely considered disastrous, triggering as it did negative changes in the school meals service, including a lower skilled workforce, loss of kitchens and debasement of the quality of food (Morgan, 2006).

All these changes meant, in short, that there was now a wide variation across the United Kingdom in the quality, price and nature of the school meal in what had become a market-led, low cost culture. The focus had moved away from ensuring adequate nutrition towards minimising waste and maximising profit. Children were now consumers, free to eat whatever they wanted, with no

restrictions or control other than their own financial limitations. The cash cafeteria, where children could select dishes, and then pay for them, had become
the system of choice in secondary schools. Most primary schools however did
(and still do) provide set meals as opposed to a cafeteria service.

By 1992 11% of local authorities were no longer providing meals for children,
and approximately 95% of secondary schools were operating a cafeteria-style
service, on a free choice basis. This resulted in an increase in the provision of
fast foods, such as burgers and chips. There were increasing concerns about
school meals being run as a commercial operation, more driven by making a profit
from cheap food than ensuring adequate nutrition. Comparisons between school
meals in 1982 and 1990 showed an increase in the percentage of energy provided by fat, together with a decrease in protein, vitamins and minerals (Noble &
Kipps, 1994). There was also a marked reduction in pupils taking school
meals – a census in 1988 found only 2.8 million children in England were eating
school meals on the day of the census, compared to 4.9 million in 1979 (White
et al., 1992). By 1991, only 42% of children were taking a school meal (Sharp,
1992). This may have been due to the sharp rise in prices following the 1980
Education Act – the cheaper the price of the meal, the greater the uptake (White
et al., 1992).

By 1992 there were calls from various quarters for the reintroduction of
nutritional standards, abolished in 1980. In 1992 around 50 different organisations came together to form the School Meals Campaign (Gustafsson, 2002). The
School Meals Campaign drew up a charter, which called for, among other things,
the reintroduction of nationally agreed nutrition standards for school meals, as
well as universal availability and affordability. In that same year the Caroline
Walker Trust – a charity *'dedicated to the improvement of public health through
good food'* – published *Nutritional Guidelines for School Meals* (Sharp, 1992), as
part of the campaign. This was widely considered to be the definitive document for
nutrient-based standards for school meals. Box 1.2 outlines the CTW nutritional
guidelines for school meals. Also in 1992, the Government published *The Health
of the Nation* (DH, 1992) in which it committed itself to drawing up voluntary
nutritional guidelines for school meals. In 1993 *Catering for Healthy Eating in
Schools* was published by the Health Education Authority (Coles & Turner, 1993).
This document initiated discussions about reintroducing nutritional standards for
school meals.

1.3.4 New Labour, new Acts

The newly elected New Labour government was sensitive to the growing
disquiet concerning the decline of the school meal service and published, in
1997, the White Paper *Excellence in Schools* (DfEE, 1997), which included a commitment to the reintroduction of nutritional standards. The government was also
aware that the profit-fixated CCT system was considered a disastrous legacy of
the Thatcher era, so replaced it with a new regime called Best Value. Best Value,
or 'continuous improvement of services', as it was referred to by the government,

Box 1.2   Summary of CTW nutritional guidelines for school meals[a].

Energy	30% of the Estimated Average Requirement
Fat	Not more than 35% of food energy
Saturated fatty acids	Not more than 11% of food energy
Carbohydrate	Not less than 50% of food energy
Non-milk extrinsic sugar	Not more than 11% of food energy
NSP ('fibre')	Not less than 30% of the calculated reference value
Protein	Not less than 30% of the Reference Nutrient Intake (RNI)
Iron	Not less than 40% of the RNI
Calcium	Not less than 35% of the RNI
Vitamin A	Not less than 30% of the RNI
Folate	Not less than 40% of the RNI
Vitamin C	Not less than 35% of the RNI

Sodium should be reduced in catering practice

[a] In June 2005 these guidelines were revised. The main changes were an increase in the proportion of the RNI that should be provided on average for calcium, vitamin A and vitamin C to *not less than 40%* of the RNI. Zinc was also added to the list, at *not less than 40%* of the RNI. Guidance for sodium was revised to *not more than 30% of the SACN* (Scientific Advisory Committee on Nutrition) recommendations. Three food-based recommendations were added: fruit and vegetables (not less than 2 portions); oily fish (on the school lunch menu at least once a week) and fried or processed potato products (not on the school menu more than once a week).

Source: *Nutritional Guidelines for School Meals* (Sharp, 1992). Reproduced with kind permission from the Caroline Walker Trust.

became law in England and Wales as part of the Local Government Act 1999, and came into effect in April 2000. The system has been in operation in Scotland since 2003 and in Northern Ireland since 2002, with some variations from the system in England. Unlike CCT, it applies to all local government services. The main thrust of Best Value was its removal of the obligation to tender the catering contract, arguably the most despised feature of CCT. Best Value has four key features:

- **Compare.** The quality and effectiveness of services are to be constantly improved, through comparisons and target-setting
- **Consultation.** Services are to be reviewed on a regulation basis, through public consultation
- **Competition.** A new approach is to be adopted, favouring neither the council nor external organisations as service providers in achieving cost effective quality services
- **Challenge.** Services are to be monitored rigorously

Although in theory the new regime carries a duty to consider quality as well as cost when considering awarding contracts, and was therefore initially widely welcomed (Davies, 2005), many consider that in reality the cheap food culture engendered by CCT was never properly addressed by Best Value. A 2005 Unison

report claimed that there remained a heavy emphasis on competition and contracting out, and local authorities were still expected to strive for improvements
in economy, efficiency and effectiveness (Davies, 2005). A 2003 report of the
school meal service from *The Regeneration Institute* described the overall result of
20 years of low cost culture and policy as:

- the reduction in the use of fresh, locally produced food
- the increase in the use of frozen, processed foods
- the loss of the kitchen infrastructure and the decline of prime cooking
- reduction in the numbers and skills of catering staff
- purchasing on the basis of lowest price
- the preference for large suppliers to reduce transaction costs (Morgan & Morley, 2003)

The 1999 Local Government Act also introduced changes to the way the school
meal budget was to be managed, via a new funding framework called Fair
Funding. This meant that after April 2000 responsibility for the school budget was
transferred from LEAs to all secondary schools, with primary schools having the
option to receive delegated responsibility if they so wished. Delegated schools
became responsible for food provision, with the right to choose another catering
contractor or run their own service. They also assumed responsibility for compliance with nutritional standards, when they came into place in 2001. Most schools
bought back into their LEA catering service, though some took control of their
own service in order to further improve standards of the school meal.

Throughout the late 1990s, the lobby for the reintroduction of nutritional
standards pressed on. Much has been made, in the media, of the introduction of
nutritional standards in September 2006 following the sustained public outcry
against the poor quality of food in schools, as exposed on television by celebrity
chef Jamie Oliver. Less well known is the fact that standards had already been
introduced, five years earlier. In 2000 the Government passed the legislation defin-
ing nutritional standards for school meals that became compulsory in England
from April 2001. The introduction of these minimum nutritional standards was
seen as a means of tackling the problem of children's deteriorating dietary habits.
They clearly failed to do so, as evidenced by comparisons of the quality of children's diets before and after these standards were introduced.

1.4 Children's diets prior to the introduction of nutritional standards in 2001

*'Nutrition is a fundamental pillar of human life, health and development across
the entire life span. From the earliest stages of fetal development, at birth, and
through infancy, childhood, adolescence and on into adulthood, proper food
and good nutrition are essential for survival, physical growth, mental development, performance, productivity, health and well-being'.* (WHO)

As recently as the early 1970s, children were more likely to be underfed at school than overfed, in sharp contrast to the state of affairs which has predominated since 1980. A survey of 48 schools in south east England carried out in 1970–1971 found that 33 of the 48 schools examined provided only 25% or less of the daily recommended intake of energy, compared with the target of 33%. Nine schools provided less than 20%. Twelve schools provided less than 25% of the recommended daily protein intake (Bender *et al.*, 1972). Yet changes in the system of provision meant that by the 1980s and 1990s, the focus of concern had switched from malnutrition to poor nutrition and its contribution to dental caries, anaemia, obesity and all the chronic diseases associated with obesity.

The Department of Health and Social Security 1989 report, '*The Diets of British Schoolchildren*' (DHSS, 1989) was commissioned to monitor the effects of the 1980 Education Act on children's dietary habits. This survey compared the nutrient intake of over 2500 children with the recommended daily amounts (RDAs) set by the Committee on Medical Aspects of Food Policy (COMA) in 1979. The results indicated that the Act had indeed had a detrimental effect on children's dietary habits. Children were found to consume meals – including lunches – high in fat and sugar, and low in fruit and vegetables. They obtained most of their dietary energy from bread, chips, cakes, puddings, biscuits and meat products. Those from manual classes were more likely than others to eat chips and less likely to drink milk. Fat intake was found to be excessive: over three quarters of children consumed more than the recommended 35% of calories from fat. Deficiencies in micronutrients were however generally low.

Less than a decade later, the 1997 *National Diet and Nutrition Survey: young people aged 4–18* (Gregory *et al.*, 2000), published in 2000, revealed that children's dietary habits appeared to have declined further. This survey found that:

- the most commonly consumed foods, eaten by more than 80% of the group, were white bread, savoury snacks, potato chips, biscuits, potatoes and chocolate;
- fizzy soft drinks were the most popular beverage;
- on average, children consumed less than half of the recommended 5 portions of fruit and vegetables a day, with around one in five eating no fruit at all in the week the survey was carried out.

Micronutrient deficiency had also become apparent. A large proportion of older children were found to have low intakes of a number of minerals, including calcium, iron and zinc. Some showed evidence of poor iron status. Low iron intakes were reported in over half the girls aged 15–18 years and low ferritin stores (a reflection of iron status) were present in 27% of this age group. A significant proportion, 13%, of 11 to 18-year-olds had poor vitamin D status. Total fat intakes were close to the population goal of 35% of food energy, but saturated fat intake was excessive. Plasma cholesterol levels in 8% of boys and 11% of girls were found to be above 5.20 mmol/l – the current recommended maximum level for adults is 5.0 mmol/l.

Matters were no better in Northern Ireland. In 1999, the Health Promotion Agency for Northern Ireland (HPA) commissioned a survey on the dietary habits of both adults and children in Northern Ireland (Health Promotion Agency, 2001). A random sample of parents of 716 children were interviewed. The survey showed that:

- 48% of children did not eat fruit every day
- 10% of children ate fruit less than once a week, or not at all
- 40% ate vegetables every day but only 12% of children aged 5–11% and 9% of 12 to 17-year-olds achieved the recommended five portions of fruit and vegetables daily
- 18% of children ate chips at least one day a week
- 73% of children ate biscuits every day
- 47% of children ate confectionery at least once a day (including chocolate bars)
- 14% of children ate cakes and buns every day.
- 38% of children drank fizzy, sugary drinks every day.

1.5   The 2001 national nutritional standards

More than twenty years after nutritional standards were abolished, and after nine years of lobbying by the School Meals Campaign, the Education (Nutritional Guidelines for School Lunches) (England) Regulations 2000 (Statutory Instrument 2000, No. 1777) were introduced on 1 April 2001 by the Department for Education and Employment (later the Department for Education and Skills (DFES) and now the Department for Children, Schools and Families). The regulations applied to all lunches provided for children during term time, at all schools maintained by LEAs in England, whether they were provided free or were paid for by the children. They applied to both hot and cold food, including packed lunches provided by the school on school trips. Box 1.3 contains an extract from the guidelines as set out by the Department for Education and Skills' *Guidance for Caterers to School Lunch Standards* (See www.dfes.gov.uk/schoollunches).

These standards were based on the five food groups set out in the *Balance of Good Health* (now *The Eatwell Plate)* – see Figure 1.3 and Box 1.4. The *Balance of Good Health* was jointly produced by the Health Education Authority, the Department of Health and the then Ministry of Agriculture, Fisheries and Farming (MAFF) in 1994. It came about as a result of recommendations made in the Government's 1992 White Paper, *The Health of the Nation* (DH, 1992) whose aim was to reduce the number of deaths from chronic disease. It was also intended to *'go some way towards assisting the general public to make these changes in their diet and enable them to choose foods for an enjoyable, interesting and healthy diet'* (Gatenby *et al.*, 1995). The *Balance of Good Health* is presented as pictorial guidelines designed to represent the types of food and their proportions which make up a healthy diet.

Box 1.3   Nutritional standards for primary and secondary schools, 2001.

Standards for primary schools
For children aged five and over a healthy diet means broadly

- a balanced diet with plenty of variety and enough energy for growth and development
- plenty of fibre-rich starchy foods such as bread, rice, pasta, potatoes and yams
- plenty of fruit and vegetables
- not eating too many foods containing a lot of fat, especially saturated fat
- moderate amounts of dairy products
- moderate amounts of meat, fish or alternatives
- not having sugary foods and drinks too often.

Primary school pupils have particularly high energy and nutrient needs in relation to their size. In their overall diets it is often difficult to achieve adequate intakes of energy, calcium, and iron.

The standards say that lunches for primary school pupils must contain at least **one** item from each of the following food groups.

- starchy foods such as bread, potatoes, rice and pasta. Starchy food cooked in oil or fat should not be served more than **three** times a week.
- fruit **and a** vegetable must be available **every day**. Fruit-based desserts must be available **twice** a week.
- milk and dairy foods.
- meat, fish and alternative sources of protein. Red meat must be served at least **twice a week**. Fish must be served at least **once a week**.

Cheese may be included in the meat/fish protein group for primary children.

Standards for secondary schools
For children aged eleven and over a healthy diet means broadly

- a balanced diet with variety and enough energy for growth and development
- plenty of fibre-rich starchy foods such as bread, rice, pasta, potatoes and yams
- plenty of fruit and vegetables
- not eating too many foods containing a lot of fat, especially saturated fat
- moderate amounts of dairy products
- moderate amounts of meat, fish or alternatives
- not having sugary foods and drinks too often.

National nutritional standards use the food groups in the Balance of Good Health. This shows the types of food which make up a healthy, balanced diet.

The standards require that at least **two** items from each of the following food groups must be available every day and throughout the lunch service.

- starchy foods such as bread, potatoes, rice and pasta. At least one of the foods available in this group should **not** be cooked in oil or fat. (For example if one option is roast potatoes, another option could be boiled rice.)
- vegetables **and** fruit.
- milk and dairy foods.
- meat, fish and alternative (non-dairy) sources of protein. Red meat must be served at least **three times a week**. Fish must be served at least **twice a week.**

Source: DfES: *Guidance for Caterers to School Lunch Standards*.

The eatwell plate

Use the eatwell plate to help you get the balance right. It shows how
much of what you eat should come from each food group.

food.gov.uk

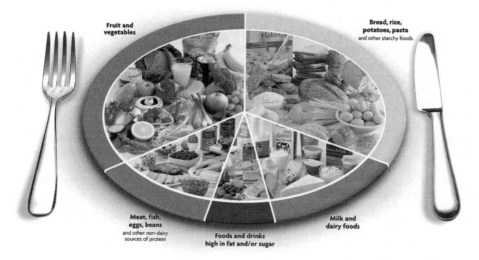

Figure 1.3   The Eatwell Plate (formerly the Balance of Good Health).

Box 1.4   The five food groups of the *Eatwell Plate*

Bread, other cereals and potatoes	Grains such as wheat, oats, barley, rice, maize, millet and rye are included. Foodstuffs include pasta, noodles and chapatis. Baked, boiled, roasted and chipped potatoes are included but snacks such as crisps are not.
Fruit and vegetables	These include fresh, frozen, chilled and canned varieties, as well as juices and dried fruit. Fruit and vegetables are considered a major source of nutrients, especially vitamins and minerals. They also provide fibre, antioxidants and carotenoids. This section also includes all root vegetables excluding potatoes which because of their starch content are considered to belong to the cereal group.
Meat, fish and alternatives	These provide a major source of protein, iron, B-vitamins, and other minerals. This section also includes eggs, pulses and nuts.
Milk and dairy foods	This section does not include butter because it is principally fat and is therefore found within the 'fatty and sugary foods' group. Milk is a major source of calcium and other nutrients, including protein and vitamin B12. It is considered preferable to eat lower fat versions of these foods, which should not affect calcium levels. Fromage frais, milkshakes and custard also fall within this food group.
Foods containing fat and foods containing sugar	This group includes butter, margarine and spreads, cream, crisps, savoury snacks, cakes, biscuits, pastries, chocolate and sugar confectionery and soft drinks.

These guidelines set out *minimum* standards for caterers. LEAs had the power to set their own, more exacting standards if they so chose. Despite the implication of the title of these regulations, they were in fact *food*-group-based rather than *nutrient*-based standards – applying only to the fat, protein and carbohydrate content of meals. There was no guidance for minimum levels of vitamins, minerals or other micronutrients.

Although not part of the regulations, the guidance also stated that drinking water should be available every day, free of charge. It was strongly recommended that some hot food should be offered, especially in winter and that milk be available as an option every day. Caterers were also urged, rather vaguely, to

- consider the likes and dislikes of the pupils
- work with the school to reinforce healthy eating messages
- encourage children to eat a balanced diet
- aim to offer a variety of food
- avoid over cooking and keeping food hot too long before serving.

1.6 Monitoring the 2001 standards

'Because I am a provider and if I go to the school and say the contractor is not doing very well, they think that I'm not being ... I've got an interest. So all I can do is make them aware of the nutritional standards and the directives. The governing body should monitor that but I don't know if or how well they do that. I can only highlight it to them ... at the end of the day, we don't have that power'.   (LACA catering officer, Storey & Candappa, 2004)

Responsibility for ensuring that national nutritional standards were met rested with the local education authority or, if the budget for the school meal had been delegated, with the individual school governing body. There was no statutory obligation for the LEA or DfES to monitor standards.

The DfES document *Guidance for caterers to school lunch standards* stated that regular monitoring of school lunches was essential in order to demonstrate that they were meeting standards, and provided a self-monitoring check list to enable this. Caterers were recommended to keep daily records of the food they provided, to monitor what was being eaten (or not eaten), and to keep a record of whether they were implementing healthier catering practices. They were advised to monitor the nutrient content of the food they provided using a computer software package (although no details of such programmes were given) or make their own approximate nutritional analysis. It was also suggested that in addition to any analysis carried out within the school, a separate analysis might be carried out by an independent expert such as a community dietitian. The DfES also recommended that a laboratory analysis should be carried out to show the level of nutrients retained in food after preparation and cooking. Although the nutritional standards in England were not based on the CWT guidelines (page 13), caterers were in effect expected to be familiar with them, understand them and use them when monitoring the nutritional value of the meals they produced.

1.7   Nutritional adequacy and meeting standards

'The statutory nutritional standards on their own, without a pricing policy to encourage healthier food choice or restrictions in food choice towards less healthy food are unlikely to catalyse the dietary changes that are so needed to ensure improved nutrient intakes amongst schoolchildren in England'.   (Gould *et al.*, 2006)

Unsurprisingly, the monitoring of school meals and nutritional standards was, in reality, a random affair. Caterers were left to monitor themselves – no audit was put in place to check whether they or their schools were compliant with require-ments. It is widely acknowledged that the standards were ineffectual, and this has been largely attributed to poor monitoring. A study into the effects of delegation of the school meal budget found lack of uniformity in monitoring of nutritional standards, with some LEAs unable to offer any monitoring service, due to not hav-ing any officer with the expertise for the role (Storey & Candappa, 2004). LEAs appeared uncertain as to their role, with some believing it to be their statutory duty to monitor standards, offering complete packages to monitor meal provision, and others believing that following deregulation to schools and governors, they had no further responsibility (Storey & Candappa, 2004). Some schools outside of central contracts were diligent in their own internal monitoring, but others had no internal or external system of monitoring (Storey & Candappa, 2004).

In the meantime, a couple of studies, commissioned by the government, looked into whether the standards were actually being met.

July 2004 saw the publication of the report *School Meals in Secondary Schools in England* (Nelson *et al.*, 2004), a nationally representative sample survey of 79 secondary schools which was commissioned to assess:

* compliance with the statutory national nutritional standards introduced in April 2001;
* food choices at lunchtime;
* what, if any, impact the standards had had on children's dietary habits.

Information was provided on lunchtime food provision, catering practice and the types of food selected by 5695 secondary school pupils aged 11–18 years. The survey revealed that 83% of the schools met all the nutritional standards for school meals every lunchtime at the beginning of service but that figure fell to 47% by the end of service, meaning that latecomers or those at the back of the queue were offered a less nutritious choice. Nine per cent of schools failed to provide any vegetables or fruit on 'most days'.

Compliance with non-statutory recommendations concerning the provision of free drinking water and available drinking milk was also studied. It was found that at the beginning of the lunch service, 82% of schools met the recommendation to provide drinking water, and 54% met recommendations for drinking milk. By the end of service 77% met the recommendation for drinking water, and 42% for drinking milk.

One third of catering managers were unaware of the government's compulsory nutritional standards for school meals. Of those who had heard of them, 39% could not describe any of the standards. There was no association between the types of contract and whether or not the catering service met the nutritional standards. Sixty-eight per cent reported that compliance with the nutritional standards was monitored, 17% said they were not monitored and 15% did not know whether they were or not.

The researchers found that the profile of foods on offer did not conform to the Balance of Good Health. The most commonly served foods, on at least four days a week, were cakes and muffins, followed by sandwiches, soft drinks and fruit. Vegetables were served on at least four days in 70% of schools, but chips cooked in oil were served in 76% of schools on four or more days. High fat main dishes, such as burgers and chicken nuggets, were served in 86% of schools on four or more days.

Of the 79 schools in the study, 48 were able to provide samples of documentation relating to healthy eating and nutrition. None of the 15 schools which provided in-house catering services provided any such documentation. Of the schools which did provide some documentation, the language, according to the study authors, was non-specific, neither measurable or time-bound. There was little reference to controlling salt content or the prevention of obesity. In most schools (two thirds) there was no evidence of healthy eating promotion in the form of posters or food labels. On the contrary; 'meal deals' that included special offers such as 10p off chips undermined any attempt at persuading children to make healthy choices. The authors suggest that many schools were only paying 'lip-service' to healthy eating and nutrition, with little translation of nutrition-related standards into meaningful specifications. The authors concluded that *'it is apparent that there has been no improvement in the profile of nutrient intake from school meals following the introduction of the National Nutritional Standards in 2001'*.

Two years later, primary schools did not prove to be any more compliant with nutritional standards than secondary schools. Indeed, they proved even less so. In June 2006 the FSA and DfES jointly published results of the survey *School Meals in Primary Schools in England* (Nelson *et al.*, 2004). Data on the food selection and consumption of 7058 primary school pupils from 151 schools were collected. The aim of the survey was to assess whether schools met the statutory 2001 National Nutritional Standards and whether the food provided met the Caroline Walker Trust guidelines. The survey also aimed to identify the food consumption and nutrient intakes of the children. Key findings included:

- Only 23% of schools met all standards at the beginning of service over 5 days. This figure fell to 17% by the end of service.
- The profile of food on offer did not conform to the Balance of Good Health.

- Nutrient analysis of meals chosen suggested that mean intakes either met or were close to CWT guidelines (Box 1.2) although saturated fat intake was higher than recommended. Intake of energy, fibre, calcium and iron were lower than recommended. Mean folate intake was low in juniors (but not in infants).
- In schools where the caterer had receive some training in healthy eating and cooking or had run healthy eating promotions, pupils chose more vegetables and salads.
- There were no associations between type of catering provider and degree of standards met.

A smaller, later study of seventy-four 11 to 12-year-olds, published in 2006, found that only one out of the three schools it examined met nutritional guidelines. Furthermore, the study found that socioeconomic deprivation was associated with worse food provision (Gould *et al.*, 2006).

1.8   Children's dietary choices – post introduction of 2001 nutritional standards

'It is clear that the National Nutritional Standards for school meals, coupled with the present model of food service and the provision of set meals that do not have to meet clearly defined nutritional requirements, failed to encourage children to select combinations of foods that were likely to contribute to a healthy diet'.   (Nelson *et al.*, 2004)

1.8.1   Opting out

School meals may not have been very healthy, following introduction of minimum nutritional standards in 2001, but neither were they very popular. Fewer than half of all children chose to eat a school lunch, the remainder bringing in food from home or buying their lunch outside the school premises (Jefferson & Cowbrough, 2003). Large number of pupils opting out of the school meal system precipitates the closure of school kitchens and withdrawal of hot meals. This can mean that those children entitled to a free meal have to make do with a bagged lunch, which may constitute the main meal of the day.

Every two years, the private catering organisation Sodexho carries out and publishes its *School Meals and Lifestyle Survey*. The 2002 survey reported that the overall frequency of eating a school meal was 2.57 times a week in 2002, compared to 2.85 times a week in 2000 (Sodexho, 2002). In 2002, 39% of children were found to never have a school meal, compared to 37% in 2000 (Sodexho, 2002). However by 2005 school meals had gained popularity, with the overall frequency of eating a school meal increasing from 2.57 times a week in 2002 to 2.79 times a week (Sodexho, 2005).

The fact that so many children choose not to eat a school meal may be due to their greater spending power. UK schoolchildren spend more than £1.3bn a year on food – almost a third of their pocket money goes on snacks eaten while travelling to and from school (Sodexho, 2002). Children spend on average £1.01 on the way to school and 74p on the way home, and spend more than £189 million more on soft drinks and confectionery than on lunch food (Sodexho, 2005).

When questioned, children have identified long queues and crowded dining rooms as main objections to taking a school meal. Other objections include price, taste, appearance and temperature of the food (Sodexho, 2005).

1.8.2 New standards, old choices

Children, when questioned, have been found to have an understanding of the basic principles of healthy eating; even primary school children have been found to have a clear perception of healthy and unhealthy foods (Noble *et al.*, 2000) and show an awareness and understanding of what constitutes a balanced diet (Edwards & Hartwell, 2002). A 2006 Ofsted study found that primary school children were more likely than secondary school children to apply their knowledge of healthy eating to their meal choices. In both primary and secondary schools, pupils' understanding of healthy eating was '*at least adequate and often good*'. (Ofsted, 2006a).

Of those children who do have a school meal, there would appear to be little difference in their dietary preferences, before and after introduction of the 2001 statutory standards. Table 1.1 shows the top five favourite main courses from 1998 to 2005, from the Sodexho 2005 survey. Pizza was the favourite main course in 2000 and 2002, followed by burger. By 2005, little had changed. In 2000, the favourite pudding was ice cream; in 2002 it was cake or bun (Sodexho, 2002). In 2005, the most popular desserts were cakes or buns and ice cream. Children were found to consume a total of 2.71 helpings of fruit and vegetables a day (in school and elsewhere). This figure rose to 3.00 where there was a food group or council in the school. Despite unchanging dietary habits, 62% of parents thought that the food provided at their child's school was healthy or very healthy, a slight increase on 2002 when that figure was 60% (Sodexho, 2005 survey).

Table 1.1 Top five favourite main courses (in order of preference).

1998	2000	2002	2005
Pizza	Pizza	Pizza	Pizza
Roast dinner	Burger	Burger	Pasta/spaghetti
Burger	Chips	Pasta/spaghetti	Burger
Sausage	Roast dinner	Roast dinner	Roast dinner
Filled jacket potato	Pasta	Curry	Turkey/chicken

Source: The Sodexho School Meals and lifestyle Survey 2005. Reproduced with kind permission from Sodexho.

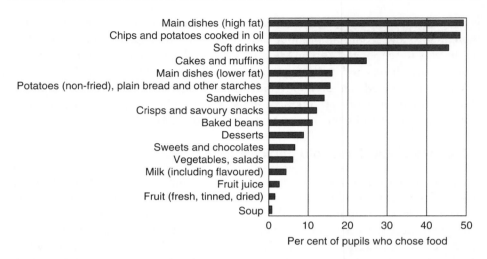

Figure 1.4 Per cent of 5695 pupils choosing specified foods in 79 secondary schools in England. From: Nelson *et al.* (2004). Reproduced with kind permission.

Children of South Asian origin, who are at greater risk of developing obesity and type 2 diabetes in adult life (McKeigue *et al.*, 1991) were found, in an earlier survey carried out in 2003, to consume diets of similar quality to their white peers. This survey of 3418 pupils of predominantly South Asian origin, using a question-naire based on food and drink consumed the previous day, found that both white and South Asian pupils made poor dietary choices; 24% ate nothing before leaving home, and only 34% had eaten vegetables the day previous to the survey. Around a third ate no fruit that day.

The 2004 *School Meals in Secondary Schools* report (page 20) also revealed that children preferred not to select healthy options. Only 6% of pupils chose a vegetable or salad option, and 2% chose fruit. Figure 1.4 shows the order of popularity of foods served. According to the authors, '*the evidence from the present study shows that if the pupils' choices are unconstrained the majority fail to make healthy choices*', and the best way to ensure healthy eating in school is '*to constrain choice to healthy options*'.

The authors make extensive recommendations, including:

- both food-based and nutrient-based compulsory national nutritional standards
- meals that meet the Balance of Good Health recommendations
- choice restricted to a range of healthier options
- documentation and monitoring to accompany provision of food
- head cooks and catering managers to have certified training in healthy catering and to ensure that nutritional standards are met.

The findings of the *School Meals in Primary Schools in England* (Nelson *et al.*, 2006) gave little scope for greater optimism. Desserts were the most commonly chosen food (78% of pupils), although vegetables did make it to second place (56% of pupils). Pupils were more likely to select vegetables in schools where the caterer had received some training in healthy eating, or where the school encouraged healthy eating. However, higher fat main dishes and chips were chosen nearly twice as often as lower fat main dishes.

In Wales the results of two studies of thirty-two schools (16 primary and 16 secondary) carried out before and then after the introduction of nutritional standards are particularly interesting because of their remarkably similar results (FSA Wales, 2002). The second study carried out in 2002 did reveal improved availability of fruit and vegetables, but that pupils – especially secondary school pupils – were still not interested in eating them. Chips were as popular as they were before the introduction of legislation, despite alternatives being widely available. Indeed, secondary school pupils were more likely to choose chips than any other food tested, with many meals consisting solely of chips – fewer than half of secondary school pupils chose any main dish. However, primary school children were found to be more likely to choose other types of potato dishes. Despite increased availability of fresh fruit and vegetables following the introduction of the statutory minimum standards, only 2% of secondary school pupils chose a stand-alone portion of vegetables, 2% selected salad and 1% chose a piece of fruit. Primary school children were more likely than secondary school children to eat vegetables, salad and fruit. Puddings with fruit were found to be unpopular: whilst 87% of primary school children selected a pudding, only 10% of these were a fruit pudding or fruit salad. Fish was also unpopular with all children, and meat cuts were generally shunned in favour of burgers and sausages. The study concluded that 'the most likely way to ensure healthy eating in schools is to constrain choice to healthy options'. The Food Standards Agency Wales felt differently and its response was that 'This school meals study underlines the need for continued action to help children choose a healthy diet' (FSA Wales, 2003).

Many schools have now adopted a 'smart card' system which pupils use to pay for meals. This system makes it possible to track the food choices made by pupils in the school cafeteria. When the food choices of 30 boys aged 8–11 were tracked over a period of 78 days, it was found that the participants 'were clearly choosing meals containing higher than the recommended maximum amounts for sugar and lower than the recommended minimum amounts of fibre, iron and vitamin A' (Lambert et al., 2005a). However protein and vitamin C levels were well above minimum requirements. High vitamin C was attributed to the popularity of drinks fortified with the vitamin, but which were also high in sugar. Overall, nutrient requirements were met 41% of the time. In the same school and using the same smart card technology, buns and cookies were found to be over 10 times more popular than fresh fruit and yoghurt, and sugary soft drinks over 20 times more popular than fresh fruit drinks and milk combined (Lambert et al., 2005b). The choices made by the boys, who generally came from affluent, well-educated families, were thought to reflect preferences in general for high sugar/fat products across most of the Western world (Lambert et al., 2005b).

Overall, studies show little difference between school meal choices before and after the introduction of standards in 2001. This is confirmed by analyses of the 1997 *National Diet and Nutrition Survey of Young People aged 4–18* and data collected in English primary and secondary schools in 2004–2005, which found that '*The introduction of food-based guidelines for school meals in England in 2001 did not improve the food choices in school meals*' (Nelson *et al.*, 2007).

1.9   Nutritional standards in Scotland

Following devolution in 1999, Scotland and Wales began to develop their own school meals policies. Scotland's health record is notoriously poor and the country has a reputation of being 'the sick man of Europe'. Concern about the health of Scottish schoolchildren led to the establishment, in 2002, of an *Expert Panel on School Meals* whose task it was to draft recommendations that would form the framework of a national strategy for school meals. The Panel's remit was to:

- establish standards for the nutritional content of school meals
- improve the presentation of school meals to increase general take up
- eliminate any stigma attached to taking free school meals.

The Panel's final report, *Hungry for Success: A Whole School Approach to School Meals in Scotland* (Scottish Executive, 2002) set out a radical, far-reaching plan to overhaul the school meals service in Scotland with recommendations linking school meals to the national curriculum as an integral part of health education. The plans included *Scottish Nutrient Standards for School Lunches,* which were expected to be in place in both primary and secondary schools by December 2006. The nutrient-based standards were based on the (revised) Caroline Walker Trust (CWT) guidelines (see Box 1.2) which cover both macro (protein, fat and carbohydrate) and micro (vitamin and mineral) nutrients and stipulate that the meal must provide roughly a third of a child's daily nutritional needs. The food-based guidelines were based on the *Balance of Good Health* (see Box 1.4 and Figure 1.3).

Although the standards went further than those introduced in England in 2001 – they were nutrient-based as well as food-based – they were not compulsory. In October 2005, HM Inspectorate of Education (HMIE) published the results of monitoring of implementation of the recommendations of *Hungry for Success*. Most but not all schools had adopted healthier menus and provided good quality food. Healthier practices had also been adopted in most schools, such as removing additional table salt from dining rooms. Some schools had made considerable effort to improve the dining environment by decorating the area with artwork, some of which related to promoting healthier eating habits. However most schools had no system of self-evaluation in place (HMIE, 2005).

The relative success of the Scottish standards may have been due to the level of investment: the Scottish Executive invested £63.5m into implementing the recommendations of *Hungry for Success*. This works out at 14p per meal. England compared poorly; with only £1.5m invested, this equated to a small fraction of a penny per meal (Sodexho, 2005).

There was still much room for improvement. Non-compulsory standards meant, inevitably, that there were wide variations in compliance levels and acknowledgement of this led to the creation of the *Schools (Health Promotion and Nutrition) (Scotland) Act 2007*. Compulsory nutritional standards, covering foods, nutrients and foods other than lunch, similar to those introduced in England from 2006 to 2009 (see page 42) came into effect in August 2008 for primary schools. Regulations governing secondary schools are due to come into effect in August 2009. Full details of the new Scottish standards can be viewed on the Scottish Government website (www.scotland.gov.uk).

1.10 Nutritional standards in Wales

In September 2001 the National Assembly for Wales introduced minimum statutory *Nutritional Standards for School Lunches (Wales) Regulations 2001*. These standards were virtually identical to those introduced in England in 2001 and like the England standards were in fact dietary standards, not nutrient standards, based on the composition of a meal.

In Wales, as in England, it soon became clear that nutritional standards introduced in 2001 were ineffective and inadequate, and in 2006 the *Food in Schools Working Group*, set up the previous year to review school food, published the consultation document *Appetite for Life*. This report proposed more stringent standards for school lunches and all other food and drink available throughout the school day, similar to those introduced in England from 2006 (see page 42). As a result, the Welsh Assembly Government published, in November 2007, the document *Appetite for Life Action Plan* (Welsh Assembly Govt, 2007). This document outlined plans to initiate a 2-year research project involving four local authorities, running from September 2008, to test the proposed standards which are both food- and nutrient-based. A training package for school caterers has also been put in place to provide qualifications in healthy eating and cooking skills (Welsh Assembly Govt, 2007). Full details of the standards can be viewed on the Welsh Assembly Government website (www.wales.gov.uk).

1.11 Nutritional standards in Northern Ireland

In 1995 the Northern Ireland *Chest Heart and Stroke Association* published the results of a survey of school food in secondary schools which showed that 46% of the calories in the meals served came from fat, and that most school meals did not normally provide enough iron, calcium or folate and in many cases vitamin C. The Association recommended that the Department of Education review its guidelines on the nutritional standards of school meals. A consultation document – *Catering for Healthier Lifestyles – Compulsory Nutritional Standards for School Meals* (Northern Ireland Assembly, 2001) was launched in December 2001. This document set out new compulsory standards for school meals, which although described as 'nutritional standards' were in fact food-based standards based on *The Balance of Good Health* food groups (see Figure 1.3) and, like the English and Welsh guidelines to which they were almost identical, gave separate recommendations for nursery, primary and secondary schools. Rather than implement the standards across Northern Ireland from a set date (originally September 2002) the standards were piloted for a period of one year, in around 100 schools, beginning on 22 March 2004. The results of the pilot were evaluated by PricewaterhouseCoopers on behalf of the Department and published in their report *Evaluation of the pilot of the 'Catering for Healthier Lifestyles Standards in Schools in NI'* (PricewaterhouseCoopers, 2005). The pilot was considered successful, despite findings of increased wastage (mainly vegetables and potatoes) and dissatisfaction from children with reduced portion sizes of chips and increased portion sizes of vegetables.

The Department of Education published consultation proposals in April 2006 in relation to new nutritional standards for school meals and food other than lunch (vending machines, tuck shops etc.) and acknowledged that a 'whole school' approach to food was necessary, which encompassed the need for training of catering staff and the need for nutrition education to form part of the curriculum. The Department also committed to increasing the spend to not less than 50p per meal in primary and special schools and 60p in secondary schools. These new standards came into effect in September 2007 with some flexibility on implementation until April 2008. Standards for food other than that provided at lunch are basically the same as those which became statutory in England in 2007 (see page 45). Standards for lunch are based on the *Balance of Good Health* food groups with additional guidance on portion sizes (Department of Education (DE), 2008). There are no nutrient-based standards in Northern Ireland where the Department is waiting to see how standards develop in England, Scotland and Wales before taking a final decision on the matter (private email correspondence, 15/01/08).

In Northern Ireland it is the responsibility of the Education and Library Board and the board of governors of each school to ensure that standards are being met. Monitoring of school meals is now carried out by the Education and Training Inspectorate. The Inspectorate appointed two 'nutritional associates' in December 2006 to monitor the implementation of the *Catering for healthier lifestyles* programme. In its 2007 report (Education and Training Inspectorate, 2007) the inspectorate reported that the majority of schools were making good or very good progress towards achieving the food-based nutritional standards. Most also had a good or very good range of appropriate food-related health initiatives in place. However a 'significant minority' did not apply efforts to meet nutritional standards to break times or breakfast clubs. Most whole-school healthy eating programmes were not monitored or evaluated effectively.

1.12   Government initiatives to improve the diets of children

'The most likely way to ensure healthy eating in schools is to constrain choice to healthy options, manipulate recipes, use modern presentation techniques with

which pupils can identify (e.g. the "fast food" approach, vending machines with healthier options), and encouragement through reward'. (Nelson *et al.*, 2004)

Since its election in 1997, the Labour government has put in place a succession of initiatives with the aim of improving the diet and health of schoolchildren. These initiatives are included in both the formal and informal curriculum. Since 2005, schools have had to demonstrate to Ofsted that they are contributing to the five national outcomes for children stipulated by *Every Child Matters* and the Children Act 2004, which are: being healthy; staying safe; enjoying and achieving; making a positive contribution; economic well-being. In order to do this, schools need to gain what the government has defined as *healthy school status*. By 2009, the government wants all schools to have achieved, or be working towards, *healthy school status*. In order to achieve this status, the *National Healthy Schools Programme* was created.

1.12.1   The National Healthy Schools Programme

'The National Healthy Schools Programme is an exciting long term initiative that helps young people and their schools to be healthy'. (See www.healthy-schools.gov.uk)

The NHSP was established in 1999 by the Department of Health (DH) and the Department for Children, Schools and Families (DCSF) (then the Department for Education and Skills) in an effort to create consistency in achieving *National Healthy School Status*. To gain this status a school must have met national criteria using a 'whole school approach' across four core themes which relate to both curricular and non-curricular school activities. These themes are:

• personal, social and health education
• healthy eating
• physical activity
• emotional health and wellbeing

The aims of the programme are:

• to support children and young people in developing healthy behaviours
• to help raise the achievement of children and young people
• to help reduce health inequalities
• to help promote social inclusion

Box 1.5 outlines the requirements regarding the *healthy eating* core theme. Each local authority has a *local healthy schools programme* to support each school to achieve *healthy school* status. Each school has to demonstrate that it complies with the new nutritional standards, the first part of which became mandatory in 2006 (see page 42). By April 2005 around 70% of all schools in England had joined the programme

---

Box 1.5   Criteria for national *Health School* status: healthy eating.

Pupils have the confidence, skills and understanding to make healthy food choices.
Healthy and nutritious food and drink is (sic) available across the school day.

A Healthy School:

  (1)   has identified a member of the senior management team to oversee all aspects of
        food in the school;
  (2)   ensures provision of training in practical food education for staff, including diet,
        nutrition, food safety and hygiene;
  (3)   has a whole-school food policy – developed through wide consultation, imple-
        mented, monitored and evaluated for impact;
  (4)   involves pupils and parents in guiding food policy and practice within the school,
        enables them to contribute to healthy eating and acts on their feedback;
  (5)   has a welcoming eating environment that encourages the positive social interac-
        tion of pupils;
  (6)   ensures healthier food and drink options are available and promoted at breakfast
        clubs, at break (if established or planned) and at lunchtime as outlined by Food in
        Schools Guidance;
  (7)   has meals, vending machines and tuck shop facilities that are nutritious and healthy
        (see Food in Schools guidance), and meet or exceed national standards, and is
        working towards the latest DfES guidance on improving school meals services;
  (8)   monitors pupils' menus and food choices to inform policy development and
        provision;
  (9)   ensures that pupils have opportunities to learn about different types of food in the
        context of a balanced diet (using the Balance of Good Health) and how to plan,
        budget, prepare and cook meals, understanding the need to avoid the consump-
        tion of foods high in salt, sugar and fat and increase the consumption of fruit and
        vegetables;
 (10)   has easy access to free, clean and palatable drinking water, using the Food in
        Schools guidance; and
 (11)   consults pupils about food choices throughout the school day using school coun-
        cils, Healthy School task groups or other representative pupil bodies.

Source: Department of Health (2005).

(15 564 schools), but only 36% (7713 schools) had achieved healthy school status. By 2006 nearly half of schools had received accreditation. To date, over 90% of schools have joined the NHSP, and 53% have achieved *healthy school status*.

Early research suggests that the NHSP has had some success, in terms of academic achievement. Government-commissioned research in 2005 (Sinnott, 2005) showed that primary schools which were part of the NHSP outperformed non-participating schools in national tests in English, mathematics and science. All 496 schools in the research study which had already achieved *healthy school status* showed greater progress over two years, in all three subjects, than those schools not involved in the NHSP. The DH has commissioned further evaluation of the NHSP and its impact on schools and children. The study is expected to be completed in 2010.

Scotland, Wales and Northern Ireland have all adopted schemes similar to the English NHSP. In Wales, the programme is called the *Welsh Network of Healthy Schools*, as part of the Welsh involvement in the *European Network of Health Promoting Schools* (see page 83). Its aim is to encourage the development of local healthy school schemes within a national framework.

In Northern Ireland, the *Health Promotion Agency* developed information and guidance materials to support the development of *healthy schools*, in the form of a toolkit. The toolkit is designed to *'assist schools to meet the requirements of the Education (School Development Plans) Regulations (Northern Ireland) 2005, which require schools to ensure that they safeguard and promote the health and wellbeing of their staff and pupils'*. (See www.healthpromotionagency.org.uk)

The Scottish Health Promoting Schools Unit (SHPSU) was established in May 2002 to help schools develop as *health promoting schools*. Every school in Scotland was set the target of achieving this by 2007. This target involves the development of a whole school approach to promoting the physical, social, spiritual, mental and emotional well-being of all pupils and staff.

1.12.2   National School Fruit and Vegetable Scheme (NSFVS)

Originally entitled the *National School Fruit Scheme* when it was introduced in July 2000 and before vegetables were included, the NSFVS is part of the government's *5-a-day programme* to reduce health inequalities in England by increasing fruit and vegetable consumption in the general population in order to reduce the level of early deaths resulting from chronic diseases.

The scheme was initially piloted in over 500 schools throughout the country in 2000 and 2001. The pilot was considered a success, and since December 2004 every child aged 4–6 years in local authority (LA)-maintained infant, primary and special schools in England has been entitled to a free piece of fruit or vegetable every school day.

The NSFVS is generally considered a success. A Department of Health evaluation of the pilot found that:

- the majority of children surveyed felt positive about the scheme
- almost all school staff considered the scheme to be a way of both improving and supplementing children's diets
- almost all schools regarded the scheme as a support to healthy eating education
- distributing fruit in class provided a social time and a time for learning
- more than half of the schools surveyed noted an improvement in class atmosphere and ethos (DH, 2001).

A 2003 Department of Health study into parents and teachers' views of the NSFS found that:

- over a quarter of children surveyed said their families ate more fruit at home as a result of the scheme
- nearly half of parents felt that the scheme had increased their awareness of the importance of fruit and vegetables

- nearly all parents reported that their child always, often or sometimes ate the fruit provided by the scheme (DH, 2003).

Although the scheme appears to work well for those children on the receiving end, there are concerns that the effect is not long-lasting. In 2007 the results of a non-randomised, controlled trial involving 3707 children aged four to six years was published. It reported that the NSFVS promoted a significant increase in fruit intake after three months. At seven months, the effect was reduced but was still significant. By the time pupils were no longer eligible for the scheme, the effect had returned to baseline (Ransley *et al.*, 2007). This suggests that although the children are willing to consume fruit when it is provided, the scheme does not induce them to develop a taste for regular consumption.

In Scotland, a similar initiative, called *free fruit in schools* started operating in 2003, with one free portion of fruit given 3 times per week during the school term to every pupil in the first two years of primary school. It forms part of the Scottish Executive's *Healthy Living Campaign* which is intended to improve the health of everyone in Scotland. An evaluation of the initiative in 2005 reported that the overwhelming consensus of both local authority professionals and school staff members perceived the initiative to be very successful, so much so that they felt it should be allowed to continue (MacGregor & Sheehy, 2005). It had resulted in an increased consumption of fruit and an improvement in healthy eating practices. It was felt that the scheme should be extended to cover more pupils, on a more frequent basis.

There is no equivalent of the English or Scottish schemes in Wales. In Northern Ireland, a successful *Fresh Fruit in School* scheme was piloted in 89 schools between October 2002 and summer 2004. It was considered a success, proving popular with both parents and children. The greatest increase in fruit consumption was observed in those who had the lowest intake at the start of the pilot, and in those schools with the highest uptake of free school meals (private email correspondence, 08/02/08). As the pilot ended, however, so did the funding. There are currently no plans to roll out the scheme across the province.

1.12.3 The Food in Schools programme

Another venture, the *Food in Schools* (FiS) programme, was launched as a joint initiative between the Department of Health and the DfES, following successful pilot schemes throughout England during 2003–2004. It involves a range of nutrition-related activities and projects designed to '*help schools implement a whole school approach to food education and healthy eating*' (see www.foodinschools.org). It was also designed to help schools work towards achieving NHSP *healthy school status*.

The eight food-related pilots were led by the Department of Health and were run in over 300 schools across the English regions. The themes of the projects were: breakfast clubs, tuck shops, vending machines, lunch boxes, cookery clubs, water provision, growing clubs and the dining room environment. In March 2005 the results of the pilots were deemed to have been 'extremely positive', with teachers reporting improved attendance, attention, behaviour and levels of concentration as a result of healthier foods being provided in the morning. It was also suggested that the pilot had contributed to improved academic performance. Successful schools were those judged to have adopted a 'whole school' approach, involving teachers, students, caterers and families.

Based on the findings of the pilot work, the Department of Health launched the *Food in Schools Toolkit* in April 2005. The aim of this toolkit, intended to be integrated into the *healthy schools* programme, is to support schools in their efforts to improve the eight areas of provision piloted, and provides guidance on how to develop a *whole school food policy* (see below). The FiS toolkit can be accessed on the FiS website at www.foodinschools.org.

The DfES strand of the programme is aimed more at teacher training and professional development and provides guidance on developing 'whole school' food policies. It also provides resources and curriculum material. Schools are encouraged to set up local food partnerships, where secondary school staff train and support their primary colleagues, helping them to work towards *National Healthy School Status*.

1.12.4 Whole school food policy

'*Most headteachers recognised that in order to adopt a coherent approach to healthier eating they needed to develop a policy towards food. However, only a minority of schools had done so*'.   (Ofsted, 2006a)

All those involved in the governance of a school are encouraged, by the government, to establish a whole school food policy, described as a document which '*expresses a common vision of the ethos, status and role of all aspects of food*' within the school. These aspects include the formal curriculum, extra curricular activities such as cookery clubs, non-lunch provision such as tuck shops and breakfast clubs, the eating environment, packed lunches, welfare issues such as free school meals and events such as the school fête. The aim of a whole school food policy is to connect with schoolchildren and put them, and food, into a broader health context. A guide to producing a whole school food policy is available on the Food in Schools website (www.foodinschools.org).

1.13 Non-government initiatives to improve food in schools

Prior to the introduction of new nutritional standards from 2006 (see page 42), many diverse individuals and organisations entered the fray over school food in the belief that government intervention had done little to reverse the decline in standards and nutritional quality since the 1980 Education Act was introduced.

Independent organisations tend to be more ambitious than government departments, demanding more than simply placing healthier options alongside options of dubious nutritional value in the school cafeteria. Their school food ideology incorporates issues such as local and organic food production and a greater understanding of food provenance. They also tend to focus more on the value of teaching children how to cook food. In addition to the main NGOs campaigning for improved school food, described below, there are numerous, independent local efforts in schools and LAs which depend on the goodwill efforts and resources of parents, teachers, governors and other stakeholders.

1.13.1   The Caroline Walker Trust

The CWT – *'dedicated to the improvement of public health through good food'* – was established in 1988 and named after the late nutritionist, writer and campaigner. It has produced nutritional guidelines for *vulnerable groups and people who need special help* – the under-5s, schoolchildren, people in residential and nursing homes and looked-after children. Its *Nutritional Guidelines for School Meals* (Sharp, 1992), formed the basis of the *Scottish Nutrient Standards for School Lunches* (page 26).

1.13.2   Soil Association – *Food for Life* campaign

'Our mission is to reach out through schools to give communities access to seasonal, local and organic food, and to the skills they need to cook and grow fresh food for themselves. We want a new generation to explore how their food choices impact on their health and that of the planet, and to rediscover the pleasure of taking time to enjoy real food'.   (See www.soilassociation.org/foodforlife)

Perhaps the most prolific NGO campaigner is the Soil Association. In 2003 it launched *Food for Life* (Soil Association, 2003), a *UK-wide alternative model to the cheap, poor quality food that is often served up today*. Since the introduction of new standards in 2006 (page 42), *Food for Life* has focussed on encouraging schools to source food locally, using seasonal, unprocessed organic ingredients. It places considerable emphasis on children developing an understanding of the link between food cultivation, the environment and food on the plate. To this end, it organises local farm visits for pupils. *Food for Life* is a partnership, led by the Soil Association, which brings together the *Focus on Food Campaign, Garden Organic* and the *Health Education Trust*. Any school in England can enrol with the *Food for Life Partnership* and work towards bronze, silver and gold 'marks' for 'good food culture'. *Food for Life* has set targets of 75% unprocessed, 50% local and 30% organic food in schools.

1.13.3   Focus on Food Campaign

The *Focus on Food Campaign* was 'set up against a background of a national decline in cooking ability and teaching coupled with rising health problems caused by poor diet and lack of food knowledge and skills' (Focus on Food Campaign website). Launched in 1998 by the RSA (Royal Society for the encouragement of Arts, Manufactures and Commerce), the *Focus on Food Campaign* aims to improve food education by teaching cooking skills in primary and secondary schools. It does this via its travelling 'cooking buses' – each one a full-sized teaching kitchen staffed by teams of experts. According to Focus on Food, 'the diet and health of the nation will not change significantly unless people are taught the basic skills to cook tasty meals from fresh ingredients and can make a connection between health messages, where food comes from and what they are eating'. The Food Standards Agency also provides cooking buses in partnership with the *Focus on Food Campaign.*

1.13.4   The Health Education Trust

The Health Education Trust (HET) is a UK registered charity formed to '*promote the development of health education for young people in the UK*'.

One of the ways it does this is by helping individual schools create a *School Nutrition Action Group* (SNAG). A SNAG is an alliance between staff, pupils and caterers, supported by health and education professionals, designed to examine and review the food and drink available to pupils in order to improve the uptake of healthier foods. This is to be achieved through the creation of a school-based food policy, considered by HET to be all the more important because of increased delegation and autonomy for individual schools (Harvey, 2000). The HET is concerned not only with the school meal but with other sources of food in the school environment: the tuck shop, vending machine and breakfast club. The action taken by a SNAG might include the removal of vending machines, or the inclusion in them of healthier snacks and bottled water.

The aims of a SNAG include:

- ensuring a match between what is taught in class and what is provided in the canteen
- promoting an image of caring and commitment to parents, especially through snacking and breakfast provision
- restricting the number of pupils leaving the school premises at midday by providing better food

The HET was involved with the School Food Trust in developing a guide to setting up a vending machine service that meets the government's new school food standards from September 2007 (A Fresh Look at Vending in Schools). Recently the HET also produced a 'Water Cooler Guidance' document for schools *to help ensure that the highest standards possible prevail in the selection, provision, installation and maintenance of water coolers in schools.*

The HET also runs a scheme called *Best in Class,* to recognise best practice in school catering provision (see page 79).

1.13.5   Garden Organic

Together with the Prince of Wales's organic food brand, Duchy Originals, Garden Organic – an organisation *'dedicated to researching and promoting organic gardening, farming and food'* – created the website *Garden Organic for Schools*. Garden Organic is part of the Soil Association's *Food For* Life partnership. The aim is to introduce pupils to gardening activities and experience cultivation of food. It provides practical help and advice to both teachers and schools and produces a document, *Growing Naturally,* which provides schools with information on how to go about starting an organic garden.

1.13.6   Sustain

Sustain – *'the alliance for better food and farming'* was the only organisation to take a parliamentary route for its campaign. It developed the Children's Food Bill, a private Bill which was presented in May 2004, which not only proposed new nutritional standards but also called for legislation to ban junk food and the marketing of unhealthy food to children. Since the introduction of new standards, starting from 2006 (page 42), Sustain has redirected its efforts into its *Children's Food Campaign* – to *'improve young people's health and well-being through better food – and food teaching – in schools and by protecting children from junk food marketing'*.

1.13.7   Feed Me Better campaign

No independent effort to improve the food served in UK schools caught the public imagination quite as much as the Channel 4 television series, screened in 2005, called *Jamie's School Dinners*. In this programme, chef Jamie Oliver took on the school meal service of a school in Greenwich where children were seen to eat, almost exclusively, cheap, processed food. This programme also revealed that kitchen staff, whose main task was to unpack and reheat containers of pre-manufactured meals, were undervalued and demoralised.

Change did not come quickly and healthy options were initially deeply unpopular. After a number of set-backs, Oliver quickly grasped the fundamental flaws which obstructed positive change: the children could still select junk food and they had no understanding of what real food was and how it was cooked. By banning all processed food, getting the children involved in food preparation and sending the dinner ladies on a catering course, Oliver was able to turn the experiment into an extraordinary success. The outcome of the series was the *Feed Me Better* campaign, which had huge public and media backing and which called for a number of changes including the return of fresh, unprocessed food, a ban on junk food options, minimum nutritional standards, vocational training for kitchen staff and greater financial investment.

Even the prime minister Tony Blair was compelled to describe the achievements of Oliver's campaign as 'remarkable' (Blair, 2005) and hasten the creation of the independent *School Meals Review Panel* and the *School Food Trust* (pages 39–42).

Since the reintroduction of nutritional standards, the *Feed Me Better* campaign now focusses on Oliver's 'manifesto', based on six points:

(1) compulsory cooking skills taught in schools
(2) the recruitment and training of cookery teachers
(3) every school to be made a 'junk food free zone'
(4) the education of parents in the basics of family cooking and nutrition
(5) adequate training and remuneration of dinner ladies
(6) commitment of a ten-year strategic plan and funding for a long-term public health campaign.

The Jamie Oliver website also produces an information pack for schools containing information on local resources and nutritionally analysed recipes for a two-week menu cycle.

1.14 The run up to the 2006 food-based standards and 2008/09 nutrient-based standards

'The current crisis in school food is the result of years of public policy failure. Financial pressures and the fragmentation of school catering, together with a lack of strict standards, have resulted in the type of school meal we see too often today'. (SMRP, 2005)

'Much more needs to be done to improve the quality of food that schools provide and also to influence the choices the pupils make'. (DfES, 2004)

In the public's imagination, Jamie Oliver is probably single-handedly responsible for instigating the changes which brought about the new food- and nutrient-based standards. The government would however rightly argue that even before Oliver came on the scene, there were plans well under way to reintroduce nutritional standards. Indeed, in September 2004 the Government unveiled its *Healthy Living Blueprint for Schools* (DfES, 2004), which set out a range of resources for schools to use to give children *'the knowledge, skills and understanding they need to lead healthy lives'* in a 'whole-school' environment. Its aim was to bring together the range of government and non-government initiatives which contribute to healthy living. The blueprint described five key objectives:

- to promote a school environment which encourages a healthy lifestyle;
- to use the curriculum to achieve a healthy lifestyle;
- to ensure that the food and drink available at school throughout the day reinforce the healthy lifestyle message;
- to provide physical education and sport in order to promote physical activity;
- to promote an understanding of all the issues which impact on long-term health.

In addition to setting out these key objectives, the *Blueprint* also announced plans to provide better training for school catering staff and to revise secondary school nutritional standards *to take account of recent advice on consumption of salt, satu-rated fats, and fruit and vegetables.*

The Government may already have had its plans in place, but these original plans were a much diluted version of what was to come instead. Furthermore, only just over £1 million had been set aside to achieve the objectives of the *Blueprint*.

Also, in 2004, the Government published its White Paper, *Choosing health: making healthy choices easier* (DH, 2004). This White Paper stated it was committed to helping schools:

- deliver clear and consistent messages about nutrition and healthy eating;
- provide opportunities to learn about diet, nutrition, food safety and hygiene, food preparation and cooking as well as where food comes from;
- actively promote healthy food and drink as part of an enjoyable and balanced diet and restrict the availability and promotion of other options.

Choosing health repeated the Government's commitment to revise primary and secondary school meal standards, reduce consumption of fat, salt and sugar and increase consumption of fruit and vegetables. These standards would cover food across the day, including food in breakfast clubs, tuck shops and vending machines. The Government also said it would improve the school meal service by providing guidance on food procurement and improving training and support for catering staff.

There can be little doubt that the government's efforts to persuade children to choose healthy food over junk were upstaged by what has since been coined the 'Jamie Oliver effect'. This effect was to precipitate a flurry of pre- general election activity designed to push through a raft of more stringent measures. *Jamie's School Dinners* compelled the government to take more radical action, and spend more money, than it had originally intended. As well as bringing to the nation's attention such culinary fare as the now notorious turkey twizzler, *Jamie's School Dinners* also revealed that some schools spent as little as 37p on ingredients per meal.

In March 2005 the government announced a package of measures to improve the provision of food in schools. The commitments that the government now made included:

- New, minimum nutritional standards for school meals. These are now in place.
- The establishment of an independent School Meals Review Panel (SMRP) and a School Food Trust (SFT) (see pages 39–42).
- Funding for authorities and schools of £220m between 2005 and 2008. This money would ensure that there was a minimum spend of 50p per pupil per day for primary schools and 60p per pupil per day for secondary schools. The government also pledged an additional £60m for the development of the new SFT. In September 2006, a new package with more funding was announced. This package, announced by the DCSF, included:
  - £240m of new funding to continue to subsidise healthy meal ingredients from 2008 until 2011 when the £220m transitional fund runs out in 2007/08.

○   £2m for the establishment of a network of regional training kitchens where school cooks can improve their cookery skills. The first Food Excellence And Skills Training (FEAST) centres were announced by the SFT in November 2007.

- New vocational qualifications for catering staff. A basic City & Guilds level 1 award (*Providing a Healthier School Meals Service*) received accreditation from 1 August 2005 by the Qualifications and Curriculum Authority and became available from September 2005. As of December 2007 more than 5000 cooks had taken this qualification. From September 2006, catering staff have been able to take units at levels 2 and 3 in food safety, preparing and cooking healthier meals, the development and introduction of recipes and controlling payments. However none of these qualifications is mandatory. Still, these basic qualifications are a good start: before the introduction of new standards, there was very little training available for catering staff.
- Arrangements for new standards to be monitored by Ofsted.
- The building and refurbishment of school kitchens so that meals could be cooked on-site from fresh ingredients.

The government, did, by and large, honour these commitments. The creation of the SMRP was to set in motion a revolution in the school meals service aimed at ending the terrible legacy of the 1980 Education Act and renewing the post-war enthusiasm for access to health for all children.

1.14.1   The School Meals Review Panel

'*The health advantages of well-cooked, well-presented meals, made from good quality ingredients to accepted nutritional standards, by school caterers who are confident in their skills and valued by the school community, are inestimable. The benefits of good school meals go beyond high quality catering. They also produce social, educational and economic advantages*'.   (SMRP, 2005)

The SMRP was set up to develop new, strict minimum nutritional standards for primary and secondary schools. The SMRP, a multi-disciplinary expert group, comprised of nutritionists, dietitians, head teachers, governors, school caterers, trade unions and other stakeholders, including representatives from the catering and food industries. Its remit was to:

- decide and recommend what form new nutritional standards should take;
- consider 'strongly' the introduction of nutrient-based standards, such as those outlined in the Caroline Walker Trust guidelines (page 13);
- advise whether food choices should be restricted, and if certain types of foods or food ingredients should be eliminated;
- advise on costs of supplying fresh, unprocessed foods and hot food.

The SMRP recommendations (which were very similar to those outlined in the research document *School Meals in Secondary Schools in England*, Nelson *et al.*,

2004 (page 20)) were described in the panel's report, *Turning the Tables: Transforming School Food,* published in September 2005 (SMRP, 2005). The panel recommended nine minimum food-based standards and fourteen nutrient-based standards. The panel believed that nutrient-based standards alone would not necessarily increase intake of fruits, vegetables and other nutrient-rich foods. Food-based standards however could, and a combination of both food- and nutrient-based standards would bring together the benefits of both approaches. The food-based standards were to be introduced in two stages: interim and final. *Turning the tables* also recommended that lunch standards should be supplemented with standards for other food and drink available throughout the school day, such as breakfast provision and items sold in tuck shops and vending machines.

Turning the tables was not only about reversing deleterious trends in children's dietary habits but also challenging one of the most fundamental ideological concepts of New Labour – choice, in this case, the unrestricted unhealthy choices available to children. The panel advised that *confectionery, pre-packaged savoury snacks and high-sugar or sweetened fizzy drinks have no place in school lunch provision and other school food outlets* (SMRP, 2005). The removal of junk food choices was recommended as a statutory requirement. According to the panel, '... *It is by constructively controlling choice that we will widen children's food experiences*'.

Turning the tables took a broad view of school food provision and recognised the need to put that provision into a holistic context – a whole school food approach. This required funds and the SMRP claimed that significant capital investment – an estimated £289m – was needed to upgrade kitchens and dining rooms to bring them up to standard. The report recommended that kitchens should be a priority under the programme. When the SMRP's report was published, the government reiterated that it would rebuild and refurbish every secondary school through its *Building Schools for the Future* programme (see page 71).

Another concern highlighted by the SMRP was the ability of schools under private finance initiative (PFI) contracts to meet the new standards. The SMRP stated that such contracts should not impose barriers to the improvement of school food. A Unison survey earlier in 2005 had drawn attention to the difficulties faced by certain schools locked into PFI contracts to provide fully operational kitchens, when the contract had provided merely for 'kitchens' which only had facilities for heating up food cooked elsewhere (Unison, 2005). According to Unison, PFI contracts were blocking schools from providing healthy meals to children – schools were being built without kitchens, and existing kitchens were badly equipped. Nearly 30% of the current 417 schools under a PFI contract were found to not have a kitchen capable of cooking a meal from fresh ingredients.

The panel made a total of thirty-five recommendations for standards, catering, school policy, financial investment and monitoring. Box 1.6 provides a summary of the main SMRP recommendations. The timetable set for introducing new standards is shown in Table 1.2. The Government accepted all the recommendations of the panel, with a few minor changes, and it then became the job of the SFT to turn these recommendations into action.

Box 1.6   A summary of the main recommendations of the School Meals Review Panel.

Standards
- Food provided at lunch time should meet both nutrient- and food-based standards.
- Compulsory standards should also be set for food other than lunch.
- Voluntary Target Nutrient Specifications should be set for processed foods provided in tuck shops or vending machines.
- Easy access to free, fresh drinking water throughout the day.

Catering
- Procurement of food should be consistent with sustainable development principles, and local suppliers used where possible.
- All relevant staff should be trained to ensure they are able to help pupils make healthy choices.
- Catering staff should be central to the whole-school approach and be represented in groups such as SNAGs.

School policy
- All schools should audit their service and curriculum and develop a whole-school food and nutrition policy.
- All children should be taught food preparation and cooking skills.
- Improve children's knowledge of food provenance and growing, through, for example, farm visits.
- Schools should aim for complete take up of free school meal entitlement.

Financial investment
- Schools and LAs should improve transparency and accountability in relation to the amount spent on school food, level of subsidy, surplus generated etc.
- The standard of kitchen provision should be a priority and investment should be made in schools which no longer have a kitchen.
- The Government should ensure that PFI contracts do not impose barriers to the improvement of school food and the provision of adequate kitchen facilities.

Monitoring
- The DfES should regularly carry out a nationwide evaluation of school food provision to assess the types of food and drink available.
- Ofsted should carry out regular monitoring and evaluation through in-depth inspections.
- Local authorities should report annually on progress in achieving healthy school standards.
- The School Food Trust should hold a database of standards-compliant menus for schools to use.

Adapted from: Turning the Tables: Transforming school food (SMRP, 2005).

1.14.2   The School Food Trust

'*It is important that school lunches contain sufficient energy and micronutrients to promote good nutritional health in all pupils and to protect those who are nutritionally vulnerable*'.   (SFT, 2007a)

Table 1.2   Timetable for implementation of new food and nutrient standards.

September 2006	The introduction of new 'interim' food-based standards for school lunches
September 2007	The introduction of food-based standards for all other school food and drink
September 2008	Deadline for all primary schools to comply with final food-based and nutrient-based standards for lunch
September 2009	Deadline for all secondary schools to comply with final food-based and nutrient-based standards for lunch

The SFT was set up in 2005 to help deliver the new standards and promote the education and health of children through improved quality of food. The SFT set itself four key goals for the following three years:

(1)   To ensure all schools meet the food-based and nutrient-based standards for lunch and non-lunch food.
(2)   To increase the uptake of school meals.
(3)   To reduce diet-related inequalities in childhood through food education and school-based initiatives.
(4)   To improve food skills through food education, and school and community initiatives.

School food is now governed by The Education (Nutritional Standards and Requirements for School Food) (England) Regulations (2007). There are four parts to the new standards: interim food-based standards, standards for school food other than lunch and nutrient-based standards. Final food-based standards will replace the interim standards by 2009 in all schools. These standards cover all food sold and served in schools and are summarised in Table 1.3. There is no requirement within the standards to provide hot meals. However, according to the SFT, the government is keen to encourage the provision of hot meals and it is a condition of the £220 transitional funding that, where local authorities do not offer a hot meals service, they develop a plan to introduce universal hot meals provision by September 2008. Standards also do not specify portion sizes, although the SFT does provide guidance on suggested portion sizes on its website (www.schoolfoodtrust.org.uk).

Although independent schools are not covered by the regulations, they are 'encouraged' to comply. All academies have to sign a funding agreement and are bound by the clauses within it. Clause 33(A) states that all food and drink provided by the academy must comply with legislation governing the provision of food and drink in maintained schools.

1.15   Interim food-based standards for school lunches

These standards (Table 1.3) apply to all local authority primary, secondary and special schools and pupil referral units in England and cover all hot and cold

Table 1.3 Interim and final food-based standards for lunches and non-lunch food.

Food/food groups	Interim food-based standards for school lunches from 2006 (revised 2007)	Food-based standards for school food other than lunches from 2007	Final food-based standards for school lunches from 2008 (primary) and 2009 (secondary)
Fruit and vegetables	Not less than two portions per day per pupil must be provided; at least one should be vegetables or salad and at least one should be fruit.	Fruit and/or vegetables must be provided at all school food outlets	Not less than two portions per day per pupil must be provided; at least one should be vegetables or salad and at least one should be fruit.
Meat, fish and other non-dairy sources of protein	A food from this group must be provided on a daily basis	No standard	No standard
Red meat	Red meat must be provided at least twice per week in primary schools and at least three times per week in secondary schools	No standard	No standard
Fish	Fish must be provided at least once per week in primary schools and at least twice per week in secondary schools	No standard	No standard
Oily fish	Oily fish such as mackerel or salmon must be provided at least once every three weeks	No standard	Oily fish such as mackerel or salmon must be provided at least once every three weeks
Meat products – categorised and restricted	A meat product (manufactured or homemade) from each of the four groups below may be provided no more than once per fortnight across the school day, providing the meat product also meets the standards for minimum meat content and does not contain any prohibited offal: **Group 1** Burger, hamburger, chopped meat, corned meat **Group 2** Sausage, sausage meat, link, chipolata, luncheon meat **Group 3** Individual meat pie, meat pudding, Melton Mowbray pie, game pie, Scottish (or Scotch) pie, pasty or pastie, bridie, sausage roll **Group 4** Any other shaped or coated meat product		

(Continued)

Table 1.3 (Continued)

Food/food groups	Interim food-based standards for school lunches from 2006 (revised 2007)	Food-based standards for school food other than lunches from 2007	Final food-based standards for school lunches from 2008 (primary) and 2009 (secondary)
Starchy food	A food from this group must be provided on a daily basis. Starchy food cooked in fat or oil should not be provided more than three times a week across the school day. Every day that a starchy food cooked in fat or oil is provided, a starchy food not cooked in fat or oil should also be provided	No standard	No standard
Bread	Bread with no added fat or oil must be provided on a daily basis	No standard	Bread with no added fat or oil must be provided on a daily basis
Deep-fried food – restricted	No more than two deep-fried items, such as chips and batter-coated products, in a single week across the school day		
Milk and dairy food	A food from this group should be available on a daily basis	No standard	No standard
Salt and condiments – restricted	No salt shall be available to add to food after the cooking process is complete. Salt shall not be provided at tables or service counters. Condiments, such as ketchup and mayonnaise, may only be available in sachets or in individual portions of not more than 10 g or 1 teaspoonful		
Snacks – restricted	Snacks such as crisps must not be provided. Nuts, seeds, vegetables and fruit with no added salt, sugar or fat are allowed. Dried fruit may contain up to 0.5% vegetable oil as a glazing agent.		
	Savoury crackers and breadsticks can only be served with fruit, vegetables or dairy food as part of school lunch	Savoury crackers and breadsticks must not be provided	Savoury crackers and breadsticks can only be served with fruit, vegetables or dairy food as part of school lunch
No confectionery	Confectionery such as chocolate bars, chocolate coated or flavoured biscuits, sweets or cereal bars must not be provided		
Cakes and biscuits – restricted	Cakes and biscuits are allowed at lunchtime but must not contain any confectionery	Cakes and biscuits must not be provided	Cakes and biscuits are allowed at lunchtime but must not contain any confectionery
Drinking water	Free, fresh drinking water should be provided at all times		
Healthier drinks	The only drinks permitted during the school day are plain water (still or sparking); skimmed, semi-skimmed or lactose-reduced milk; fruit juice; vegetable juice; plain soya, rice or oat drinks enriched with calcium; plain fermented milk (e.g. yoghurt) drinks; combination drinks; flavoured milk. Tea, coffee and low-calorie hot chocolate are also permitted.		

Source: School Food Trust (2007a).

food and drink provided, on and off school premises, including school trips. Food provided for special occasions and events and cookery lessons are exempt from regulations.

Interim food-based standards were announced in May 2006 and the SFT produced a guide to these standards for caterers, cooks and schools in June 2006, which was revised in 2007 to take account of some small changes. When the nutrient-based standards become law, in 2008 and 2009, schools will be required to move to final food-based standards. The SFT guidance document provides advice only how to incorporate some of the more challenging aspects of the standards, such as persuading pupils to eat oily fish.

Packed lunches provided by the school must also meet the food-based standards for school lunches, but do not apply to packed lunches brought in from home.

1.16 Food-based standards for all other school food and drink

There is now a wide range of food served in schools, outside the lunch hour. Table 1.4 provides an indication of the proportion of primary and secondary schools providing various services. Whereas in the pre-1980 school setting, the meal served in the middle of the day was usually the only opportunity to eat, post-1980 the school lunch has had to compete with other commercial enterprises, such as the vending machine. Indeed, if a child so wished he or she could derive every morsel consumed during the school day from such a machine. These alternative sources of food provide revenue to the school and more choice to the pupil. But they are also in direct competition with the school meal and until September 2007 were not subject to control.

Standards for non-lunch food and drink did not become statutory until September 2007 but schools were expected to start complying from September 2006. This means that:

- no confectionery, including chocolate, sweets and cereal bars, may be sold in schools

Table 1.4 The proportion of primary and secondary schools providing non-lunch food.

Type of service	Primary (%)	Secondary (%)
Breakfast	31	67
Caterer-run mid-morning break service	15	96
Snack vending	1	57
Cold drinks vending	2	69
Hot drinks vending	1	16
Tuck shop	22	8
After school food	No data	No data

Source: School Food Trust (2007b).

- no bagged snacks may be sold, other than unsalted, sugar-free nuts and seeds
- a variety of fruits and vegetables be made available in all school food outlets
- only water, milk (skimmed or semi-skimmed), fruit juices, yoghurt and milk drinks, low calorie hot chocolate and tea and coffee are to be provided as beverages.

Cakes, buns, pastries and biscuits may be provided only as part of the lunch provision.

1.16.1 Breakfast clubs

A breakfast club is a scheme whereby children arriving at school before the start of formal lessons can be served food on a drop-in basis. It is becoming increasingly common for primary school pupils in particular to arrive at school before the start of classes, in order to eat the first meal of the day. However still less than 10% of primary schools provide a breakfast service (LACA, 2007).

For many children, the breakfast club is potentially one way of ensuring that they start the day well nourished. Although it is frequently referred to as the most important meal of the day, breakfast is also the meal most likely to be skipped, especially by teenagers. The *Sodexho School Meals and Lifestyle Survey 2005* (Sodexho, 2005) found that 8% of schoolchildren ate nothing before going to school. This figure rose to 12% for 15 to 16-year-olds. Other children skip breakfast in favour of grazing along the school route: on average children spend £1.01 on the way to school, 40% of which is on drinks, 38% of which is on confectionery, 29% on crisps and other savoury snacks and 19% on chocolate (Sodexho, 2005).

Breakfast clubs started appearing throughout the UK in the 1990s, partly as a way of addressing these issues, but also because of parental demands for supervised before-school childcare (Street & Kenway, 1999). What the children are served, and by whom, depends on the individual school, and the usual school caterer may be involved, but not necessarily. They typically serve toast with spreads, cereals, fruit and sometimes hot food. The club may have been developed by staff or by a charitable organisation or be part of a local authority initiative. Food provided may be free or subsidised, and staff are usually, but not always, paid. Most clubs have an average daily attendance of between 10 and 15 children (Street & Kenway, 1999).

Not only can the breakfast club contribute to a child's daily nutritional requirements within a safe environment (depending on what's provided), it can also help tackle inequalities in health by improving access to healthy food. Furthermore, the breakfast club has been shown to have a positive effect on children's attention, concentration, behaviour and motivation to learn, with improved punctuality and school attendance also observed (Harrop & Palmer, 2002).

Until September 2007 what was provided at breakfast fell outside legislation and not all clubs served food which was nutritious and well-balanced (Harrop & Palmer, 2002). One study of 11 children in three schools found that children who attended breakfast clubs had significantly great intakes of fat, saturated fat and sodium than those who did not (Belderson *et al.*, 2003). The main obstacles to creating and maintaining a successful – and healthy – breakfast club are funding and staffing (Street & Kenway, 1999). More deprived areas are unlikely to be able to charge enough to cover their costs and fund-raising can be time-consuming and difficult. Staffing can be problematic because of the difficulty in finding volunteers – not all staff are paid. Schools cannot afford to waste good food and will often cut back on fresh foods and offer only popular, less healthy foods which they know the children will eat (Street & Kenway, 1999).

The Food in Schools *Healthier Breakfast Club* (see page 32) was piloted in 2003–2004 with the aim of improving the nutritional content of food and drink provided. The pilot was judged a success on a number of levels: schools successfully rose to the challenge of identifying ways to introduce healthier foods, through games and prizes, for example, and at the same time managed to create a positive atmosphere and strengthen relations between teachers and pupils. As a result, a guide to setting up and running healthier breakfast clubs is included in the Department of Health's *Food in Schools* Toolkit.

1.16.2   Breakfast clubs in Scotland

In Scotland, as many as 42% of 11 to 15-year-olds do not eat breakfast on a daily basis (Cassels & Stewart, 2002). Breakfast clubs were introduced to help improve this figure. They have become increasingly popular since the mid-1990s, mainly in primary schools (Food Commission, 2001). However, HM Inspectorate of Education reported in early 2008 that less than half the 165 primary schools it had inspected had a breakfast club initiative in place. Those that did were found to offer a variety of foods, both healthy and unhealthy, including cereals (including sugar-coated varieties), toast, fruit juices, fresh fruit, yoghurts, milk, hot chocolate and tea (HMIE, 2008). Most secondary school catering services sold food and drink each morning before the start of school (HMIE, 2008).

To assist schools in Scotland with the practicalities of setting up and running a healthy breakfast club, Community Food and Health (Scotland), formerly called the Scottish Community Diet Project, produces a downloadable, step-by-step toolkit, *Breakfast Clubs: More of a Head Start* (available at www.community-foodandhealth.org.uk).

1.16.3   Breakfast clubs in Wales

Keenest of all UK countries to get more children to eat their breakfast is Wales, where, since January 2007, all pupils in primary schools have been entitled to a free breakfast at school. However it is not obligatory for all schools to participate, nor is the club intended to replace breakfast if it is already provided at home. By March 2007 around 50% of primary schools in Wales had signed up to be part of the free breakfast initiative, even though it had been hoped that full participation would be achieved by January 2007.

It is intended that the food provided should be 'healthy and nutritionally balanced', and sourced locally, wherever possible. According to the Welsh National Assembly, the initiative is intended to help improve the health and concentration of pupils, thereby raising standards of learning and attainment. An evaluation of the service published in March 2007 found that in the schools that had availed themselves of the service, *'There was general agreement that it had impacted on pupil dietary behaviour, learning, school behaviour and health and well being. Effects were also noted for improvements in social interactions with peers and teachers and the social skills of pupils'* (Lynch & Murphy, 2008).

1.16.4   Breakfast clubs in Northern Ireland

Since 2006, schools in disadvantaged areas and those with a free school meal entitlement of 37% or more have been able to apply for 'extended schools' funding. This money can be used to fund a number of activities – including breakfast clubs – which help raise standards in schools. In 2004 a Department of Education report stated that breakfast club provision was offered by 16% of secondary schools and only very few primary schools (DE, 2004). However, in 2005, an evaluation of the effects of piloting compulsory nutritional standards for school meals found that the numbers of participating primary and secondary schools offering breakfast clubs and other healthy initiatives had increased significantly (PricewaterhouseCoopers, 2005).

1.16.5   Vending machines

A hitherto somewhat contentious source of both sustenance and revenue, vending machines are commonplace in secondary schools throughout the UK, as well as many other countries. Although subject to strict regulation since September 2007, they typically sold, prior to that date, carbonated, sugared drinks and foods high in fat, sugar and salt, and low in fibre and nutrients. A survey carried out by YouGov in 2003 found that 81% of parents wanted vending machines selling junk food removed from schools and a number of concerned organisations called for a ban. However, some head teachers expressed their opposition to any such ban, on the grounds that children would still buy junk food from elsewhere, and thus deprive the schools of much-needed funds (Frewin, 2004). Vending machines provide a source of revenue which can be used to pay for equipment and resources and can be worth up to £20 000 a year to a school (Food Commission, 2001).

The Food in Schools *Healthier Vending Project* (see page 32) which was piloted in secondary schools in England and Wales, produced 'extremely positive' results (Harvey, 2004). Although the pilot involved selling drinks only, with no food options, it revealed that children would choose healthy drinks (water, fruit juice, milk) from a 'healthier' vending machine, even when that machine was positioned alongside a more traditional vending machine with the usual soft drinks options (Harvey, 2004). According to the Health Education Trust, which carried out the pilot, vending machines should not be seen as inherently evil as they can play a role in encouraging healthier consumption habits, reduce queues and keep pupils on site during the day.

Since legislation was introduced, vending machines may provide milk drinks, but these must contain at least 90% milk (skimmed, semi-skimmed or lactose-reduced). They may contain added vitamins and minerals and less than 5% added sugar or honey. They may also contain additives and flavourings permitted by EU law. Combination fruit drinks must contain at least 50% juice and no added sugar. They may contain permitted additives and flavourings, but schools are 'strongly encouraged' to provide drinks that are additive free.

1.16.6   Tuck shops

Like vending machines, these can provide additional revenue for a school. Prior to the introduction of mandatory controls in September 2007, they too were frequently criticised for selling branded, high fat, high sugar and high salt snacks. However, a trend for healthier tuck shops, selling fruit in particular, had already emerged a few years before legislation was introduced.

As a result of the positive findings of the Food in Schools *Healthier Tuck Shop* project (see page 32) the Food in Schools toolkit was produced which provides guidance on setting up and running tuck shops. During the pilots, schools offered fruit, yoghurt, vegetables and filled rolls, and found that a healthier tuck shop could be both popular and profitable. Furthermore, they were found to help keep pupils on-site during break-time. One further appeal of setting up such an initiative is that the tuck shop can be run almost entirely by pupils, once the initial planning and organising has been completed.

1.17   Nutrient-based standards

Table 1.5 outlines the fourteen minimum nutrient-based standards, to be introduced by 2008 (primary schools) and 2009 (secondary schools). These standards are derived from UK nutrient recommendations (dietary reference values). Separate nutrient-based standards are given for single sex secondary schools as it was considered that there are sufficiently large differences in the energy and nutrient requirements of girls and boys aged 11–18 years to warrant different sets of values. Nutrients have either minimum or maximum standards and apply to an average school lunch.

1.18   Final food-based standards

These come into effect in September 2009 and are outlined in Table 1.3. Although there are standards for red meat, fish, milk, dairy and starchy foods in the interim standards, these have not been included in the final standards because, the SFT states, iron, protein and calcium are covered in the nutrient-based standards (private email correspondence, 08/01/08), a claim that runs contrary to the recommendations of the SMRP (see page 40).

Table 1.5 Nutrient-based standards for the average lunch meal – primary and secondary schools.

Nutrient	Min/max	Primary	Secondary		
			Mixed	Girls only	Boys only
Energy (kJ)		2215 ± 5%	2700 ± 5%	2412 ± 121	2985 ± 149
(kcal)		530 ± 5%	646 ± 5%	577 ± 28.9	714 ± 35.7
Carbohydrate (g)	min	70.6	86.1	77.0	95.2
Non-milk extrinsic sugars (g)	max	15.5	18.9	16.9	20.9
Fat (g)	max	20.6	25.1	22.5	27.8
Saturated fat (g)	max	6.5	7.9	7.1	8.7
Protein (g)	min	7.5	13.3	12.7	13.8
Fibre (g)	min	4.2	5.2	4.6	5.7
Sodium (mg)	max	499	714	714	714
Vitamin A (µg)	min	175	245	210	245
Vitamin C (mg)	min	10.5	14.0	14.0	14.0
Folate (µg)	min	53	70	70	70
Calcium (mg)	min	193	350	280	350
Iron (mg)	min	3.0	5.2	5.2	4.0
Zinc (mg)	min	2.5	3.3	3.2	3.3

Taken from: School Food Trust (2007a).

1.19   Diverse diets and special dietary needs

The new standards do not make provision for children following religious or other diverse diets, or those with food allergies. However, the SFT states that it is up to the individual school to decide whether it is feasible to cater for individual needs, and it should consider adopting a policy and procedure to ensure that special requests are handled appropriately (SFT, 2007a). In its *A guide to introducing the Government's food-based and nutrient-based standards for school lunches,* the SFT outlines the dietary requirements of the main religions and provides basic information on common allergies.

1.20   Target Nutrient Specifications

When the government announced the creation of the SMRP it also announced its intention to introduce ingredient specifications for processed foods such as sausages and burgers. Product specifications were originally developed in Scotland to help meet the standards outlined in the Scottish document *Hungry for Success* (page 26), and raise the quality of manufactured products used in school lunches.

The result was the publication, by the Food Standards Agency in May 2006, of target nutrient specifications (TNS) for a range of manufactured foods used in school meals throughout the UK, to assist caterers in meeting the wider standards for school lunches.

These specifications – which are voluntary only – set maximum levels for total fat, saturated fat, salt and sugar content and apply to thirty-eight categories of manufactured products including bread, poultry products, soups and burgers. Minimum levels for protein in certain vegetarian products were also set. No information is available on whether manufacturers have reformulated their products to meet standards.

1.21   Monitoring the new standards

Each local authority in England is responsible for ensuring that school food provision meets the new standards, unless the budget has been delegated to the school, in which case the governing body is responsible. Each school must be able to demonstrate that the service provided complies with standards, by providing evidence in the form of menus, portion sizes and graphs and tables (SFT, 2007a). The SFT's *A guide to introducing the Government's food-based and nutrient-based standards for school lunches* (SFT, 2007) gives further advice to schools on ensuring compliance. The Trust has also developed an on-line interactive tool, the *School lunch checklist*, to assist schools in their self-assessment of compliance, which is downloadable from their website.

It is now the responsibility of Ofsted to monitor the new standards and examine the evidence presented by each school. Inspections were conducted during 2006/07 whose aim was to evaluate the progress schools were making in achieving compliance. Her Majesty's Inspectors visited 18 primary/middle schools and 9 secondary schools in 12 local authorities. The inspectors found that in all the schools visited, the food provided met the new interim standards, and all pupils with special dietary requirements had those needs met. However, religious requirements were not always accommodated – for example, not all the schools with Muslim pupils provided halal meat every day. Most schools cooked food on site, from fresh ingredients, except where no kitchen existed or food had to be cooked in a microwave or prepared elsewhere. In all the schools, menus were planned in advance, in cycles of 3–6 weeks, and the schools ensured that pupils and their families saw the menus in advance. In those schools running breakfast clubs and tuck shops, those services were found to provide a range of healthy foods (Ofsted, 2007).

1.22   Current system of meals provision

'*School caterers are currently being expected to provide what is essentially a welfare service whilst still endeavouring to operate as a commercial venture*'. (LACA, 2007)

Just as the nature of the food served to children today has evolved beyond anything comparable to pre-1980 years, so too has the way in which it is served. Today, the dining environment is where young consumers make decisions about how to spend their money. Commercial interests compete for their loyalty with other, less material interests.

In primary schools and special schools, a standard set meal is the most common form of provision, whereas the cash cafeteria is the system of choice of most secondary schools (Unison, 2002). The cash cafeteria, where each food item is priced separately, came about largely as a result of the 1980 Act. For children making the transition from primary school to secondary school, the cafeteria can be an exciting opportunity to choose their own food, possibly for the first time. However it also means that children as young as 11 are expected to take responsibility for their diet – and therefore health – as well as their budget.

1.22.1   The dining environment

'Improving children and young people's meal experience will have a positive impact on the take-up of school meals, and the wider school day'.   (SFT 2007c)

'In the best instances, schools recognised the contribution that a good dining experience could make. In these cases, teaching staff often ate in the dining room with the pupils and the atmosphere was warm and friendly, with sufficient time for all to eat their lunch comfortably and to enjoy socialising'. (Ofsted, 2007)

The *Food in Schools Dining Room Environment* project (see page 32), which was piloted in 10 schools in the Yorkshire and Humber region in 2003–04, found, perhaps not surprisingly, that pupils would prefer to *'eat, relax and socialise in an environment as stylish, efficient and up to date as can be found off campus on the high street'*, rather than in the often rather rigid settings of the school dining room. They preferred décor which resembled popular high street 'café culture'. However, the real dining experience does not always meet aspirations: in 2006 Ofsted reported that dining conditions in secondary schools were variable, and at times poor. A minority of schools were found to have such short lunch breaks that pupils (and staff) were unable to eat their food in comfort (Ofsted, 2006a). A year later, Ofsted reported that the environment in secondary schools remained unchanged: in none of the schools visited for inspection were dining arrangements good (Ofsted, 2007). Overcrowding, excessive queueing and considerable noise characterised the meal experience. Few teachers ate with pupils and pupils eating a school lunch could not sit with friends who brought a packed lunch. Ofsted reported that pupils were more likely to eat a school meal when queues were short and they could sit with friends who brought packed lunches. According to Ofsted, the quality of the dining area was a determinant of whether pupils ate a school meal; one reason given by pupils for taking a packed lunch to school was precisely that sandwiches could be eaten quickly where and when they chose (Ofsted, 2007).

Conditions in primary schools however, appear to be much better. The quality of the dining environment was found by Ofsted to be good (Ofsted, 2007). Primary schools were found to make more of an effort in terms of decorating the dining room, using vibrant displays and information on healthy eating. There was sufficient room for those taking a school lunch to sit with friends who had brought a packed lunch.

1.22.2   The cashless payment system

Many secondary schools have now adopted smart card technology and cashless payment systems (LACA, 2004). Around 69% of LAs in England and 61% in Wales now have some form of cashless payment system in their secondary schools, based on a swipe card (sometimes called an e-card) which contains credits which have been paid for in advance by parents or carers. This smart card technology has a number of advantages. It is an effective means of monitoring children's dietary habits, without the need for researchers and questionnaires. The results are also likely to be more accurate as they do not rely upon children to complete questionnaires honestly. This system can also be used to encourage healthier choices – all the cards contain a chip which stores information about purchases, and can be used to automatically reward children with, for example, free cinema tickets or money-off vouchers (DfES, 2006). For catering companies, it is a useful marketing tool and can be used to monitor changing trends and inform menu planning.

One of the greatest benefits of the system is improved uptake of free school meals, as it prevents identification of pupils with entitlement (see page 60). Reduced cash handling also reduces the risk of money being lost or stolen. Children are therefore less likely to spend money on snacks en route to and from school. In its 2007 report, Ofsted cited one particular school where all parents received a detailed record of what their children had eaten during the month. They were then able to identify food they did not wish their children to eat and put an electronic block on this. The school had found that take-up was high, because it removed any stigma attached to receiving a free school meal and had resulted in a dramatic reduction in bullying and theft. It is not known how the pupils felt about their parents' invisible presence controlling their food choices.

1.23   Catering contracts

Under Fair Funding, which began in 2000 (see page 14) all secondary schools have been delegated responsibility for their own budget and the provision of food to pupils. Primary schools have the option to accept delegation if they so wish (DfES, 2006). As well as being responsible for their own budget, delegation also meant that the school became responsible for supplying free school meals to eligible pupils, paid meals on request and compliance with nutritional standards (Storey & Candappa, 2004). It is estimated that over 80% of LAs have universal delegation of funding to all secondary and primary schools in England (Storey & Candappa, 2004).

A local authority secondary school can choose from one of the four main types of catering contract, as outlined below.

1.23.1 Local authority in-house catering

This is the most common form of delivery and was, before the delegation of budgets, the standard method. Opting for this system means that the local authority is responsible for the full delivery of the service. One main disadvantage is that the service offers no protection against poor performance (DfES, 2006). Poor performance can lead to reductions on the amount spent on ingredients, and greater dependence on processed foods, in order to make ends meet. The school has little choice in what is provided.

The benefits of this option include economies of scale – greater buying power for ingredients at better prices. The local authority catering service is generally a non-profit making organisation and if a profit is made it is returned to the schools (DfES, 2006). It also means that the school does not have to concern itself with the risk and responsibility of adhering to external standards and requirements such as health and safety and nutritional standards.

1.23.2 Local authority contract with a private catering company

Outsourcing the contract means the local authority can concentrate on developing and improving specifications, managing policy issues and negotiating contracts. Catering companies often have greater expertise and experience in buying food than the local authority. Contractors can offer lower prices to schools who have more chance of making a profit (DfES, 2006). On the other hand, it is harder for the school to deal with poor performance or dissatisfaction. Contractors, if left unchallenged by the local authority, often source the cheapest food (DfES, 2006).

1.23.3 School contract with its own private catering company

The main advantage of the school selecting its own private contractor is that the contractor takes full responsibility for the delivery of the service, as well as for compliance with external requirements such as nutritional standards and health and safety. However, the school should have considerable negotiation and procurement skills and may have to pay for costly external advice.

1.23.4 In-house school meals provision

This means that the school runs the service in-house. This system gives the school total control of the school meals service, which can be a liberating experience but also a very daunting one. Knowledge of budgeting, staffing, menu planning, standards and other issues is essential. However, it can be highly advantageous, as the school is able to respond directly to the requirements of children, parents and the school community.

Local authority catering managers in England, Wales and Scotland are represented by the Local Authority Caterers Association (LACA), which regularly carries out surveys of school meals in England. The 2007 LACA school meals survey

(LACA, 2007) found that 60% of local authorities provide catering to schools themselves. Only 3% of catering services are self-operated by schools. In Wales nearly all (97%) of primary school contracts, and 95% of secondary school contracts are operated by the LA. By contrast, almost all catering contracts in Scotland and Northern Ireland are operated in-house (LACA, 2004).

The most widely used catering firm is Scolarest, followed by Initial Catering Services and Sodexho (Unison, 2002). All three contractors are multinational companies, enjoying a lack of competition from smaller operators and for whom industrial food processing methods on economies of scale make considerable financial sense.

Some schools gained from delegation and others lost out. Many found that taking responsibility for operating and staffing the school kitchen was an overwhelming experience – some LAs offered guidance documents to schools on managing their own budget but others offered only ad hoc support. Kitchen repair and maintenance proved a difficult aspect of delegation, especially as budgets do not always stretch to major repairs. Many schools and governors, finding themselves unprepared for this, opted to close the kitchen (Storey & Candappa, 2004). Kitchens also closed because of fears of having to deal with the quagmire of health and safety legislation. Other schools responded to delegation by increasing prices, a reaction which could carry serious implications for the take-up of meals (Storey & Candappa, 2004).

For some schools, however, assuming responsibility for the provision of meals provided an opportunity to negotiate the supply of healthier, more nutritious meals. They were able to source new suppliers or embark on an in-house service offering meals that exceeded the minimum legal nutritional standards. However after delegation there was an overall greater focus on the commercial viability of the meal service with schools tending to offer more popular but not necessarily nutritious meals (Storey & Candappa, 2004).

Some schools which saved money on the budget redirected those savings towards the general school budget (Storey & Candappa, 2004). According to LACA savings of around £154 million per year that were made from school catering budgets, after delegation, were not been ploughed back into the school meal service, but instead used to subsidise other education costs (LACA, 2004). Had they been returned to catering, LACA estimates that an extra 25p per head spend on the food cost of a school meal could have been added (LACA, 2004).

1.24 Catering staff

'There is good evidence that pupils in schools with well-trained catering staff eat healthier food, but there is little training available for catering staff'. (DfES, 2004)

'The best food was provided in those schools with experienced, well qualified and appropriately trained cooks'. (Ofsted report, 2007)

It wasn't just the school meal which was overhauled by the 1980 Education Act: so too were conditions for those employed to produce it. Until 1980, all catering staff were employed on national pay terms and conditions, but following the introduction of the Act, these terms and conditions have varied from one authority to another. Where contracts have been won by the private sector, staff are employed on the company's own pay rates, terms and conditions. After 1980 many local authorities cut staffing numbers, or hours, or even did away with the service completely. In 2000, the Local Authority Caterers Association identified '*a huge range of pay rates, terms and conditions in existence across the British Isles*' in this sector of employment. Rates of pay could be locally determined, or in line with private sector rates, or even vary within the same workforce. In 2006/07 the average rate of pay for a school cook was £7.02 per hour. For a primary school head cook the average hourly rate was £7.76 and for a secondary school head cook/catering manager, £8.46 (LACA, 2007).

In excess of 87 000 staff are employed in the industry. When surveyed, LACA members identified a number of difficulties in recruitment, most notably that '*the rates of pay are at the lower end of the market rates*' (LACA, 2004). The survey also identified that most staff who join the school catering services are mothers with school-aged children who found the working hours conveniently fitted into their children's school day. The school catering service is made up of at least 95% women.

Despite low rates of pay, catering services staff can play a valuable role in the provision of better food – in its 2007 inspection, Ofsted found that some schools involved catering staff in finding effective ways of making healthier choices more attractive. They could also help young children with the practicalities of social dining. Ofsted inspectors identified some primary school children as being unable to manage a knife and fork or make conversation during a meal, but were helped by staff who showed the children how to hold their cutlery and eat properly (Ofsted, 2007). Inspectors found that the number of catering and supervisory staff, and the extent to which they had been trained, had an impact on the quality of the dining experience.

1.25 Expenditure

The retail price of a school meal can vary quite considerably and is met by a combination of expenditure by local authorities, schools and parents. The cost of a free school meal is met by the school or local authority. It is the local authority or school that sets the price of a meal, which includes the cost of the food, labour and direct overheads. There is no specific allocation for school food within the budget allocated to local authorities or schools by the Department for Children, Schools and Families (DCSF). The government has not subsidised school meals since 1967, when financial responsibility for the provision of meals passed from government to individual LA. In 56% of local authorities, the meals provided in primary schools are subsidised, either by the council or the school. The average subsidy is 43p (LACA, 2007).

1.25.1   School meal expenditure, pre- new standards

In 1995 the price of a school meal was found to range from 65p to £1.25 in primary schools and from 65p to £1.50 in secondary schools (Unison, 2002). In 2002 a Unison survey found the average retail cost of a school meal to be £1.37 in England and £1.35 in Wales. Overall, highest prices were found in Edinburgh (£1.85 in secondary schools and £1.65 in primary schools). However, other Scottish Authorities such as Dumfries and Galloway were able to produce much cheaper meals (£1.00 in secondary schools and 95p in primary schools). Unison found meal prices in primary and secondary schools to be, on average, 4p cheaper in authorities which subsidised the cost, and the greater the subsidy the lower the cost. Although the Unison survey found that most LAs subsidised the school meal – fifty-nine per cent – there was an indication that authorities were moving away from subsidies completely.

1.25.2   School meal expenditure, post new standards

The LACA National School Meals Survey 2007 (LACA, 2007) reported that the average retail price of a primary school meal, as at April 2007, was £1.64. That figure represented a mean average increase of 20% from 2003/04 and ranged from £1.40 (in Sefton and Greenwich) to £1.95 (Wandsworth). These findings are similar to those reported by the SFT survey which found that the cost of a primary school meal rose from £1.56 in 2005–2006 to £1.63 in 2006–2007 (Nicholas *et al.*, 2007).

The average cost of ingredients, per meal, was 57p in 2006–2007, up from 52p in 2005–2006 and representing about a third of the meal price (Nicholas *et al.*, 2007). The labour cost of a primary school meal, in 2007, was £1.09, 67% of the total meal cost. This represents an average labour cost increase of 34% compared to the 2005–2006 survey where the labour cost was £1.03.

In secondary schools the cost of a meal also rose – from £1.64 in 2005–2006 to £1.72 in 2006–2007. This represents a 5% increase (Nicholas *et al.*, 2007).

According to the SFT, these increases are probably due to the catering practices required to meet the standards introduced in 2006, as well as training and increased hours of work and increases in hourly wages. Increases in costs make it harder still for catering services to make a profit. Using better ingredients has also proved costly: the average cost of ingredients for a school meal was 40p in 2003/04 and 60p in 2006/07 (LACA, 2007). In 2003 nearly all LA caterers either made a profit or broke even; by 2007 over 91% of LAs were either losing money or just breaking even. The situation is furthermore explained by the fall in take-up of the school meal since the introduction of standards: the average spend in cash cafeterias in secondary schools dropped from £1.18 in 2003/04 to 97p in 2006/07 (LACA, 2007).

1.26   Procurement of school meals

'*By 2020 ... we would like all schools to be models of healthy schools, with local and sustainable food and drink produced and prepared on site (where possible), with strong commitments to the environment, social responsibility and animal welfare, and with increased opportunity to involve local suppliers'.* (DfES, 2006)

The public sector in England spends £2 billion on food and catering services, and school food represents 20–25% of that spend. Recent years have seen not only a strong drive to improve the quality of food in schools, and other institutions, but also a desire to put that food into a context which respects the wellbeing of both the producer and the natural environment. School food, it is now recognised, can no longer be viewed as a discrete operation, but as part of a 'whole school' process. The *School Meals Review Panel*, in its document *Turning the tables* (page 40) as well as making recommendations for food and nutrient-based standards, also recommended that the procurement of food served in schools should be consistent with sustainable development principles. The panel advised that schools and caterers should look to local farmers and suppliers for their produce wherever possible. The impetus for sustainable procurement methods relates to all public sector catering. In acknowledgement of this, Defra launched, in 2004, the Public Sector Food Procurement Initiative (PSFPI), which has six priority objectives:

• promote food safety, including high standards of hygiene
• increase the consumption of healthy and nutritious food
• improve the sustainability and efficiency of production, processing and distribution
• increase tenders from small and local producers and their ability to do business
• increase cooperation among buyers, producers and along supply chains
• improve the sustainability and efficiency of public food procurement and catering services

At the moment schools are a long way off achieving this aim, with three large firms – Scolarest, Initial and Sodexho – dominating the market, with little competition and operating mainly centralised supply chains. Between them they supply over 200 local authorities in the UK, as well as individual schools (DfES, 2006). In order to assist the public sector procurement agencies in achieving the six objectives it set, the PSFPI publishes a number of guidance documents which are downloadable from the Defra website (www.defra.gov.uk). These include:

• *Putting it into practice*
• *Best practice in sustainable public sector food procurement*
• *Guide to implementing the PSFPI – advice for practitioners*
• *How to increase opportunities for small and local producers when aggregating food procurement – guidance for buyers and specifiers*
• *Providing meals in primary schools*
• *Guidance for procuring school lunches.*

The National Audit Office also published its own guide, *Smarter food procurement in the public sector* in 2006, identifying areas with scope for delivering efficient sustainability in public sector food procurement. The advice is more general than specific, focussing on suggestions such as schools working together to share procurement costs, using cheap seasonal produce and adopting good practice in contracting, by ensuring that specifications are clear and unambiguous.

Most would argue in favour of prioritising local, seasonal produce, and although the advice offered by the NAO is useful, no catalogue of practical tips can circumvent the EU Treaty of Rome which protects the free movement of goods and services and prevents public bodies from discriminating in favour of domestic producers. The Treaty means that public sector buyers cannot restrict purchases to specific locations or suppliers. Currently it is not known what percentage of UK-produced food is supplied to schools.

Writing of the differences between school meal procurement in the UK and in Italy, Professor Kevin Morgan and Dr Roberta Sonnino of Cardiff University's Regeneration Institute define a sustainable school meal service as one that *delivers fresh and nutritious food; conceives healthy eating as part of a socially negotiated 'whole school' approach; and, wherever feasible, seeks to source the food as locally and as seasonally as possible* (Morgan & Sonnino, 2007). Aware of the legalities which appear to obstruct the creation of a truly sustainable school meal service, Morgan and Sonnino advocate what they call a *creative procurement policy.*

The perception of EU regulations is one of tension between sustainability and free trade. As Morgan and Sonnino point out, the principle of 'non-discrimination' presents the biggest problem to the implementation of local procurement initiatives. In the 1990s the decision to allocate contracts had to be based either on the lowest cost or 'the most economically advantageous tender' (Morgan & Sonnino, 2007). 'Cost' did not include environmental costs. However all that changed in 2004 when the European Parliament endorsed two new directives on public procurement which were enshrined in law in early 2006. These introduced a 'revolutionary' change in the European regulatory context of public procurement by stating that:

> 'Contracting authorities may lay down special conditions relating to the performance of a contract ... The conditions governing the performance of a contract may, in particular, concern social and environmental considerations'.
> (European Parliament and Council 2004 in Morgan & Sonnino, 2007)

Earlier, in 1999, the EU Council of Ministers had also agreed that contracting authorities should be allowed to take into consideration production methods of the bidder – meaning authorities could select environment-friendly food over cheaply produced food (Morgan & Sonnino, 2007). These changes in regulation mean that institutions, including schools, have been given the opportunity to be 'creative' when it comes to interpreting the EU Treaty of Rome.

In the UK, public sector procurement departments have been slow – or unwilling – to grasp the opportunities for creativity presented to them. Yet some European countries had already managed to manoeuvre around European legislation in order to secure more local and even organic produce (Morgan & Sonnino, 2007). It is not surprising that Italy, where good quality, fresh food is central to the nation's cultural identity, *is the country where public procurement strategies establish the clearest priority for local and organic food* (Morgan & Sonnino, 2007). Indeed, because school meals are considered an integral part of a child's right to education and health, the Italian system allows the possibility of discriminating in favour of local operators. This system also allows contractors to retain complete control over the system. In 1992 the State Council stated that it is legal for a municipality to restrict the participation in a public competition to companies located in the province (Morgan & Sonnino, 2007). It also makes a creative interpretation of the term 'best value' which in the UK is often taken to mean lowest price but in Italy assesses other issues such as the nutritional and educational aspects of the proposed service (Morgan & Sonnino, 2007) As Morgan and Sonnino astutely observe, the Italian system opens up a legal way to 'creatively' interpret EU directives on public procurement and *emphasize the territorial 'rootedness' of the school meal service over and above the European principle of 'non-discrimination'.*

1.27   Free school meals

'Within low-income families children cannot always rely on healthy, nutritious meals at home'.   (SMRP, 2005)

'The capacity of schools to provide a supportive environment for children, particularly those experiencing disadvantage, has been eroded over the past 15 years, through such measures as the deregulation of school meals of a minimum standard and subsidised price, (and the) reduction of entitlement to free school meals'.   (Acheson, 1998)

School meals in England, Wales and Scotland are free to pupils whose families receive any of the following:

• income support
• income-based jobseeker's allowance
• support under part VI of the Immigration and Asylum Act 1999
• child tax credit, provided they do not receive working tax credit and have an annual income that does not exceed £14 495 (as of 6 April 2007)
• the Guarantee element of State Pension Credit.

Children who receive income support or income-based job seekers allowance in their own right are also eligible to receive free school meals. Although local authorities are not obliged to provide milk to pupils, they can choose to do so and if they do, it must be free to those pupils who qualify for free meals.

In Northern Ireland, the Education and Library Board (ELB) is obliged to provide a free lunchtime meal to pupils if:

- either parent is in receipt of income support
- either parent is in receipt of income-based job seeker's allowance
- either parent is in receipt of pension credit
- the family are in receipt of child tax credit with an annual taxable income of less than £13 000 and they are not in receipt of Working Tax Credit

Currently 1.8 million children in the UK are eligible for free school meals, but almost one in five fails to claim this (Storey & Chamberlain, 2001). Stigma is thought to be a principle reason for this – research has found embarrassment and fear of being teased to be main obstacles to uptake (Storey & Chamberlain, 2001).

The *School Meals in Secondary Schools in England* report (Nelson *et al.*, 2004) revealed that in over three-quarters of the schools surveyed, those pupils receiving free school meals were easily identifiable by other pupils. The 2007 Ofsted inspection survey of 27 schools in 12 local authorities also found that the visibility of payment methods deterred entitled pupils from taking a free meal (Ofsted, 2007).

Children with free entitlement can often be easily identified, because they may have to hand in their free meal tickets, or give their names, or stand in a different queue. In Northern Ireland, pupils receiving a free school meal may not get the same meal as paying pupils. In schools where no cooked meal is provided, eligible pupils are given packed lunches which are also sometimes identifiable as 'free'. The meal ticket does not necessarily meet the cost of the meal, requiring extra money and often causing embarrassment at the till (McMahon & Marsh, 1999). There are also cases of parents not claiming eligibility because they were unaware of their entitlement or did not know how to apply for it (Storey & Chamberlain, 2001).

The cashless 'smart card' (see page 53) has been identified as an effective way of addressing the problem of poor take-up but it is not used universally, and the problem of entitled children being easily identified has by no means been eliminated.

1.27.1 Poverty

Universality had been a central theme in welfare since the 1944 Education Act which introduced compulsory free secondary education for all children under the age of 15 (Morelli & Seaman, 2004). Child poverty went into decline after the Second World War, but rose rapidly from the late 1970s (Morelli & Seaman, 2004). The rising cost of welfare saw the gradual increase in means testing throughout the 1950s and 1960s but it wasn't until the late 1970s that a rapid reversal of the mainly universal system was undertaken in order to avoid a 'dependency culture'. Since Labour came to power in 1997, means tested tax credits have shaped welfare provision, alongside a sharp rise in levels of child poverty in Britain.

Children living in poverty are at increased risk of malnutrition. Children from lower income families tend to be shorter than children from higher income

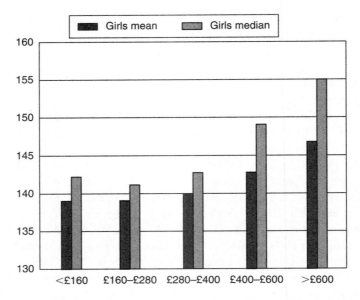

Figure 1.5   Height (cm) by family income, girls aged 5–15. (*Source*: The Food Commission, 2001. Reproduced with kind permission.)

families, but do not tend to be underweight (Food Commission, 2001) – see Figures 1.5–1.7. This suggests that although poorer children may get enough energy (calories) to maintain body weight, they do not get enough nutrients to grow adequately.

Many, including the Child Poverty Action Group (CPAG), regard school meals as an important anti-poverty measure, providing the only hot meal received by one in four children in the UK. Free school meals are seen by many parents as providing the 'one good meal a day' (McEvaddy, 1988). According to the CPAG, one in three school children in the UK lives in poverty, yet only one in five is eligible to receive a free school meal. There have been calls for universality of free school meals, with child benefit cited as a positive example of the success of universality – take up of child benefit stands at 98% (Unison, 2002).

1.27.2   The Hull experience

In England, the City of Hull became the first local authority in the UK to provide universal free school meals by initiating a three-year pilot to provide free meals for all pupils in primary and special schools. Hull received permission from the Secretary of State to provide free meals from April 2004 and rollout was completed in February 2005.

The focus of the scheme, which was called *Eat well do well* was health as well as free provision. It was introduced in order to tackle the underachievement and

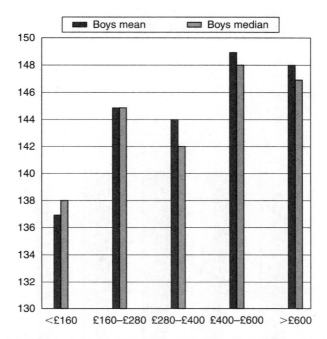

Figure 1.6 Height (cm) by family income, boys aged 5–15. (*Source*: The Food Commission, 2001. Reproduced with kind permission.)

health inequalities, as well as deprivation, the city faced. Hull languishes near the bottom of league tables in terms of pupils who achieve good GCSE results, and the council hoped universal free school meals would raise educational attainment. Hull also has the highest concentration of type 2 diabetes and has been labelled the UK's 'fat capital'.

Most of the food was produced fresh and on-site. There were four strands to the scheme: breakfast, fruit, lunch and after-school refreshments. Breakfast consisted of low sugar cereals, high fibre toast, low fat spread and reduced sugar jam or marmalade. Fruit juice was also provided. Hull City Council also decided to extend the existing free fruit and vegetables in schools scheme to all pupils in primary schools, instead of just those aged 4–6 years. The after-school refreshment consisted of two digestive biscuits and either a carton of fresh milk or orange juice.

The scheme was considered a great success, with take-up almost doubling in just two years from 36% to 64% (see www.cpag.org.uk). High take-up was credited in part to the removal of stigma attached to claiming free meals – before the scheme, only around half of the children eligible for free school meals were claiming them. Despite this success, and to the disappointment of many, the new Liberal Democrat leadership of Hull City decided, in the summer of 2006, to scrap the scheme once the pilot ended in 2007, on the grounds that the policy

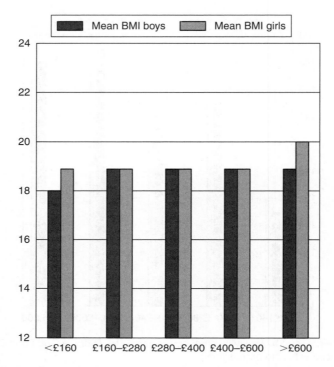

Figure 1.7 Body mass index by family income. Children aged 5–15. (*Source*: The Food Commission, 2001. Reproduced with kind permission.)

was unaffordable, even though the estimated £3 million cost of providing free meals represented just over 1% of the council's education budget (Green, 2006). In September 2007, charging was reintroduced. Take-up quickly fell from 64% to around 40%.

In North Tyneside, a pilot scheme to introduce free school meals for children of primary school age was introduced in September 2007. Eight schools took part and, as expected, the scheme is now being rolled out across all primary schools in the region, with full implementation expected by the end of 2008.

1.27.3   The Scottish free school meals campaign

Scotland has one of the worst child poverty rates in Europe, with around 29% of Scottish children living below the Government's poverty line (Brown & Phillips, 2002). Despite this, only 17% of children are entitled to a free school meal. Many children living in poverty have no right to free school meals because their parents are working, but on low wages.

Take-up of free school meals entitlement varies from region to region – from 88.8% in Shetland to 36.7% in Edinburgh City (Brown & Phillips, 2002). Of pupils not entitled to a free meal, many (21% of primary and 31% of secondary school pupils) are deterred from buying a meal because of the cost (CPAG).

An ongoing campaign for universal free school meals has highlighted the debate between universality and targeted welfare provision. Research at the University of Dundee examined universality versus targeted welfare provision with regard to school meals, and found that the best way to ensure that the poorest children receive the greatest benefits from free school meals was to make them available to all (Morelli & Seaman, 2004). The researchers found that the current system of free school meal provision did not reduce inequality because it failed to benefit large numbers of the very poorest. The report suggests that free school meals would promote greater equality for 90% of families with children – of the remaining wealthiest 10%, many send their children to private school anyway. At the time of the research – 2004 – it was estimated that universally free school meals would cost the Scottish executive £170 million a year (Morelli & Seaman, 2004).

The Campaign for Free School Meals was launched in Scotland in 2001, with support from many organisations including Unison Scotland, in response to the levels of child poverty and diet-related ill-health in Scotland. The School Meals (Scotland) Bill was launched to provide every child in a Scottish state school (primary and secondary) with a free, nutritious school meal every day, and had three main aims: reducing stigma, tackling poverty and improving health (Scottish Executive, 2003). Despite widespread popularity, the Scottish Parliament rejected the bill.

The campaign started up again in March 2004, with considerable public, media and celebrity support. A new free school meals bill was launched, successfully, in 2006 and in October 2007 the Scottish Government began a free school meals pilot scheme for primary 1 to 3 pupils in Borders, East Ayrshire, Fife, Glasgow and West Dunbartonshire at a cost of £5 million. Pupils were entitled to a free school meal during the 2007–2008 academic year and the Scottish Government has said that it hopes to roll the scheme out to all pupils in the first three years of primary school if an evaluation of the pilot shows it to have been a success. A report of the evaluation is expected to be published at the end of 2008.

1.28   The lunch box

'Having little involvement with the school meals service, and virtually no knowledge of it, some parents, for example, over-reacted to the recent and very successful Jamie Oliver series by withdrawing their children from school meals and providing them with a packed lunch instead – an alternative that was sometimes of less nutritional value than the school meal it had replaced'. (Morgan & Sonnino, 2007)

By law, each local authority or governing body is required to provide facilities for pupils to eat their own food, free of charge. Schools are not required, however, to provide refrigerated storage for lunch boxes.

Whereas a considerable amount of criticism has been levelled at the quality of the school meal, much the same can be said for children's lunch boxes brought in from home. The Food Standards Agency 2003 survey into the lunch boxes of children across the UK found that nine out of ten contained too much saturated fat, salt and sugar and inadequate fruit and/or vegetables (Jefferson & Cowbrough, 2003). Ham or cheese sandwiches made with white bread were the most popular item, followed by crisps, chocolate bar or cake. The most popular drinks were fruit squashes. Other surveys have found similar results. The *Sodexho 2005 School Meals and Lifestyle Survey* found that crisps and savoury snacks, meat sandwich or roll and a chocolate bar were the top three favourite items (Sodexho, 2005).

The Food Standards Agency survey found that only 21% of packed lunches met the 2001 minimum standards set for primary school meals (Jefferson & Cowbrough, 2003). A later study of 621 pupils in south west England, published in 2007, compared the nutritional values of the school meal and packed lunch and found the packed lunch to be 'worse', although both meals compared unfavourably with dietary guidelines (Rogers *et al.*, 2007). Only around half of the recommended amount of fruit and vegetables was eaten by children having either type of school meal.

Children who take a packed lunch from home are at greater risk of overeating because they still have the option of buying additional food and have been found to supplement their meal with food and drinks purchased from the canteen (Brannen & Storey, 1998). This puts them at greater risk of developing obesity. It also appears to puts them at great risk of developing other chronic diseases: when researchers examined whether markers of nutrition, cardiovascular health and type 2 diabetes differed between pupils who ate school dinners and those who brought in a packed lunch, they found that anthropometric markers of adiposity were slightly, but not significantly, lower among pupils who ate school meals. However, other markers – leptin, systolic blood pressure, total cholesterol, glucose and insulin were significantly lower in the school meal group. The researchers of the study, published in 2005 in the *British Medical Journal,* suggest that the average health status of pupils eating school meals is no worse and may actually be better than those who bring in a packed lunch (Whincup *et al.*, 2005).

There are around 10 million pupils, aged 5–18, currently attending school in the UK. The biggest threat to the school meal service, from a commercial point of view, is the packed lunch; almost half of schoolchildren take a packed lunch with them to school every day. About 5% of children buy their lunch from outlets outside the school and 2% go home to eat. The social group AB – thought to be the group most likely to be concerned about healthy eating – is also the group most likely to have a packed lunch. This is believed to be because their parents like to have more control over what their children eat (Mintel, 2003). They might also be influenced by costs: in 2005 the average amount spent on a school meal was £1.68, whereas the average cost of providing a packed lunch was £1.35 (Sodexho, 2005).

1.28.1   Additional snack foods

As well as the lunch box options, there are other ways for pupils to supplement their diets with snacks of their own choosing. The new regulations governing food provided in schools other than lunch (page 45) may have removed unhealthy snacks from vending machines and tuck shops but cannot prevent children from buying these products from outside the school gates. The *Sodexho School Meals and Lifestyle Survey 2005* found a disturbing increase in spend on the way to and from school. The average amount spent on the way to school increased from 54p in 1998 to 77p in 2002 and £1.01 in 2005. Of this amount, 38% is spent on confectionery, 29% on crisps and other savoury snacks and 27% on canned or fizzy drinks. The average amount spent on the way home increased from 63p in 2002 to 74p in 2005, with much the same sort of purchases made (Sodexho survey, 2005).

1.29   Food and cooking in the national curriculum

'We want schools to think carefully about the food offered during the school day – before school, at break and lunch time and after school – and ensure it reflects the healthy eating messages taught in the Curriculum'.   (DfES, 2004)

'Most pupils in the schools visited had a good understanding of what constituted healthy eating through food technology lessons and other subjects, notably personal, social and health education, physical education and science. In too many instances, however, pupils' knowledge had little bearing on the food they chose'.   (Ofsted, 2007)

For children brought up on a poor diet at home, the school setting may provide the only opportunity they have to learn about the value of good food and nutrition and develop healthy eating habits. Many blame the absence of cookery lessons – written out of the national curriculum in 1992 – for the apparent ignorance of many children of where food comes from and how it is produced. If a child's perception of food is of something highly processed and packaged, then produce such as fruit and vegetables may fall outside that child's range of acceptable food items. When surveyed, 78% of parents and 56% of children said they would like to see cooking taught in schools (Sodexho, 2005).

The national curriculum (see Box 1.7) was introduced in 1988 under the Education Reform Act. Learning about food and nutrition is incorporated into the subjects *science, design and technology* and *personal, social and health education*. It is also woven into cross-curricular themes such as geography (looking at food production and distribution); history (understanding the evolution of the role of food in society) and religious education (looking at food customs and beliefs). In Wales, children aged 5–16 learn about food and nutrition through the statutory *science* subject. In Scotland, nutrition education for children aged 5–14 features in *science, environmental studies* and *technology and health education*. In Northern Ireland, children between the age of 11 and 16 learn about food and nutrition through the subjects *science* and *home economics*.

Box 1.7   Nutrition in the national curriculum.

Key stages 1 & 2 (5–11 years)
Key stage 1: Pupils should be taught 'that humans need food and water to stay alive'.

Key stage 2: Pupils should be taught 'that food is needed for activity and for growth, and that an adequate and varied diet is needed to keep healthy'.

Key stages 3 & 4 (11–16 years)
Key stage 3: Pupils should be taught 'that balanced diets contain carbohydrates, proteins, fats, minerals, vitamins, fibre and water; the sources of the main food components in the diet; the principles of digestion, including the role of enzymes; that food is used as a fuel during respiration to maintain the body's activity and as a raw material for growth and repair; that the products of digestion are absorbed and waste material egested.'

Key stage 4: Pupils should be taught 'the structure of the human digestive system and the processes involved in digestion, including the roles of enzymes, stomach acid and bile'.

Since September 2000 it has been a statutory requirement that primary school children in England learn some basic cooking skills, though to what extent depends on the individual school. *Food technology*, as part of the subject *design and technology*, is compulsory at primary school level. This gives children the opportunity to learn about where food comes from through practical work, that is, food preparation and *designing and making healthy sandwiches*. Food technology as a subject is offered by most secondary schools, but is not statutory.

There have been concerns that food has been placed in a commercial and industrial context only. Projects include *exploring ingredients for a ready-prepared meal* and *pasta production*, with the emphasis on the technical aspect of food production rather than cooking skills, nutrition or health. According to Ofsted's 2006 report *Food technology in secondary schools*, there is concern among many about the nature of *food technology*, and its value is unclear. The Ofsted report recognised the conflict between the need for children to learn to cook and the requirements of the design and technology curriculum, but concluded that achievement across all aspects of *food technology* was rarely better than satisfactory.

The SMRP, in its document *Turning the tables* (see page 40), claimed that cooking was an essential life-skill which all children should acquire before leaving school. As part of the overhaul of the provision of food in schools, which began in September 2006, the Government promised a review of the curriculum at key stage 3 to introduce basic cooking skills. In September 2006 the government announced plans to introduce entitlement to school cookery lessons for all 11 to 16-year-olds in England and Wales, from 2008. The course, called *licence to cook*, is intended for schools not offering food technology, and is to be run in after-school cooking clubs or neighbouring schools. Similar such schemes, or cooking clubs, have been in existence for a number of years across the UK. What's Cooking? (formerly Cook-It) currently has 92 clubs across north east England. What's Cooking is intended as a guide to setting up and running community and school food clubs. Another scheme, called Let's Get Cooking is a national network of cooking clubs led by the SFT and funded by the Big Lottery Fund. It aims to set up a network of 5000 cooking clubs across England over 5 years.

In January 2008 the Government bowed to pressure and announced that cookery lessons were to be made compulsory for all 11 to 14-year-olds, from 2011. The emphasis is to be on how to make cheap healthy dishes from simple, fresh ingredients. Pupils will also be taught diet, nutrition, hygiene and healthy food shopping. The Government also promised an extra £2.5 million a year to cover or subsidise the cost of cooking ingredients for pupils receiving free school meals. Around 800 new *food technology* teachers are to undergo training until the compulsory cookery lessons are introduced.

1.30   School food – post new standards

1.30.1   Meal uptake

'I like school meals but my mum says I can't have them because they cost too much'.   (Child quoted in Ofsted, 2007)

There is clear evidence that the introduction of new standards, which began in 2006, led to fewer children taking a school meal. LACA (the Local Authority Caterers Association), in its 2007 survey, reported a 10% decline in the uptake of school meals in the first year of food-based standards. There was a decrease in meal numbers in over 75% of authorities, with some schools experiencing as much as a 30% drop. In secondary schools the national average drop was 17%. However, the report also expressed optimism that meal uptake in primary schools was slowly recovering.

Similar results were reported by the School Food Trust, which since the introduction of the new standards carries out annual surveys of school meal uptake. The Trust set a target to increase uptake by four percentage points by March 2008 and ten percentage points by autumn 2009. Its 2007 survey revealed that uptake of meals in primary schools was 41%, down 1% from 2005 to 2006 (42%). This figure varied from 28% in the south east to 55% in the north east. In secondary schools, uptake was 38%, down 5% from 2005 to 2006 (43%). This figure varied from 26.8 in the south west to 41.9 in the north west. The SFT 2007 survey also suggested that although the downward trend in secondary schools was continuing (only 12 out of 53 secondary school services showed an increase in uptake), the downward trend in primary schools may have ceased – one half of primary services showed an increase in uptake between 2005–2006 and 2006–2007 (Nicholas *et al.*, 2007). Only 17% of primary school services and 1% of secondary school services thought there was a good to high likelihood of meeting the SFT 4% uptake target by March 2008 (Nicholas *et al.*, 2007).

That target was not met, but the SFT's provisional findings for 2008 suggested a positive turnaround in uptake (Nicholas *et al.*, 2008). This survey found a 2.3% increase in take-up amongst primary school pupils. In secondary schools, uptake declined by only 0.5% – which equates to roughly 50 000 extra pupils per day taking a school lunch, compared to the previous year.

This turnaround was much needed. Low uptake of school meals is a real concern: being a commercial operation, the service relies on high demand, and if the number of meals provided declines, less money is rung through tills. The SFT (2007) survey found that in both primary and secondary schools, the most common explanation for the decline was that children were opting for packed lunches rather than taking a 'healthy' meal option. Other factors considered important were media coverage of school meals and increased prices, the shorter lunch break and poor organisation of lunch arrangements (Nicholas *et al.*, 2007).

The 2007 survey found that where there had been increased demand for meals in primary schools, this was attributed to the marketing of meals to both pupils and parents, providing more healthy options and adopting whole school food policies. Holding the price of the meal was another important factor. Similar explanations were given by the few secondary schools which had seen an increase in uptake, where improvements in dining facilities were also considered an important factor. The strongest positive influences on uptake were considered to be the introduction of a whole school food policy and the reorganisation of the school meals service. Interestingly, many local authorities mentioned the adoption of a locked gate policy as being highly important (Nicholas *et al.*, 2007).

In October 2007 Ofsted, responsible for monitoring the new school food standards, published its report into the progress schools were making in meeting new standards. When surveyed, the reasons for the decline in uptake given by the schools were:

- lack of consultation with pupils and parents about the new arrangements in schools;
- poor marketing of the new menus;
- the high costs for low income families who are not eligible for free school meals;
- lack of choice in what was offered.

Headteachers at the surveyed schools felt that the cost of a meal was prohibitive, especially for those parents on low incomes but not eligible for free meals. For them, the cost of a packed lunch could be absorbed into the weekly shop, so it was a better option even if the quality of the packed lunch was sometimes poor. According to Ofsted, '*If this trend continues, the impact of the government's food policies will have limited effect. This will be particularly the case for children from more vulnerable families*'.

1.30.2   Catering facilities

One of the more detrimental effects of the 1980 Education Act (page 10), which saw the removal of the statutory duty to provide school meals, was the concomitant removal or stripping of kitchens so that they could be converted for other purposes. Dining rooms were also subsumed into other projects. Primary schools seemed to have suffered the most – The SFT 2007 survey found that 69% of primary schools had full-production kitchens, compared with 99% of secondary schools. Over a fifth of primary schools had no facilities either for cooking or reheating. Of these, 1.9% transported hot food from another source and 3.7% provided sandwiches and cold food only (Nicholas *et al.*, 2007).

Even where a school has a full-production kitchen, the standard of facilities is often low. According to the LACA National School Meals Survey 2007, over 50% of school kitchens need capital investment and over 10% need to be completely rebuilt (LACA, 2007). It has been estimated that it would cost around £289 million to upgrade all schools in England to the required standard. The average cost of upgrading school kitchens is estimated to be £13 000 in primary schools and £23 000 in secondary schools, and dining room refurbishment is estimated at £6000 in primary schools and £12 000 in secondary schools (SMRP, 2005). Estimates do not include the cost of reinstating kitchens in schools which operate a cold packed lunch service only (SMRP, 2005). The Government's *Building schools for the future* programme is a multi-billion pound investment in school buildings, which began in 2005–2006. The aim is to rebuild or renew nearly every secondary school in England by 2015. The Government has stated that new or upgraded school kitchen facilities where fresh food can be cooked from scratch will be made a priority.

The state of the school kitchen is likely to impact significantly on meal uptake. A 2006 Ofsted report found that a lack of on-site cooking facilities was a particular problem for primary schools – food delivered to schools could be lukewarm and unappetising (Ofsted, 2006a). A later Ofsted report, published in 2007, found that food which was cooked on the school site tended to be '*well presented and appetising*'. Food prepared off-site '*tended to look unattractive and, in several cases, was cold by the time the pupils ate it*'. (Ofsted, 2007)

1.30.3   What children choose now

Whereas the new standards have had an undeniably positive impact on the nutritional quality of the school lunch, they appear to have had little influence on packed lunches. The SFT surveyed 136 8-to-10-year-olds in six primary schools in Sheffield in February and March 2007 (SFT, 2007d). Table 1.6 outlines comparisons made between the lunchtime choices of those taking a school meal and those who brought in a packed lunch. Those who ate a school lunch clearly made healthier choices. Those taking a school lunch were more likely to have more vegetables and fruit, drink healthier drinks and have

Table 1.6 Food choices: school lunch versus packed lunch following the introduction of food-based standards.

Food item	School lunch (%)	Packed lunch (%)
Vegetables	72	6
Fruit (including fruit-based desserts with ≥50%	23	31
Savoury snacks (e.g. crisps)	0	65
Confectionery (e.g. chocolate)	0	65
Drinks not meeting standards	0	31
Freely available bread	37	0

Source: School Food Trust (2007d).

no confectionery and snacks. Of those children who brought in a packed lunch, 65% had a food item from the confectionery and snacks categories, with 28% eating both a confectionery and savoury snack item. Thirty-one per cent of packed lunches contained a drink which did not meet the food-based standards. However, more children with a packed lunch chose fruit (31%) than pupils who ate a school lunch. The mean content of energy, carbohydrate, non-milk extrinsic sugars, total fat, saturated fat and sodium were lower and fibre content significantly higher for school lunches compared with packed lunches. More school lunches than packed lunches met the 2008 standards (not statutory at the time of the survey) for individual nutrients with the exception of saturated fat, calcium, iron and zinc (SFT, 2007d).

1.31   Determinants of choice

'Encouraging take-up of healthy food is a complex task, because ultimately the pupils (particularly in secondary schools) have a choice about what to eat'. (DfES, 2006)

'Adults do not make healthy choices, as is evident from the latest National Diet and Nutrition Survey – why should we expect school children to behave differently? They are even less well equipped than adults in terms of knowledge and understanding of the health consequences of poor dietary choices'. (Nelson *et al.*, 2004)

1.31.1   Education

The Government's agreement to the recommendations made by the SMRP in its report *Turning the tables*, which included limiting meal options to healthy choices only, marked a massive turning point in policy. It came after endless failed government campaigns to 'educate' children to make healthier choices. Educating children about healthy eating, and then providing them with a range of options in the hope that they will make the choices that concerned adults want them to make, ignores a raft of literature regarding the key psychological factors influencing children's food choices. There are many reasons why children choose what they do, and good health is not usually one of them. Nutrition education would appear to be entirely academic: school nutrition campaigns have been shown to increase children's knowledge of healthy eating but have little or no impact on what they eat (Baer *et al.*, 1987). A Food Standards Agency report (2001) into the promotion of food to children found that although children understood the basic principles of healthy eating, they had little interest in putting healthy eating principles into practice. Of the 11 to 12-year age group, most displayed a 'profound' lack of interest in applying healthy eating principles to dietary choices. A later FSA report into pupils' views on school food also found that, in general, there is a good understanding of what constitutes a balanced diet (FSA, 2007a). An earlier study had shown that television programmes, designed to educate five to six-year-olds about the nutritional value of certain foods, were effective in improving children's knowledge, but had no effect on what children actually ate, or their stated preferences (Peterson *et al.*, 1984). The 2007 Ofsted report confirmed all previous findings that most schoolchildren have '... *A good understanding of healthy eating but too often this had little bearing on the food they chose*'. Food choices were found to be worse when there were alternative sources for buying food near the school, and when the school canteen did not market itself (Ofsted, 2007). The catering company Sodexho in its 2005 school meals survey states that '*It's clear from the 2005 survey that children have an understanding of what a healthy lifestyle entails, but are failing to put it into practice*'. One reason for this, as the authors note, is that children find it difficult to relate to adult health messages concerning heart disease, diabetes and obesity.

1.31.2 School Nutrition Action Groups

These groups appear to have a positive influence over children's dietary choices: the 2005 Sodexho survey found that the average daily consumption of fruit and vegetables rose from 2.71 portions to 3.00 portions in schools where there was a food group or council (Sodexho, 2005). Figure 1.8 suggests that pupils are more enthusiastic about ideas to encourage healthy eating when there is an active food group at the school. Another 2005 study, devised to determine the effectiveness of a SNAG, found that these groups can significantly increase sales of main meals and snacks. Although the food sales data did not show qualitative changes, they did show that SNAG activities influenced pupils' choices (Passmore & Harris, 2005).

1.31.3 Peer influence

Peer emulation is a major factor in children's food choices. Children will change their preferences to fit in with others: they have been found to make a significant shift from their preferred vegetable to the preferred vegetables of their peers, after eating with them (Birch, 1980). The Food Standards Agency, in a study into

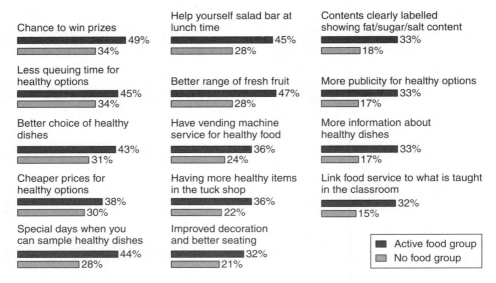

Figure 1.8   Ideas which would make children eat more healthy foods at school. (*Source*: Sodexho, 2005. Reproduced with kind permission.)

the promotion of food to children (FSA, 2001) found that by age 4–5 years, peer group influence was manifest and children made requests for items seen in other children's lunch boxes. These results confirmed the findings of an earlier, much smaller study of four children aged 4–6 years who consistently refused to eat several types of fruits and vegetables (Lowe *et al.*, 1998). Before each meal, they were shown videos of older children –'Food Dudes'[1] who enthusiastically ate the target fruits and vegetables and encouraged viewers to do the same, in order to fight the evil 'Junk Food Junta'. Viewers were offered gifts if they did so. Consumption of all the target foods rose immediately to 100% following the intervention. Following the video, one child, who had previously claimed to 'hate' kiwi fruit, remarked that they were 'nice'. The authors found that combining the Food Dudes video with a reward was the most effective way to influence the food choices of children.

1.31.4   Family influence

Parental meal practices may also influence children's eating patterns (Koivisto *et al.*, 1994). Children have been found to be more likely to eat certain foods if prompted to do so by one or both of their parents. If parents liked a food, and demonstrated this liking to their children, children were found to be more likely to favour that food (Casey & Rozin, 1989). The relationship between mother and child has been found to be stronger than that between father and child (Oliveria *et al.*, 1992). The way that the family eats also appears to be influential. Children from families who normally watched television while eating have been found to consume significantly fewer fruits and vegetables, and more snack foods, pizzas and soft drinks than children from families who do not watch television while eating (Coon *et al.*, 2001).

If children have poor dietary habits at home, those habits are likely to be replicated at school. Children's consumption of fruits and vegetables were found, in telephone interviews with family members, to be related to home availability and accessibility (Hearn *et al.*, 1998). The extent to which fruits and vegetables are made available and accessible to children may shape children's liking and consumption of that food.

1.31.5 Advertising

Advertising has been found in many studies to have a profound effect on children's dietary habits. A survey undertaken with the aim of determining what food products children chose, using their purchase requests to parents as an indicator, showed that breakfast cereals, the largest group, made up 18% of requests, followed by biscuits and cakes (11%) and fruit and vegetables (11%), sweets and chocolate (10%) and drinks 10%. Thirty-nine per cent of the products requested by the children had been advertised in the 6-month period prior to the study, and in some cases, the frequency of requests matched the frequency of advertising of those products (Donkin *et al.*, 1993). In another study (Taras *et al.*, 1989), it was observed that foods that children requested most frequently were the foods most often advertised on television.

The more children watch television commercials, the greater the number of purchase-influencing attempts directed at the mother at the supermarket are made (Galst & White, 1976). Younger children appear to be more likely than older children to believe that TV advertisements are truthful (Clancy-Hepburn *et al.*, 1974). Even brief exposures to televised food commercials can influence children's food preferences. When children viewed a video of a popular cartoon either with or without advertisements embedded in it, it was found that those children exposed to the commercials were significantly more likely to choose the advertised items than children who watched the same cartoons without the embedded commercials, which were for sweet snacks, fast food and breakfast cereals. The greatest preference appeared for products promoted by two commercials rather than one – suggesting that multiple exposure has even stronger effects on preferences (Borzekowski & Robinson, 2001).

In 2001, the Food Standards Agency published commissioned research into the promotion of food to children (FSA, 2001). Television was regarded as a very powerful medium: by age 4–5 years, children were aware of products and brands. Breakfast cereals were the most frequently remembered food advertisements. Children were beginning to recall promotions and sometimes asked for items they had seen advertised on TV. Pestering reached a height around the age of 7–8 years, when children were found to be 'brand-driven' and highly motivated by peer pressure.

Obese children appear to have heightened alertness to food-related cues. In 2004, researchers published the results of a study into the effects of food and non-food advertising on lean, overweight and obese children. They found that obese children recognised significantly more food advertisements. Although exposure to advertisements induced increased food intake in all children, it was found that the overall snack food intake of the obese and overweight children was significantly higher than that of the lean children (Halford *et al.*, 2004).

Many, including children's food campaigning organisation Sustain, have long called for a ban on the advertising of junk food to children. On 1 April 2007 restrictions on TV advertising of foods to children under 10 years of age came into force. These restrictions apply to advertisements for foods high in energy, saturated fats, salt and sugar shown during children's TV schedules. These regulations were introduced by the communications regulator Ofcom and in January 2008 were extended to programmes of 'particular appeal' to children under the age of 16. However, this means that other programmes which may be popular with children but intended for an adult audience are not affected. For this reason, Sustain and others have called for the introduction of a 9 p.m. watershed for all television advertising of unhealthy food.

1.31.6   What children say

'The food is not very healthy but that's good, because normally teenagers don't want healthy food'.   (Schoolchild in Brannen & Storey, 1998)

Children have always had plenty to say about school food and it would be unwise to ignore their opinions if the school meal service is to survive. The 2005 Sodexho survey asked pupils what they thought about the food provided. Even before the introduction of new standards, it was clearly losing popularity: 77% said they quite liked school meals or liked them a lot, compared with 84% in 2002 and 2000, and 81% in 1998. When asked what they wanted their school to provide, there were clear differences between what children wanted and what their parents wanted, as shown in Table 1.7. There were also gender differences, with girls wanting more healthy options. Children were presented with a number of ideas and asked which

Table 1.7   Foods parents and children want schools to provide (in order of preference).

Children overall	Boys	Girls	Parents
Pizza	Pizza	Pasta dishes	Fresh fruit
Fresh fruit	Burgers	Pizza	Healthy meals
Pasta dishes	Fresh fruit	Fresh fruit	Vegetables
Burgers	Fizzy drinks	Salad	Salad
Salad	Pasta dishes	Filled jacket potatoes	Pasta dishes
Fizzy drinks	Chicken	Baked potatoes	Filled jacket potatoes
Chicken	Curries	Fruit juices	Baked potatoes
Baked potatoes	Hot pudding	Sandwiches/filled rolls	Milk
Hot puddings	Roast dinner	Sausage rolls	Fresh fruit juice
Filled jacket potatoes	Baked potatoes	Hot puddings	Roast dinner

Source: Sodexho (2005). Reproduced with kind permission.

were most likely to make them choose healthier meals, and their responses are shown in Figure 1.8. It is interesting to note that where there is a food group or council, more children are enthusiastic about the idea.

Children (and presumably their parents) are increasingly opting for a packed lunch in favour of a cooked school meal. The 2005 Sodexho survey revealed that 51% preferred a packed lunch, compared with 45% in the previous survey (2002). The reasons stated for this were: too expensive (12%); didn't like the food (10%); parents preferred that they had a packed lunch (10%); poor food (9%); queues too long (8%); no reason given (2%). The dining environment was also strongly criticised. Crowding and cramped seating were considered by 35% of respondents to be a considerable problem. In many schools the lunch break has been much shortened and children are reluctant to spend their little free time queuing for food. Ofsted has recommended that secondary schools with very short lunch breaks should evaluate their meal provision to take into consideration whether pupils have enough time, in pleasant surroundings, to eat their food properly and experience the social benefits of eating together (Ofsted, 2006b).

In the school cafeteria, children are consumers making choices in the same way that adults do. They have stated that balancing the cost of food items was more important to them than balancing their diet in terms of health (Brannen & Storey, 1998). They will save money on food expenditure in order to have spare cash for other purchases. Therefore, cheap food – and processed food usually is cheap – has an additional attraction.

Children are not only aware of what constitutes a healthy diet, they also prove to be surprisingly canny when asked for suggestions on how to improve their own diets. The Food Standards Agency published, in January 2006, a report by a school council network which it set up 'to gain a better insight into what children and young people think about a range of food issues' (FSA, 2006). Apart from demonstrating, again, that children have a good knowledge of healthy eating, this report revealed that children ate unhealthy food simply because they had the choice to do so. Indeed some children were aware of an internal struggle between what they knew and what they chose. Although the report covered only nine schools (five primary schools and four secondary) the children's suggestions for improving their own diets were similar to those made by concerned organisations: restrict choice, limit chips and other fried foods and provide bonus points and incentive schemes for healthy choices. Children also felt that making healthy food more 'fun' and 'attractive' and using celebrities to talk about or promote healthy food would be helpful. There was 100% agreement with the suggestion that unhealthy items such as poor quality burgers and nuggets be removed from the school menu. Children, it would appear, are like adults: they know what's good for them but are prey to market forces.

1.32   Diet and behaviour

'The Panel repeatedly heard head teachers and others from schools where food had already been improved speak of associated improvements in behaviour: of

calmer, better behaved children, more ready to learn. Improving food in schools may contribute to improved attainment and behaviour'.   (SMRP, 2005)

As the School Food Trust has pointed out, improving school food brings clear benefits to children's health, growth and development. There may also be wider educational benefits in terms of learning ability, mood and behaviour. Following the introduction of food-based standards, the SFT carried out a study to determine whether improvements in food provision and the dining environment enhanced pupils' concentration and made them more alert in the classroom in the learning period after lunch (SFT, 2007e). Six primary schools in Sheffield took part in the study, which measured 'on-task' behaviour (i.e., concentration) and 'off-task' behaviour (i.e. disengagement/disruption) over a 12-week period. There were two intervention groups (nutrition-first, with introduction of healthier food first, and environment-first, with changes in the dining environment first) and a control group (no intervention). The researchers found that pupils were over three times more likely to be on-task with the teacher in the intervention schools than in the control schools. However, and surprisingly, pupils who engaged with other pupils, but not a teacher, were less likely to be on-task and more likely to be off-task in the intervention schools compared with the control schools. The researchers concluded that a combined nutrition – environment intervention in primary schools had a beneficial impact on pupils' behaviour in a setting in which teachers engage directly with pupils. The nutrition-first intervention was more powerfully associated with perceived differences in behaviour compared with the control schools.

An earlier report, published jointly by Business in the Community and the Soil Association in 2004 also found that changes in diet resulted in better behaved, more alert pupils. Pupils who ate fresh, unprocessed foods and had access to drinking water had better concentration and improved concentration spans, according to the report which recorded the views of education chiefs from thirteen local authorities and two schools in England and Wales following improvements to the quality of food served.

The hypothesis that diet can directly affect behaviour and cognitive function has a strong case. The brain is metabolically a highly active organ and accounts for about 20–30% of the body's resting metabolic rate (Garrow *et al.*, 2000). Therefore its nutrient requirement is high, especially its requirement for energy – about one fifth of the glucose in arterial flow to the brain is used for metabolism (Garrow *et al.*, 2000). Studies suggest that the brain can be sensitive to short-term variations of glucose availability (Bellisle, 2004), which is why the consumption of breakfast is thought to be so important. Eating breakfast has been found to impact on a child's learning capability and behaviour (Dani *et al.*, 2005) and poor performance in the classroom has been attributed to skipping breakfast and being unable to find enough energy in the morning to cope with classroom demands. Children who are already malnourished are more likely to be affected by skipping breakfast than those who are generally well-nourished (Bellise, 2004).

A 2006 review of dietary influences on cognitive development and behaviour found that the range of behaviour affected by food is wide and includes attention, conduct disorder and mood (Stevenson, 2006). It is well established that essential fatty acids are crucial to brain development and function. This review found some evidence that omega-3 supplementation (fish oil) may improve behaviour in some children, but possibly only those with learning disabilities. Indeed, the journal *Pediatrics* reported in 2005 that when children suffering from developmental coordination disorder (which is associated with difficulties in learning and behaviour), were given supplements of omega-3 fatty acids over a period of three months, significant improvements were found in reading, spelling and behaviour (Richardson & Montgomery, 2005).

The concentration of vitamin C is 4–10 times higher in the brain than in plasma (Garrow *et al.*, 2000). An adequate supply of vitamins and minerals is essential for normal brain function (Garrow *et al.*, 2000) and any deficiency of essential nutrients is likely to impact on its ability to function optimally. Thiamin (B1) deficiency interferes with neurotransmitter synthesis and is associated with behavioural problems (Benton *et al.*, 1997). Pyridoxine (B6) deficiency is associated with fatigue, irritability and insomnia. Zinc deficiency is associated with mental lethargy (Garrow *et al.*, 2000). It is well established that iron-deficiency anaemia is associated with impaired cognitive development and function in children.

It would appear that it is not only the availability of nutrients which affects behaviour and learning. Parents and teachers have long reported anecdotal evidence that certain foods induced hyperactive, unruly behaviour in children, and in 2007 the Food Standards Agency advised parents of children showing signs of hyperactivity to cut out certain artificial colours from the diet. This advice was based on research carried out by Southampton University and commissioned by the FSA which linked certain artificial colours, namely sunset yellow (E110), quinoline yellow (E104), carmoisine (E122), allura red (E129), tartrazine (E102) and ponceau 4R (E124) with a negative effect on children's behaviour (FSA, 2007b).

1.33 Good practice

Examples of best practice in school catering abound in individual schools which have recognised the value of providing their children with quality, nutritious meals and made their catering service a priority. Prioritisation of the meal service is contingent on the enthusiasm and commitment of head teachers, governors and parents. The charity the Health Education Trust publishes, on its website, details of a scheme called *Best in Class*, designed to give recognition to examples of best practice across the school catering system. The HET gives a listing of schools who have achieved success in one or more areas of their school meals service, and provides details of how they have done this, with sample menus. Table 1.8 provides a sample menu from St Peter's Church of England primary school, in East Bridgford, Nottinghamshire which is perhaps the best known example of best practice. This menu was in place before compulsory standards were introduced. Because of the desserts on offer this menu would not now meet current standards, but it is interesting to note that choice is very limited, and fresh vegetables are always

Table 1.8   Sample menu from St Peter's Church of England Primary School.

Monday	Tuesday	Wednesday	Thursday	Friday
Macaroni Cheese or Chilli	Homemade cheese or ham and pineapple pizza	Roast lamb or Vegetarian option	Meatballs in tomato sauce or Cauliflower cheese	Sausage or Cheese and tomato pasta bake
Rice or bread roll	Homemade jacket wedges	Mashed potatoes, gravy and mint sauce	Pasta or bread roll	Mashed potatoes or bread roll
Carrots & sweetcorn	Baked beans	Country mixed vegetables	Peas & roasted cherry tomatoes	Carrots & sweetcorn
Iced buns	Chocolate or blueberry muffins	Mandarin sponge with custard	Date slice	Blackberry sponge with custard

Source: Health Education Trust website. Reproduced with kind permission from the HET.

available. The then catering manager at St Peter's, Jeanette Orrey, is credited with being the main influence behind Jamie Oliver's successful television series, *Jamie's school dinners* (page 36). St Peter's changed its catering system by opting out of the local authority catering service in order to have *greater freedom and flexibility for creativity, better food, better menus, complete ownership for staff and for catering staff to feel part of the school* (see www.healthedtrust.com).

The changes took place over a five-year period, prior to the introduction of the new standards, and involved a 'whole school approach' using School Nutrition Actions Groups, catering committees and a school food policy. The aim of this policy was

- to enable pupils to make healthy food choices through the provision of information and development of appropriate skills and attitudes;
- to provide healthy food choices throughout the school day.

Box 1.8 outlines the phased programme which led to the introduction of changes to the school meal service. Prior to the changes, school meal uptake was 61%; after the changes were introduced, uptake increased by a third to 80%. This meant that more income was generated, which could be ploughed back into the catering service. This aspect was monitored by the school governors. The school became the first primary school to serve a fully organic meal, which was achieved with support from the local Post Office which sold the school organic, fresh produce from its own allotment. St Peter's and Jeanette Orrey (who later became involved in the Soil Association's Food for Life programme, page 34) were awarded the Observer Newspaper National Award for 'Best Contribution to the Food and Drink Industry' 2004; Midlands Woman of Achievement of the Year 2004; BBC Radio 4 Public Caterer of the Year 2003; Soil Association National Award for Local Food Initiative of the Year 2002.

Box 1.8 Best Practice: How St Peter's primary school introduced changes to its school meals service.

Phase 1

More money was available to be put towards the food service – this allowed menus to be more varied and creative, for example, custard was made with real milk, and there was more fresh fruit as a daily option.

Communications improved between the school and the parents, with children taking menus home as part of better marketing of the school meals service. Parents then had the freedom to opt in or out of the meals service. Parents were invited and positively encouraged to come into school and eat with their children on a regular basis (this facility has continued and has become an integral part of the school routine).

Phase 2

Beef was sourced locally, in direct response to the BSE concerns. Other meats are also now locally sourced.

Phase 3

Other foods were incorporated in the local sourcing policy, including vegetables and potatoes. This meant moving back to cooking with fresh produce (as opposed to pre-peeled/pre-prepared varieties). This move has enabled more fresh produce to be included on the menu as well as providing knowledge about where the food is sourced from.

The amount of food cooked on site started to increase, for example, freshly made pizzas. Cooking such meals has given the catering staff greater job satisfaction.

Phase 4

The use of organic produce increased, such as flour, sugar, pasta, milk, butter and eggs.

Phase 5

The school joined the Government's National Free Fruit scheme. This enabled an extension of the healthy eating policy from lunchtimes into the curriculum. This also stimulated changes in the snacks brought in from home, with increased awareness of parents and children of the importance of healthy eating and what this involves, allowing them to make more informed choices. Using the National Free Fruit scheme as the lever enabled the school to state that they would prefer all snacks brought into school to be fruit and vegetables, and drinks to be water.

Phase 6

The catering service was professionalised by giving it a name and identity – Primary Choice Catering. A leaflet was produced for all parents with a mission statement to introduce them to the new caterers. It was important for the school to establish Primary Choice Catering as a fundamental part of the school, with a genuine partnership between the school, governors, parents, pupils and the local community. Of particular importance for the success has been the partnership between the Head and the Catering Manager.

At this stage the school began to focus on the social side of eating – etiquette, the introduction of table cloths and plates replaced the flight trays that were used previously.

Phase 7

The school's view of health was broadened to encompass physical activity as well as food and this has involved extracurricular sporting activities.

Assorted fresh salad, seasonal vegetables and jacket potatoes are served daily alongside the main meal with fresh fruit, yoghurt, cheese and biscuits available for dessert.

Source: The HET website. Reproduced with kind permission.

1.34   School meals in Europe and the US

1.34.1   Dietary habits

Childhood obesity is not peculiar to the United Kingdom but is, rather, a global concern. Nor are the dietary habits of UK children unique. The food choices of 11-, 13- and 15-year-olds of thirty-five European and North American countries were examined in the most recent Health Behaviour in School-Aged Children study carried out in 2001/02 (Currie *et al.*, 2004). This study suggested that children generally across Europe and North America do not follow nutrition advice, and their consumption of fruit and vegetables is low. Only 30% of boys and 37% of girls reported eating fruit on a daily basis. In all, 45% of boys and 51% of girls reported eating fruit five or more days a week. In sixteen countries young people reported eating fruit once a week or less. Consumption of fruit decreases with age in every country, with the exception of Italy. All countries, with the exception of Belgium-Flanders, reported less than 50% of all young people eating vegetables every day, with girls consuming more vegetables than boys.

Soft drink consumption is high, especially in the Netherlands, Malta, Slovenia, Scotland and the US, and is lowest in certain Scandinavian countries (Denmark, Finland and Sweden), Greece and some Baltic states. More boys than girls consume soft drinks. Almost one third of young people eat sweets or chocolate once or more a day, with Malta having the highest percentage of daily consumers, followed by Scotland and Ireland (Currie *et al.*, 2004). Breakfast is skipped by a significant number of children: on average, 69% of boys and 60% of girls eat breakfast.

1.34.2   Overweight and obesity

The World Health Organization describes the prevalence of obesity in children as a global epidemic. Ten per cent of the world's school-aged children are estimated to be carrying excess body fat, and a quarter of these are obese. The prevalence of overweight is much higher in economically developed countries, but is rising significantly in most parts of the world (Lobstein *et al.*, 2004).

Overweight and obesity are a serious health concern throughout Europe. Figure 1.9 shows the percentage of schoolchildren, aged 7–11, reported in 2005 to be overweight or obese in 20 countries (figures for Italy and Sicily are given separately). There is a greater prevalence of overweight children among the southern countries of Europe. Lower levels of overweight are found in central and Eastern Europe, where economic recession and a decline in per capita prosperity during the 1990s occurred alongside a decline in the prevalence of overweight children and a rise in the prevalence of underweight children. Non-eastern bloc countries around the Mediterranean have been found to have rates for overweight children in the range of 20–40%. Those in northern areas have been found to have rates in the range of 10–20% (Lobstein & Frelut, 2003).

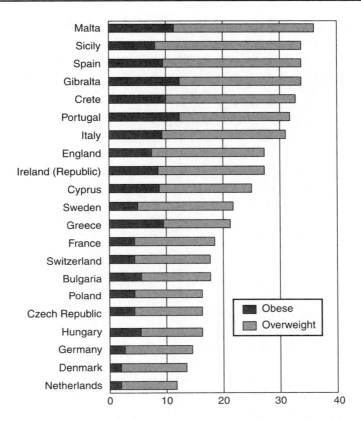

Figure 1.9 Percentage of schoolchildren aged 7–11 either obese or overweight. (*Source*: International Obesity Task Force (2005). Reproduced with kind permission.)

1.34.3 School meal provision – Europe

The European Network of Health Promoting Schools (ENHPS), a joint project of the European Commission, the World Health Organization (WHO) Regional Office for Europe and the Council of Europe is working towards the integration of health promotion into all aspects of school life, including food provision. In 1999 the ENHPS produced a manual – *Healthy Eating for Young People in Europe – a School-based Nutrition Education Guide* – the aim of which was to 'encourage the further development of nutrition education in European schools' by placing nutrition education within the concept of the health promoting school (Dixey *et al.*, 1999).

In November 2003 a forum was held by the Council of Europe in collaboration with the WHO entitled *The European forum on eating at school – making healthy choices* (Chauliac, 2003). The forum considered different European approaches to school meals and was designed to promote healthy eating in schools and encourage cooperation between those responsible for meals and those involved in nutrition. The results of a survey, undertaken on behalf of the Council of Europe and the WHO (European Office) were presented at the forum. The aim of the survey was to explore and compare the provision of food in schools across Europe, to explore the links between nutrition education and provision and to examine to what extent provision and education are grounded in the 'whole school' approach. Participating countries included: Albania, Belgium, Croatia, Cyprus, Czech Republic, Denmark, France, Finland, Germany, Ireland, Latvia, Lithuania, Luxembourg, Moldavia, the Netherlands, Poland, Portugal, Scotland, Slovakia, Slovenia, Spain, Switzerland, Turkey and Wales, with case studies from England.

The study revealed similarities across Europe with regard to dietary habits and physical activity. It also highlighted another global phenomenon: the strong presence of multinational companies in schools, either through the provision of food or through commercial sponsorship. This resulted in the promotion of fast foods at odds with policy and curricula. Overall it was found that primary schools tend to provide school meals within a traditional school meal system, whereas secondary schools tend to have a variety of systems, including cash cafeterias, vending machines, kiosks and so on. Many schools reported that vending machines were not allowed in primary schools. Vending machines have a much higher presence in secondary schools throughout Europe. There is often competition between the school meal and outside food options, such as snack bars, depending on the amount of access the pupils are allowed during the lunch break.

Seventeen out of the 24 countries responded that there were nutrition-based regulations for food served in school, and in general these regulations were based on national healthy eating guidelines. However there was greater emphasis on food safety and hygiene than on healthy eating. Many countries cited low funding as a major barrier to the implementation of healthy nutrition policies in schools. There was no indication that, where they existed, nutritional guidelines were effectively implemented and monitored, with the exception of Luxembourg (Young *et al.*, 2005).

Thirteen countries were found to have fruit and vegetable programmes in schools, with the majority of these interventions aimed at primary schools. Many of these were pilot schemes. Some countries, such as Lithuania, already served large portions of fruits and vegetables as part of the school meal (de Boer, 2003).

The forum concluded by emphasising the need for a 'whole school' or 'health promoting school' approach, and the development of policies and strategies to facilitate healthy choices (Young *et al.*, 2005). In September 2005 the Committee of Ministers of the Council of Europe passed a resolution on healthy eating in schools. It recommended that member countries:

- review food provision in schools to determine to what extent they comply with or are integral to a health promoting school approach
- consider the elaboration of national provisions and nutritional standards for food in schools which:
  - acknowledge the changing health situation and lifestyles of young people in Europe
  - take into account the good practices in European schools as demonstrated at the Forum on Eating at School

- ○   contribute to the promotion of the health of young people
- ○   involve the pupils and all stakeholders in this process
- ○   are integrated into the health-promoting school approach
- ○   have in-built systems of monitoring and evaluation
- consider the development of assistance measures at national and regional level to support schools in adopting and implementing healthy eating policies.

1.34.3.1   France

In 2001 the Ministry of Health launched the National Nutrition and Health Programme (PNNS), which listed nine objectives, one of which was to halt the rising prevalence of childhood obesity. One way of achieving this was to improve school meals. Childhood obesity is rising sharply in France (currently around 15%), alongside the emergence of a preponderance for 'le snacking' and a taste for processed food (Coudyser, 2003). The current nature of the school meal in France is determined by a circular issued by the French education ministry on 25 June 2001 – 'Composition of school meals and food safety' which was designed to 'structure meals to ensure that they include fish or meat and that priority is placed on green vegetables, cheese and fruit'. It emphasised the need for fewer fats, more iron, calcium, fibre, fruit and vegetables (Coudyser, 2003). Although the French guidelines are non-compulsory, much more money is spent per meal in France than in Britain – the cost can be anything up to £3 and is subsidised according to parents' income. Children do not receive the same choice as their British counterparts and about half of schoolchildren take a school meal. Each municipal authority is responsible for premises, equipment and operation of kitchens in nursery and primary schools. The municipal authority can choose to manage the school meal service itself, or bring in a private supplier. The education ministry is responsible for the operation of kitchens in secondary schools, which are staffed by state employees.

In 2004 the French Parliament approved a ban on vending machines in schools selling soft drinks and sweets which came into effect on 1 September 2005. As a result, around 8000 vending machines were removed from schools.

1.34.3.2   Italy

In Italy, the school meal is not unlike any other meal, in terms of how it is valued. The Italian model is a working version of the English 'whole school' initiative. Perhaps it is because food is central to Italian culture that it is very much a feature of school life, with meals served at the table by pupils themselves who eat alongside their teachers. A typical meals consists of pasta, meat with vegetables, bread, fruit, water (Walker, 2004). An average of 90p is spent on ingredients for each school meal, with parents paying according to income. Meals are free for low-income families. The maximum charge is £2.37 (2004 figure). There is virtually no choice offered, and uptake is 100%. Each school must appoint a *Commissione Mensa* (canteen commission), which involves the child's family in the monitoring and evaluation of food provided. Parents are appointed to make unannounced visits to the school any time during term time. They produce a check list which is given to a nutritionist, appointed by the municipality, for evaluation (Morgan & Sonnino, 2007).

Italy has one of the most progressive approaches to school meals in the world. In the UK, the focus has, in recent years, been on improving the nutritional quality of food provided and eliminating the cheap, fast foods which had come to dominate the school meal service. In Italy, where nutritional standards are already high, the drive to raise standards has focussed on providing local, traditional and organic produce. For example, as early as the mid-1980s the municipality of Cesana in northern Italy designed an organic school meal system which now provides approximately 2400 school and council cafeteria organic meals every day. In 1999 an Italian law was created which stipulated that use should be made of organic and traditional products in school and hospital canteens (Morgan & Sonnino, 2007). In 2003, 68% of Italian schools made some use of organic ingredients, with 3% offering entirely organic meals. The number of organic school canteens rose from 70 in 1997 to 561 in 2003. In Milan, 65 000 organic school meals are provided every day and in Rome that figure reaches around 140 000 (Morgan & Sonnino, 2007).

1.34.3.3 Finland

Some Scandinavian countries, such as Finland and Sweden, have a long established history of providing free school meals, with limited (if any) choice. Finland in particular has shown that a universal free school meal system based on nutritional standards can be an effective legislative measure to improve public health. Finland's attempts to deal with soaring levels of heart disease in the 1990s are impressive. At that time, Finland's record on heart disease was similar to Scotland's. Since the 1990s, Finland has seen a reduction of about 60% in mortality rates from heart disease (Vartiainen et al., 1994). This is due to radical policy change and public health campaigns, including the introduction of free school meals to all children. Take-up is very high, at 90%. Since 1948 primary school children have received a free lunch, consisting of a main dish, side salad, crispbread and milk (Roos et al., 2002). Today, all pupils attending comprehensive school also receive a free meal every day, with each meal based on children's nutritional requirements and designed to cover a third of a child's nutritional requirements. Many schools also offer healthy snacks, with junk food banned from school grounds (Ministry of Social Affairs and Health, 1999). Each municipality is responsible for food served in its schools, and the State subsidises around 70% of the costs.

1.34.3.4 Sweden

In Sweden, all children in state schools have been entitled to receive a free and nutritious school meal since 1973, although this only became statutory in 1998.

Upper secondary schools (for pupils aged 17–19) may charge for a meal. In 2001 Sweden adopted guidelines for school meals, but these are not compulsory. As a result the quality of meals varies between local authorities and from school to school. Half of Sweden's 290 local authorities lack a nutritional policy objective for school meals. However, uptake is good at around 85%, even though most pupils consume just 70% of their nutritional requirements. The average cost of producing a meal is around the equivalent of 60p, with costs ranging from 50p to £1.00. There is currently a campaigning organisation, the School Meals supporters, which was founded to ensure quality and standards of school meals and promote breakfast in schools (Wesslén).

1.34.3.5 Norway

The story is very different in Norway and Denmark, where school meals, free or otherwise, are not provided at all. Children have to bring in a packed lunch and eat it at their desks, and often have only around 20 minutes in which to do so. The consumption of fruit and vegetables among Norwegians in general is comparatively low, with approximately only 10% of the adult population consuming 5-a-day in 1997. Few students bring in fruit with their packed lunch, which usually consists of an open-sandwich (Owren Aarum, 2003). A school fruit pilot scheme was launched in 1996, and by 2003 a fruit and vegetable programme was running in 18 of Norway's 19 counties. Each subscribing pupil receives a piece of fruit or a vegetable daily, but has to pay for it (the equivalent of €0.30 in 2003 which includes a €0.13 subsidy). In 2003, about 28% of Norways' primary and lower secondary schools were involved, with about 35% of the pupils from participating schools subscribing to the scheme. A 2003 survey found that half of parents would like the price to be lower or free of charge, and that no parents were willing to pay more than the then current price (Owren Aarum, 2003).

1.34.4 United States

The National School Lunch Act, which came into force in 1946, mandates that school meals 'safeguard the health and well-being of the nation's children'. In the US, the *School Meals Initiative for Healthy Children* (SMI) was launched in 1994 by the United States Department of Agriculture (USDA) and took effect in 1996. This meant that all school meals had to meet the recommendations of the *Dietary Guidelines for Americans*. The SMI stipulates that:

- no more than 30% of calories should come from fat
- less than 10% of calories should come from saturated fat
- lunch must provide one-third of the recommended daily amount (RDA) of protein, vitamins A and C, iron, calcium and energy (calories)
- meals must include decreased levels of salt and cholesterol
- breakfast must provide a quarter of the daily RDA.

The SMI guidelines require that records be maintained of all menus to show that nutrition standards are met when averaged over each school week. An audit is conducted at least once every three to five years by state nutrition officials.

Although school meals must meet federal nutrition requirements, it is up to the local school food authority to decide what specific food is served and how it should be prepared. Schools can choose a system of menu planning, based either on a computerised nutritional analysis of the week's menu or based on minimum component quantities of meat (or meat alternative), vegetables, fruits, grains and milk. Alternatively, the school must develop a 'reasonable approach' to meeting the guidelines, based on menu planning guidelines provided by the USDA.

Standards are nutrient-based – food-based standards are not in place. This means that unhealthy food options can still be made available. Monitoring of the standards appears to be weak and there is a strong presence of commercial interests in the form of snack bars, shops and vending machines which compete with the school meal. Of particular concern are 'pouring rights', in relation to soft drinks sold in vending machines. School districts give vendors exclusive rights to sell their products in schools, a contractual agreement which is increasingly common across the US. In exchange for exclusivity, schools receive financial and non-monetary benefits, including upfront payments. Because of the inevitable controversy surrounding 'pouring rights' contracts, some school districts have banned them completely, notably Los Angeles, San Francisco and Seattle. Schools need to generate revenue for school activities and this can conflict with nutrition education programmes (Cline & White, 2000). Participation in school meals programmes is declining in the US, and a study of the impact of 'competitive foods' served in schools, which do not have to meet nutrition standards, found that healthy school meals programmes were being jeopardised by these foods (USDA, 2001). The report states that 'competitive foods undermine the nutrition integrity of the programs and discourage participation'. Sales of competitive foods have continued to increase as student participation in the National School Lunch Program (described below) has decreased. It was also found that competitive foods could stigmatise participation in these programmes: only children with money could afford competitive foods, so school meals could be seen as primarily for poor children.

There have been accusations of a corporate takeover of school food provision, with heavy selling of brand-name fast foods items. Products from companies such as Pizza Hut and Taco Bell are sold in schools, and it is to the school's advantage to do so. Whereas a student may pay only 40 cents for a reduced-cost federal meal, a fast-food meal could be sold for $2–$3 in the late 1990s (Nestle, 2002). Fast food does not meet the USDA guidelines and therefore is not eligible for federal reimbursement. The availability of competitive foods is also thought to convey a mixed message with regard to what children are taught in the classroom about good nutrition. The contrast between what they is taught and what they see available in snack bars and vending machines is thought to make nutrition education merely an academic exercise. Students themselves have expressed intense dislike of school meals, citing taste, appearance and portion size as key issues (James *et al.*, 1996). Meals are 'notoriously' lacking in taste and nutritional quality and participation rates (58% of eligible children) are low (Nestle, 2002).

1.34.5   The National School Lunch Program (NSLP)

This programme was established in 1946 under the National School Lunch Act to provide nutritionally balanced, low-cost or free lunches. It is a federally assisted meal programme which currently operates in almost 101 000 public and non-profit private schools and residential child care institutions. It is administered by the USDA through its Food and Nutrition Service. School districts and independent schools which take part in the NSLP receive cash reimbursement from the USDA for each meal they serve. They also receive donated commodities known as 'entitlement' foods from the USDA as well as surplus agricultural stock. These entitlement foods include fresh, canned and frozen fruits and vegetables, meats, fruit juices, peanut products, vegetable oil, flour and other grain products.

Any child attending a participating school may buy a meal through the NSLP. Only those from families with incomes at or below 130% of the poverty level are eligible for free meals. Children from families between 130% and 185% of the poverty levels are entitled to reduced price meals at a cost of no more than 40 cents. Higher income families pay the full price which is set by the local school food authority, which must operate their meal service on a non-profit basis. As of July 2008, 130% of the poverty level stood at $27 560 for a family of four. The National School Lunch Program is available in almost every school, and around 92% of all pupils have access to meals through the programme. About 58% of these children take a meal on a typical day, which equates to around 26 million children.

In 1998 the NSLP was extended to include reimbursement for snacks served to children in after-school activities. These snacks are provided on the same eligibility basis as school meals. In areas where at least 50% of pupils are entitled to free or reduced-price meals the school may serve all their snacks for free. To qualify for reimbursement, the snack must contain at least two of the following four components: milk or meat (or alternative); a serving of fruit or a vegetable, fruit or vegetable juice; a serving of whole grain or enriched bread or cereal.

1.34.6   School Breakfast Program (SBP)

The SBP operates in the same manner as the National School Lunch Program and is a scheme which provides cash subsidies to states to operate breakfast programmes in schools on a non-profit basis. These breakfasts must meet federal requirements and be offered free or at a reduced price to eligible children. Originally a pilot scheme in 1966, the programme became permanent in 1975. In 2007, the SBP served a daily average of 10.1 million children.

1.35   Discussion and conclusion

The year 2006 marked one hundred years of school meal provision. School meals were introduced as a means of producing fighting-fit men and a strong workforce and ended up as a means of profiteering from overweight children heading for chronic disease. But there was a glorious period somewhere in-between when the focus was simply on providing children with the nutrition they needed to grow and thrive. Indeed, school food was once considered to be one of the foundation stones of the British welfare state (Morgan, 2006). War-time ministers, who had plenty of other matters to think about, recognised the importance of giving the school meal service priority in the supply of rationed foods. Time was even found to introduce the first nutritional standards, helping to turn around the patterns of ill-health during the difficult war years.

The history of school food provision is also a history of the welfare state. During the 1980s and 1990s, the service was lost in a political wilderness, driven by the desire for deregulation and privatisation and based on a cheap food policy. For the best part of twenty years, the parlous state of school meals went largely ignored. All that was to change in 2005, when the school meal service was, quite suddenly, thrust back onto the political agenda. Although much of this has been attributed to the 'Jamie Oliver effect', there had been much agitation for change, albeit with limited success, for many years before. The 'effect' was to force the issue which New Labour had dallied over and intensify political commitment. Thanks to the power of television and the celebrities it espouses, the school meal service was catapulted to the top of the political agenda, with people suddenly outraged by facts that had long been in the public domain. If the wartime government was able to recognise its responsibilities to children whose mothers had been enlisted in employment to support the war effort, one has to wonder why the government was so slow to recognise this need when it launched policies to get single parents back to work.

Having said that, there can be no doubting the commitment and enthusiasm behind the new nutritional standards, the first part of which were introduced in 2006. In policy terms, *Turning the tables* is the most radical school meals policy statement since the founding of the welfare state. It was certainly overdue: as the SMRP commented in the report, '*The current crisis in school food is the result of years of public policy failure*'. The Government's new nutritional standards represent the opportunity to reverse a deeply entrenched culture of neglect. The food- and nutrient-based standards are radical and far-reaching, and easily meet the recommendations made by the Council of Europe in its 2005 *resolution on healthy eating in schools* (Council of Europe, 2005). The new standards represent sweeping changes to the English school meals service.

There is much to learn from one hundred years of school food history, and at least some of the more disastrous legacies offer up some interesting insights into what constitutes best practice in school meal provision. With some considerable certainty it can be said, from lessons learnt, that:

- Children thrive on a healthy diet
- The more a meal is subsidised, the greater the uptake
- Children entitled to a free school meal will not take their entitlement if it means they are easily identifiable
- The dining environment is an important influential factor in uptake
- Nutritional standards must not only be compulsory, they have to be properly monitored.
- Schools with a SNAG often provide a better, more popular service
- The most successful meal services are those embedded within a 'whole school' approach
- When given the choice, children usually choose unhealthy food over healthy food, even when they have been well educated on the composition of a good diet.

The new Conservative government of 1979 regarded health as a personal rather than social issue, and food choices the responsibility of the individual. It chose to ignore the recommendations of the 1980 Black report (*Inequalities in health*) which presaged:

> 'To leave school children, especially young school children, to make their own free choices of (meal) would be wrong ... (This would be) likely to lead to increases in obesity and in dental caries'.   (Black et al., 1980)

New Labour took up the free choice ideology of the Conservatives with gusto. In one hundred years of school meals history, successive policy changes concerning what children eat at school created a fragmented approach, with responsibility passed from central control to LEA, from LEA to individual school and from school to child. In areas beyond commercialism, Labour has frequently been accused of 'nannying', and interfering with people's private lives. Yet children constitute one of the few population groups which society, and above all the Government, is morally bound to nanny. Minding what children eat is as crucial to their wellbeing as monitoring every other aspect of their lives, yet this duty has been woefully neglected.

The question of monitoring children's dietary habits brings up the matter of perception of responsibility. Who, exactly, is responsible for what children eat? The answer depends on where children are. At home, and beyond the school gates, parents or guardians are responsible for their children, but when away from parental vigilance that duty falls to the Government, and the school itself. The 2005 Sodexho school meal survey found that 53% of parents think that working parents need schools to provide the main meal of the day for their child. That belief is justified in view of Government policies to get as many parents back to work as possible. The Sodexho survey also found that only 14% of parents were prepared to pay more for school meals, despite claiming that it was important, or very important that the school provide a healthy meal at lunchtime.

The mantra of the processed food industry is that there is no such thing as a bad food, only a bad diet. This conveniently absolves the industry of responsibility and shifts blame to the consumer, that is, the child, for choosing an unhealthy diet. It does not help when politicians make pronouncements on subjects they know very little about. In the foreword to the 2001 Northern Ireland document, *Catering for Healthier Lifestyles*, Martin McGuinness, then education minister, wrote:

> '*In recognising that there are no healthy or unhealthy foods, only healthy or unhealthy diets, the proposed Standards do not ban any particular foods ... The key, as is borne out in the document, is to have more healthy options available*'. (Northern Ireland Assembly, 2001)

UK Governments have come to understand that there are indeed unhealthy foods and that these foods should not be made available as components of the school lunch. In the long-term, we all benefit from ensuring that children eat a healthy diet. Serving cheap food of poor nutritional quality is in itself costly when the burden on the NHS of chronic disease, the effect on the local economy and the impact of environmental damage are also taken into consideration. Furthermore, it is generally accepted that getting children to eat healthier produces better behaved children. The SMRP, when preparing its document *Turning the Tables: Transforming School Food* (SMRP, 2005) claimed that they '*repeatedly heard head teachers and others from schools where food had already been improved speak of associated improvements in behaviour*'.

Good nutrition is also required for cognitive function. When compulsory education was introduced in Britain in 1880, it brought to light the extent of underfed children too malnourished to be able to learn. Who knows how many children are malnourished today to the extent that their learning capability is impaired?

It is too early to assess the effects of new food- and nutrient-based standards on the health of schoolchildren, in terms of obesity and other chronic disease. The introduction of standards may have been essential, but they have not come without their own problems, in particular that of falling levels of uptake. Improving uptake must now be the focus of activity. Experience has shown a number of methods which can greatly increase uptake. These include:

- **Reduction of the cost of the meal through subsidisation.** The school meal is doomed if it continues to be cheaper for parents to give their children a packed lunch alternative. Prices are likely to increase further to cover the costs of meeting standards. The new lunch standards should not exist solely to improve the health of those who can afford them. Unless the government agrees to expand eligibility of free school meals, and subsidise existing costs, higher prices could further reduce uptake.

- **Improving the dining experience.** It has been shown that pupils are more likely to eat a school meal when queues are short and they can sit with friends who brought packed lunches. According to Ofsted, the quality of the dining area is a determinant of whether pupils eat a school meal; one reason given by pupils for taking a packed lunch to school is precisely that sandwiches could be eaten quickly where and when they chose (Ofsted, 2007).

- **Introduction of a whole school food policy and a school nutrition action group (SNAG).** Schools which have such a policy have better meal uptake. As the SMRP said in its report *Turning the tables*, successful school food improvements require a partnership approach, with input from pupils, caterers, parents and everyone who is in some way involved with child care. '*Evidence heard by the Panel indicates that the most successful way of bringing about significant changes to the picture set out above is for schools to develop 'whole-school' food and nutrition policies*'. (SMRP, 2005)

- **Introduction of a cashless payment system.** Smart card technology has been shown to increase uptake by removing the stigma attached to claiming a free school meal by making entitled children hard to identify.

- **Universality of free school meals.** Universality has been shown in Finland and (for a short while) Hull to greatly increase uptake of free school meals. The current system is clearly failing poor children who suffer embarrassment and risk bullying by being identified as claimants. Means testing results in too many children falling through the net. The cost of providing free school meals is not prohibitive to the fourth largest economy in the world and indeed in the long run may help reduce the cost to the NHS of treating chronic disease.

- **Fair pay and conditions for catering staff.** The school meals service needs to be provided by staff on fair pay and conditions. Caterers play a huge role in encouraging children to try healthy foods, and are part of a whole school approach. Their role continues to expand: school catering is becoming an all-day service, starting with breakfast and including snacks, lunch and after-school meals.

Finally, there can be no lasting improvement without a change in collective mindset on the role of food in society. The UK needs to develop a good food culture, similar to the one in Italy. '*Had there been a greater cultural attachment to the quality of food, as there is in Italy, there might have been more opposition to the debasement of school meals; but, in the event, the combination of a cheap food culture and a neoliberal government proved to be a noxious cocktail from a nutritional point of view*' (Morgan & Sonnino, 2007). The development of a food culture is an evolving process but there are already signs of a revival of interest in real, traditional and local food. If adults change the way they value food, there is hope that the effect will trickle down to their children.

Note

1   The Food Dudes is an intervention, devised by the Bangor Food Research Unit at the University of Wales, incorporating video adventures of hero figures who enjoy eating fruit and vegetables and who provide role modules for children to emulate. The initiative also involves rewards in the form of small gifts for children who experiment with fruits and vegetables.

References

Acheson, D. (chair) (1998) *Independent Inquiry into Inequalities in Health Report*. London: TSO.

Baer, J.R., Blount, R., Detrich, R. & Stokes, T. (1987) Using intermittent reinforcement to program maintenance of verbal/nonverbal correspondence. *Journal of Applied Behavior Analysis*, **20**:179–184. In: Murcott, A. (1998) (ed.) *The Nation's Diet: The Social Science of Food Choice*. London: Longman.

Belderson, P., Harvey, I., Kimbell, R., O'Neill, J., Russell, J. & Barker, M.E. (2003) Does breakfast-club attendance affect schoolchildren's nutrient intake? A study of dietary intake at three schools. *British Journal of Nutrition*, **90**(6):1003–1006.

Bellisle, F. (2004) Effects of diet on behaviour and cognition in children. *British Journal of Nutrition*, **92**(S2):S227–S232.

Bender, A.E., Magee, P. & Nash, A.H. (1972) Survey of school meals. *British Medical Journal*, **2**:383–385.

Benton, D., Griffiths, S. & Haller, J. (1997) Thiamin supplementation, mood and cognitive functioning. *Psychopharmacology*, **129**:66–71. In: Bellisle, F. (2004) Effects of diet on behaviour and cognition in children. *British Journal of Nutrition*, **92**(S2):S227–S232.

Birch, L.L. (1980) Effects of peer models' food choices and eating behaviours on preschoolers' food preferences. *Child Development*, **51**:489–496.

Black, D., Morris, J., Smith, C. & Townsend, P. (1980) *Inequalities in Health: Report of a Research Working Group*. London: DHSS.

Blair, T. (2005) Serving them a better future. *The Observer*, 20th March.

Booth, C. (1970) *Life and Labour of the People in London, First Series: Poverty*. New York, NY: AMS Press. In: Colquhoun, A., Lyon, P. & Alexander, E. (2001) Feeding minds and bodies: The Edwardian context of school meals. *Nutrition & Food Science*, **331**(3):117–125.

Borzekowski, D. & Robinson, T. (2001) The 30-second effect: An experiment revealing the impact of television commercials on food preferences of pre-schoolers. *Journal of the American Dietetic Association*, **101**(1):42–46.

Brannen, J. & Storey, P. (1998) School meals and the start of secondary school. *Health Education Research*, **13**(1):73–86.

Brown, U. & Phillips, D. (eds) (2002) *"Even the Tatties have Batter!" Free Nutritious Meals for all Children in Scotland*. Glasgow: CPAG in Scotland.

Business in the Community & the Soil Association (2004) *Looking for innovation in healthy school meals*. www.bitc.org.uk/rural

Casey, R. & Rozin, P. (1989) Changing children's food preferences: Parent opinions. *Appetite*, **12**:171–182.

Cassels, J. & Stewart, R. (2002) *Breakfast Service Provision for School Aged Children: A Mapping Exercise*. Edinburgh: Health Education Board for Scotland.

Chauliac, M. (2003) National inter-agency co-operation regarding nutrition in schools. *Proceedings of the European Forum on Eating at School – Making Health Choices*, 20–21 November 2003. Strasbourg: Council of Europe.

Child Poverty Action Group (Scotland) *Free school meals: a briefing from CPAG in Scotland*. www.cpag.org.uk. Accessed February 2008.

Clancy-Hepburn, K., Hickey, A.A. & Nevill, G. (1974) Children's behaviour responses to TV food advertisements. *Journal of Nutrition Education*, 6(3):93–96.

Cline, T. & White, G. (2000) Local support for nutrition integrity in schools. *Journal of the American Dietetic Association*, 100:108–111.

Cole, T.J., Bellizzi, M.C., Flegal, K.M. & Dietz, W.H. (2000) Establishing a standard definition for child overweight and obesity worldwide: International survey. *British Medical Journal*, 320:1240–1243.

Coles, A. & Turner, S. (1993) *Catering for Healthy Eating in Schools*. London: Health Education Authority.

Coon, K.A., Goldberg, J., Rogers, B.L. & Tucker, K.L. (2001) Relationships between use of television during meals and children's food consumption patters. *Pediatrics*, 107(1):E7.

Coudyser, R. (2003) Healthy eating in the traditional school meals system. The role of the private food operator. *Proceedings of the European Forum on Eating at School – Making Health Choices*, 20–21 November 2003. Strasbourg: Council of Europe.

Council of Europe (2005) Committee of Members (2005) Resolution ResAP(2005)3 on healthy eating in schools. www.wcd.coe.int.

Currie, C., Roberts, C., Morgan, A., Smith, R., Settertobulte, W., Samdal, O., Barnekow Rasmussen, V. (eds) (2004) Young people's health in context. Health Behaviour in School-Aged Children (HBSC) Study. *International Report from the 2001/2002 Survey, Health Policy for Children and Adolescents*. Copenhagen: WHO European Regional Office.

Dani, J., Burrill, C. & Demmig-Adams, B. (2005) The remarkable role of nutrition in learning and behaviour. *Nutrition & Food Science*, 35(4):258–263.

Davies, S. (2005) *School Meals, Markets and Quality*. London: Unison.

De Boer, F. (2003) Eating at school – a European study. *Proceedings of the European Forum on Eating at School – Making Health Choices*, 20–21 November 2003. Strasbourg: Council of Europe.

Department for Education and Employment (DfEE) (1997) *Excellence in Schools*. London: TSO.

Department for Education and Skills (2006) *Guidance for procuring school lunches*. www.teachernet.gov.uk.

Department for Education and Skills (DfES) (2004) *Healthy Living Blueprint for Schools*. Nottingham: DfES.

Department for Education and Skills (DfES). *Guidance for Caterers to School Lunch Standards*. www.dfes.gov.uk/schoollunches. Accessed October 2005.

Department of Education (DE) (2004) Out of schools learning provision and school improvement in Northern Ireland. Research briefing 2/2004. DENI.

Department of Education (DE) (2008) *New nutritional standards for school lunches and other food in schools*. DENI.

Department of Health (DH) (2001) *The National School Fruit Scheme*. Evaluation Summary. www.5aday.nhs.uk. Accessed August 2005.

Department of Health (DH) (2003) *A Study into Parents' and Teachers' Views of the National School Fruit Scheme*. www.5aday.nhs.uk. Accessed August 2005.

Department of Health (DH) (2004) *Choosing Health: Making Healthy Choices Easier*. London: TSO.

Department of Health (DH) (1992) *The Health of the Nation: A Strategy for Health in England*. London: HMSO.

Department of Health (DH) (2005) *National Healthy School Status. A Guide for Schools*. London: DH.

Department of Health (DH). *Dining room environment*. www.dh.gov.uk. Accessed January 2008.

Department of Health and Social Security (DHSS) (1989) The diets of British schoolchildren. *Report on Health and Social Subjects*, 36. London: HMSO.

Department of Health, DCSF & The Information Centre (2008) National Child Measurement Programme: 2006/07 school year, headline results.

Dixey, R., Heindl, I., Loureiro, I., Pérez-Rodrigo, C., Snel, J. & Warnking, P. (1999). *Healthy Eating for Young People in Europe – A School-Based Nutrition Education Guide*. Copenhagen: WHO Regional Office for Europe.

Donkin, A.J.M., Neale, R.J. & Tilston, C. (1993) Children's food purchase requests. *Appetite*, **21**:291–294.

Ebbeling, C.B., Pawlak, D.B. & Ludwig, D.S. (2002) Childhood obesity: Public-health crisis, common sense cure. *Lancet*, **360**:473–482.

Education and Training Inspectorate (2007) *Progress made in the implementation of 'Catering for healthier lifestyles'*. Executive summary. Department of Education for Northern Ireland.

Education and Training Inspectorate (2007) *Progress made in the implementation of 'Catering for healthier lifestyles'*. Executive summary. Department of Education for Northern Ireland.

Edwards, J.S.A. & Hartwell, H.H. (2002) Fruit and vegetables – attitudes and knowledge of primary school children. *Journal of Human Nutrition & Dietetics*, **15**(5):365.

Fisher, P. (1987) History of school meals in Great Britain. *Nutrition and Health*, **4**:189–194.

Food Commission (2001) *Children's Nutrition Action Plan*. London: The Food Commission.

Food Standards Agency (2001) *Promotion of food to children*. Report on qualitative research RS 4922. www.food.gov.uk

Food Standards Agency (2006) *Report from the school council network*. www.food.gov.uk.

Food Standards Agency (2007) *Agency revises advice on certain artificial colours*. www.food.gov.uk.

Food Standards Agency Wales (2002) *School meals report*. July 2002.

Food Standards Agency Wales (2003) *Healthier fruit and vegetable options on the school menu but children's choices haven't changed yet*. Press release 21 October 2003.

Frewin, A. (2004) Head teachers claim victory over vending machines, 16 June 2004. www.caterersearch.com.

Galst, J.P. & White, M.A. (1976) The unhealthy persuader: The reinforcing value of television and children's purchase-influencing attempts at the supermarket. *Child Development*, **47**:1089–1096.

Garrow, J.S., James, W.P.T. & Ralph, A. (2000) (eds) *Human Nutrition and Dietetics*. Edinburgh: Churchill Livingstone.

Gatenby, S.J., Hunt, P. & Rayner, M. (1995) The *National Food Guide*: development of dietetic criteria and nutritional characteristics. *Journal of Human Nutrition and Dietetics*, **8**:323–334.

Gillard, D. (2003) Food for thought: Child nutrition, the school dinner and the food industry. *Forum*, **45**(3):111–118.

Gorn, G. & Goldberg, M. (1982) Behavioural evidence of the effects of televised food messages on children. *Journal of Consumer Research*, **9**:200–205.

Gould, R., Russell, J. & Barker, M.E. (2006) School lunch menus and 11 to 12 year old children's food choice in three secondary schools in England – are the nutritional standards being met? *Appetite*, **46**(1):86–92.

Green, K. (2006) Bring back free school meals. *The Guardian*, 9 June, 2006.

Gregory, J.R., Lowe, S., Bates, C.J., Prentice, A., Jackson, L.V., Smithers, G., Wenlock, R. & Farron, M. (2000) *National Diet and Nutrition Survey: Young People Aged 4 to 18 years. Volume 1: Report of the Diet and Nutrition Survey*. London: TSO.

Gustafsson, U. (2002) School meals policy: The problem with governing children. *Social Policy & Administration*, **36**(6):685–697.

Halford, J.C., Gillespie, J., Brown, V., Pontin, E.E. & Dovey, T.M. (2004) Effect of television advertisements for foods on food consumption in children. *Appetite*, **42**(2):221–225.

Harrop, A. & Palmer, G. (2002) *Improving Breakfast Clubs: Lessons from the Best*. London: New Policy Institute.

Harvey, J. (2000) *The Chips are Down. A Guide to Food Policy in Schools*. Stockport: The Health Education Trust.

Harvey, J. (2004) *A Feasibility Study into Healthier Drinks Vending in Schools*. London: Food Standards Agency.

Health Education Trust (HET) website. www.healthedtrust.com Accessed February 2008.

Health Promotion Agency (HPA) (2001) Eating for health? A survey of eating habits among children and young people in Northern Ireland. HPA.

Health Promotion Agency for Northern Ireland. *How healthy is your school? A toolkit to assist school development planning for health*. www.healthpromotionagency.org.uk. Accessed January 2008.

Hearn, M.D., Baranowski, T., Baranowski, J., Doyle, C., Smith, M., Lin, L.S. & Resnicow, K. (1998) Environmental influences on dietary behavior among children. *Journal of Health Education*, **29**(1):26–32.

HM Inspectorate of Education (HMIE) (2005) *Monitoring the implementation of Hungry for Success: A whole school approach to school meals in Scotland*. Report on progress. HMIE.

HM Inspectorate of Education (HMIE) (2008) *Hungry for success – Further food for thought*. HMIE.

International Obesity Task Force (2005) EU platform on diet, physical activity and health. *EU Platform briefing paper*. March 15, 2005. Brussels.

James, D.C., Rienzo, B.A. & Frazee, C. (1996) Using focus group interviews to understand school meal choices. *School Health*, **66**(4):128–131.

James, W.P.T., Nelson, M., Ralph, A. & Leather, S. (1997) Socioeconomic determinants of health: The contribution of nutrition to inequalities in health. *British Medical Journal*, **314**:1545.

Jamie Oliver (2008) *Feed Me Better*. www.jamieoliver.com/schooldinners.

Jefferson, A. & Cowbrough, K. (2003) *School Lunch Box Survey*. London: Food Standards Agency & Community Nutrition Group.

Koivisto, U.K., Fellenius, J. & Sjoden, P.O. (1994) Relations between parental mealtime practices and children's food intake. *Appetite*, **22**(3):245–257.

LACA (2004) *School Meals Survey 2004*. Woking: Local Authority Caterers Association.

Lambert, N., Plumb, J., Looise, B., *et al.* (2005a) Using smart card technology to monitor the eating habits of children in a school cafeteria: 2. The nutrient contents of all meals chosen by a group of 8- to 11-year-old boys over 78 days. *Journal of Human Nutrition and Dietetics*, **18**:255–265.

Lambert, N., Plumb, J., Looise, B., *et al.* (2005b) Using smart card technology to monitor the eating habits of children in a school cafeteria: 3. The nutritional significance of beverage and dessert choices. *Journal of Human Nutrition and Dietetics*, **18**:271–279.

Le Gros Clark, F. (1942) The school child and the school canteen. Hertford: Hertfordshire County Council. In Welshman, J. (1997) School meals and milk in England and Wales 1906–45. *Medical History*, **41**: 6–29.

Lobstein, T. & Frelut, M.L. (2003) Prevalence of overweight among children in Europe. *Obesity Reviews*, 4(4):195.

Lobstein, T., Baur, L. & Uauy, R. (2004) Obesity in children and young people: A crisis in public health. *The International Association for the Study of Obesity. Obesity Reviews*, 5(Suppl. 1):4–85.

Local Authorities Caterers Association (2007) *National School Meals Survey 2007*. Woking: LACA.

Lowe, C.F., Downey, A.J. & Horne, P.J. (1998) Changing what children eat. In: Murcott, A. (ed.) *The Nation's Diet: The Social Science of Food Choice*. London: Longman.

Lynch, R. & Murphy, S. (2008) *A process evaluation of the Welsh Assembly Government's primary school free breakfast initiative.* Cardiff Institute of Society, Health and Ethics, Cardiff University.

MacGregor, A. & Sheehy, C. (2005) *Evaluation of Free Fruit in Schools Initiative.* The Scottish Government. www.scotland.gov.uk/publications/2005.

McCarthy, H.D. & Ellis, S.M. (2003) Central overweight and obesity in British youth aged 11–16 years: Cross sectional surveys of waist circumference. *British Medical Journal,* 326:624–626.

McEvaddy, S. (1988) *One Good Meal a Day – the Loss of Free School Meals.* London: Child Poverty Action Group.

McKeigue, P.M., Shah, B. & Marmot, M.G. (1991) Relation of central obesity and insulin resistance with high diabetes prevalence and cardiovascular risk in South Asians. *Lancet,* 337:382–386.

McMahon, W. & Marsh, T. (1999) *Filling the Gap: Free School Meals, Nutrition and Poverty.* London: Child Poverty Action Group.

Ministry of Social Affairs and Health (1999). Finnish Family Policy. Helsinki. In: Scottish Parliament. *School meals (Scotland) Bill.* (2001) Policy memorandum. Edinburgh: TSO.

Mintel (2003) *Children's School Meals – UK 2003.* London: Mintel International Group Ltd.

Morelli, C. & Seaman, P. (2004) Universal versus Targeted Benefits: The distributional effects of free school meals. Working paper No. 173. Department of Economic Studies, University of Dundee.

Morgan, K. (2006) School food and the public domain: The politics of the public plate. *The Political Quarterly,* 77(3), July–September 2006.

Morgan, K. & Morley, A. (2003) *School Meals: Healthy Eating and Sustainable Food Chains.* The Regeneration Institute, Cardiff University.

Morgan, K. & Sonnino, R. (2007) Empowering consumers: The creative procurement of school meals in Italy and the UK. *International Journal of Consumer Studies,* 31(1):19–25.

National Audit Office (NAO) (2001) *Tackling Obesity in England.* Report by the Comptroller & Auditor General HC 220 session 2000–2001, 15th February. London: TSO.

National Audit Office (NAO) (2006) *Smarter Food Procurement in the Public Sector: Case Studies.* Report by the Comptroller and Auditor General HC963-II session 2005–2006, 30 March 2006. London: TSO.

Nelson, M. (2000) Childhood nutrition and poverty. *Proceedings of the Nutrition Society,* 59:307–315.

Nelson, M., Bradbury, J., Poulter, J., McGee, A., Msebele, S. & Jarvis, L. (2004) *School Meals in Secondary Schools in England.* Research Report RR557. London: FSA/DfES.

Nelson, M., Lowes, K. & Hwang, V. (2007) The contribution of school meals to food consumption and nutrient intakes of young people aged 4–18 years in England. *Public Health Nutrition,* 10:652–662.

Nelson, M., Nicholas, J., Suleiman, S., Davies, O., Prior, G., Hall, L., Wreford, S. & Poulter, J. (2006) *School meals in primary schools in England.* Research report RB753. Food Standards Agency/Department for Education and Skills.

Nelson, M. & Paul, A.A. (1983) The nutritive contribution of school dinners and other mid-day meals to the diets of schoolchildren. *Human Nutrition: Applied Nutrition,* 37(2): 128–135.

Nestle, M. (2002). *Food Politics. How the Food Industry Influences Nutrition and Health.* California: University of California Press.

Nicholas, J., Wood, L., Morgan, C., Russell, S. & Nelson, M. (2008) *Third annual survey of take up of school meals in England. Provisional findings.* School Food Trust/LACA.

Nicholas, J., Wood, L. & Nelson, M. (2007) *Second annual survey of take-up of school meals in England.* School Food Trust.

Noble, C. & Kipps, M. (1994) Implementing quantified guidelines for school meals. *International Journal of Hospitality Management,* 13(4):361–374.

Noble, C., Corney, M., Eves, A., Kipps, M. & Lumbers, M. (2000) Food choice and school meals: Primary schoolchildren's perceptions of the healthiness of foods and the nutritional implications of food choices. *Hospitality Management*, 19:413–432.

Northern Ireland Assembly (2001) *Catering for Healthier Lifestyles*. Compulsory Nutritional Standards for School Meals: A consultation document. Department of Education.

Ofsted (2006a) Healthy eating in schools. www.ofsted.gov.uk. March 2006.

Ofsted (2006b) Food technology in secondary schools. www.ofsted.gov.uk March 2006.

Ofsted (2007) Food in schools. Encouraging healthier eating. October 2007.

Oliveria, S.A., Curtis Ellison, R., Moore, L.L., Gillman, M.W., Garrahie, E.J. & Singer, M.R. (1992) Parent–child relationships in nutrient intake: The Framington Children's Study. *American Journal of Clinical Nutrition*, 56:593–598.

Owren Aarum, A. (2003) How to provide healthy food in schools: school fruit programmes as a short cut to promoting healthy eating in schools – The Norwegian experience. *Proceedings of the European Forum on Eating at School – Making Health Choices*. 20–21 November 2003. Strasbourg: Council of Europe.

Passmore, S. & Harris, G. (2004) Education, health and school meals: A review of policy changes in England and Wales over the last century. *British Nutrition Foundation Nutrition Bulletin*, 29:221–227.

Passmore, S. & Harris, G. (2005) School Nutrition Action Groups and their effect upon secondary school-aged pupils' food choices. *Nutrition Bulletin*, 30:364–369.

Peterson, P.E., Jeffrey D.B., Bridgewater, C.A. & Dawson, B. (1984) How pronutrition television programming affects children's dietary habits. *Developmental Psychology*, 2:55–63. In: Murcott, A. (1998) (ed.) *The Nation's Diet: The Social Science of Food Choice*. London: Longman.

PricewaterhouseCoopers (2005) *Evaluation of the pilot of the 'Catering for healthier lifestyles' standards in schools in NI*. Department of Education for Northern Ireland.

Private email correspondence with Department of Education NI, 15 January 2008.

Private email correspondence with Department of Education NI, 8 February 2008.

Private email correspondence with the School Food Trust, 8 January 2008.

Ransley, J.K., Greenwood, D.C., Cade, J.E., Blenkinsop, S., Schagen, I., Teeman, D., Scott, E., White, G. & Schagen, S. (2007) Does the school fruit and vegetable scheme improve children's diet? A non-randomised controlled trial. *Journal of Epidemiology and Community Health*, 61:699–703.

Richardson, A.J. & Montgomery, P. (2005) The Oxford–Durham study: A randomized, controlled trial of dietary supplementation with fatty acids in children with developmental coordination disorder. *Pediatrics*, 115:1360–1366.

Rogers, I.S., Ness, A.R., Hebditch, K., Jones, L.R. & Emmett, P.M. (2007) Quality of food eaten in English primary schools: School dinners vs packed lunches. *European Journal of Clinical Nutrition*, 61:856–864.

Roos, G., Lean, M. & Anderson, A. (2002) Dietary interventions in Finland, Norway and Sweden: Nutrition policies and strategies. *Journal of Human Nutrition & Dietetics*, 15:99–110.

School Food Trust (SFT) (2007a) *A guide to introducing the Government's food-based and nutrient-based standards for school lunches from the School Food Trust*. www.schoolfoodtrust.org.uk.

School Food Trust (SFT) (2007b) *A guide to introducing the Government's new food-based standards for all school food other than lunches*. www.schoolfoodtrust.org.uk.

School Food Trust (SFT) (2007c) *A fresh look at the school meal experience*. www.schoolfoodtrust.org.uk.

School Food Trust (SFT) (2007d) *What are we eating? School lunch versus packed lunch following the introduction of food-based standards for school lunch*. www.schoolfoodtrust.org.uk.

School Food Trust (SFT) (2007e) *School lunch and behaviour: Systematic observation of classroom behaviour following a school dining room intervention*. Available from www.schoolfoodtrust.org.uk.

School Meals Review Panel (SMRP) (2005) *Turning the Tables: Transforming School Food.* London: DfES.

Scottish Executive (2002) *Hungry for Success: A Whole School Approach to School Meals in Scotland.* Final Report of the Expert Panel on School Meals. Edinburgh: TSO.

Scottish Executive (2003) Press Release. 19 February 2003. In: Hurley, C. & Riley, A. (eds), *Recipe for Change. A Good Practice Guide to School Meals.* London: CPAG.

Sharp, I. (1992) *Nutritional Guidelines for School Meals. Report of an Expert Working Group.* London: Caroline Walker Trust.

Sinnott, J. (2005) *Healthy Schools and Improvements in Standards.* London: Health Development Agency.

Sodexho (2002) *The Sodexho School Meals and Lifestyle Survey 2002.* Kenley: Sodexho Limited.

Sodexho (2005) *The Sodexho School Meals and Lifestyle Survey 2005.* Kenley: Sodexho Limited.

Soil Association (2003) *Food for Life.* Bristol: Soil Association.

Soil Association. *Food for Life.* www.soilassociation.org/foodforlife. Accessed January 2008.

Stevenson, J. (2006) Dietary influences on cognitive development and behaviour in children. *Proceedings of the Nutrition Society,* 65:361–365.

Storey, P. & Candappa, M. (2004) *School Meals Funding Delegation.* Institute of Education, University of London. Research Report RR512. London: DfES.

Storey, P. & Chamberlain, R. (2001) Improving the take up of free school meals. *Research Brief 270.* London: DfEE.

Street, C. & Kenway, P. (1999) *Food for Thought: Breakfast Clubs and their Challenges.* London: The New Policy Institute.

Taras, H.L., Sallis, J.F., Patterson, T.L., Nader, P.R. & Nelson, J.A. (1989) Television's influence on children's diet and physical activity. *Journal of Developmental and Behavioral Pediatrics,* 10(4):176–180.

The Information Centre (2006) *Statistics on obesity, physical activity and diet: England, 2006.* www.ic.nhs.uk. IC/NHS.

The National Healthy Schools Programme. www.healthyschools.gov.uk. Accessed January 2008.

Unison (2002) *School Meals in the 21st Century.* London: Unison Educational Services.

Unison (2005) PFI contracts blocking decent school meals. Press release 12/09/05.

USDA Food & Nutrition Service (2001) *Foods sold in competition with USDA School Meals Programs: A report to congress, January 12, 2001.* Washington DC: USDA.

Vartiainen, E., Puska, P., Pekkanen, J., Toumilehto, J. & Jousilahti, P. (1994) Changes in risk factors explain changes in mortality from ischaemic heart disease in Finland. *British Medical Journal,* 309:23–27.

Walker, B. (2004) School meals around the world. *Caterer & Hotelkeeper,* 193:4316.

Welsh Assembly Government (2007) *Appetite for life action plan.* Information document 026/2007. Issued November 2007.

Welshman, J. (1997) School meals and milk in England and Wales, 1906–45. *Medical History,* 41:6–29.

Wesslén, A. School meals in Sweden. http://www.skolmatensvanner.org. Accessed July 2005.

Whincup, P.H., Owen, C.G., Sattar, N. & Cook, D.G. (2005) School dinners and markers of cardiovascular health and type 2 diabetes in 13–16 year olds: Cross sectional study. *British Medical Journal,* 331:1060–1061.

White, J., Cole-Hamilton, I. & Dibb, S. (1992) *The Nutritional Case for School Meals.* London: School Meals Campaign.

Woolton, Lord (1945) Speech made to the Warwickshire Women's Institute. In: Fort, M. *Hold The Two Veg. The Guardian,* 3rd December 1999.

World Health Organization (WHO) (2003) *Diet, Nutrition and the Prevention of Chronic Diseases*. WHO Technical Report Series 916. Geneva: WHO.

World Health Organization. Child and Adolescent Health and Development. www.who.int/child-adolescent-health/nut.htm. Accessed January 2008.

Young, I., de Boer, F.A., Mikkelsen, B.E. & Rasmussen, V.B. (2005) Healthy eating at school: A European forum. *British Nutrition Foundation Bulletin*, 30:85–93.

2 Hospitals

Barbara MacDonald

2.1 Introduction

Today, anybody who has been inside a hospital building cannot have failed to notice the vending machines, fast food outlets and the often pervading smell of food in corridors, emanating from kitchens, canteens, restaurants and wards. For many people, this is their first experience of hospital catering, an experience which might have added to their opinions on hospital food in general, opinions which might have been already influenced by press reports or hearsay from visitors, former patients and hospital employees. All this could add to future patients' expectations of the type of food they could be expected to eat after their admission to hospital. The actual experience of hospital food might be very different from any expectations: it could be a pleasant surprise or disappointingly inadequate and these experiences reflect the anomalies that exist throughout the NHS in the UK.

For many years hospital food has been viewed as an 'add on' to the many excellent services that the NHS provide, despite the fact that the link between nutritious food and good health is well recognised and very much in the public domain. Indeed, there is a certain irony in the fact that although the treatment of ill health from poor diets costs the NHS at least £4 billion a year (Department of Health (DH), 2005a), in some circumstances, the NHS seems to be contributing to these statistics.

Back in the 1800s, the provision of hospital food was reportedly fraught with problems of inadequate supplies and standards, coupled with kitchens that were often unhygienic, poorly located and run by people who were less than sympathetic towards their diners. It seemed that hospital catering in general just evolved in a haphazard fashion with little or any forethought.

During the further evolution of hospital catering in the 1900s, catering managers steered their way through various methods of food service, dietitians concentrated on specialised diets and reports on all aspects of hospital catering were not encouraging. The role of nurses in the delivery of food was challenged and it seemed that all the staff involved in hospital food, in whatever guise, fragmented into their own blinkered roles without seeming to realise that there was a common goal to provide nutrition for their patients. Little wonder that in the 1970s some patients were found to be suffering from malnutrition (Hill *et al.*, 1977).

In the 1980s the hospital catering system underwent massive changes with Compulsory Competitive Tendering putting huge financial pressures on catering departments while the issue of poor hygiene practices in kitchens was finally resolved by the lifting of Crown Immunity, whereby hospitals were no longer exempt from prosecution (Deer, 1985). There were numerous calls for more education on the importance of hospital food and plenty of advisory documents were published to support this notion. Eventually in the 1990s nutrition guidelines were introduced to raise standards of food but, yet again, nobody seemed to be taking responsibility for the actual feeding of the patients.

Then in 2001, there were great expectations about improvements to hospital food through the Better Hospital Food programme, which had set criteria to be adhered to, with help and advice easily accessed via the internet (NHS Estates, 2001a). In addition, hospital food standards were to be regularly inspected with the results made public. As a result, many hospitals have vastly improved on all aspects of their catering, some veritably flourishing but for some, malnutrition is still in evidence. It should also be remembered that it is not only the United Kingdom that has problems with hospital food: similar problems are to be found across Europe and there are currently many organisations involved in trying to tackle these issues which are too often compounded by both a laissez faire attitude and a lack of funding.

Thus, this chapter attempts to trace the evolution of hospital catering from its beginnings in the workhouses[1] to the present day. Many of the relevant documents and reports have been included, others have not, but the outcome is a reflection of the many difficulties and many hurdles that have and still have to be overcome in the provision of nutrition in these very public institutions.

2.2   The development of workhouses

Knatchbull's Act of 1722 authorised parishes to construct workhouses in an attempt to limit the cost of assisting the poor in their own homes by trying to provide them with some sort of work. In 1782, Gilbert's Act allowed adjacent parishes to combine into unions, building workhouses for the exclusive use of the sick, aged and children. Despite the fact that many parishes thought it was more economical to look after the poor in their own homes, it is likely that in the early nineteenth century there would have been a considerable number of sick people accommodated in workhouses, exceeding those in hospitals: by 1861 there were 50 000 'sick persons' under the care of workhouse medical officers – many of the patients were of 'a type' which the voluntary hospitals would not accept (Abel-Smith, 1964).

The rapid growth of workhouses was the result of the Poor Law Commission of 1832 and the subsequent Poor Law Amendment Act of 1834 which deterred people from claiming benefits from the Poor Law authorities (Abel-Smith, 1964). The workhouses were referred to as 'bastilles' by the poor and effectively imprisoned the sick, unemployed, disabled and insane (Richardson & Hurwitz, 1989). During the latter part of the nineteenth century, there was an increase in the level of medical care provided for workhouse inmates. The hospital wings of workhouses increased in size and patients were admitted to workhouse hospitals for treatment rather than being admitted as workhouse inmates. After about 1913, many workhouses changed their name to 'institutions' to reflect this change in their role but also because the very name 'workhouse' carried such a social stigma. Workhouses were officially abolished by the Local Government Act of 1929, which from 1 April 1930 abolished the Unions and transferred their responsibilities to the County Councils and County Boroughs. The workhouses officially became known as hospitals at this time or shortly thereafter but the association with the workhouse remained, which would explain why some people would have been reluctant to ask for free care at these hospitals. The remaining responsibility for the Poor Law was given to local authorities before final abolition in 1984 when both the voluntary and public hospitals came into the ownership of the National Health Service placing them under the management of local hospital management committees.

2.3 Food provision

2.3.1 Workhouse food

The Poor Law Commissioners did not insist on national uniformity in diet but believed in 'similarity' as *'the habits of the people and mode of living being different in different places'* (Nicholls, 1898), with regional variations in the types of food served encouraged:

> *'In Cumberland and some of the northern counties, milk is generally used where beer is used in the southern counties. The requisite equality in diet would probably be obtainable without forcing any class of the inmates of the workhouses in the northern counties to take beer or those of southern counties to take milk'.* (Johnson, 1985)

Subject to approval from the Commissioners, workhouses provided their own 'dietaries' (Parliamentary Papers), monitored by audits and periodic inspections. However, these were seldom made more than once a year with, often, advance warnings of a visit. In addition auditors were not always trained so could not always judge whether the diet served was 'official' (Johnson, 1985).

They were later advised that they had to consider factors of both health and economy: this did not mean buying the cheapest food available but finding the most nutritious foods available at a low cost. What was important was that the food was actually eaten and the importance of the need for good cooking and palatable food was stressed. Guardians were urged to remove foods such as rice pudding and pea soup, which were particularly disliked by paupers and replace them with extra milk and fresh vegetables. It was also recommended that meals should be served hot and eaten in cheerful surroundings to ensure that the paupers not only ate their food but also digested it. Issues of food wastage were also in evidence:

> 'The food should be plain and wholesome, the quantity sufficient without being excessive, and the composition and cooking such as to render it palatable so that waste may be avoided, either from the allowance being more than the inmate requires, or from the food being distasteful to them'.   (Parliamentary Papers)

The realities of the standard of the food were very different from what might have been expected via the guidance: the Lancet doctors thought *'the infirm and chronic patients decidedly require a diet of their own'* and heard *'many bitter complaints of the pea soup as causing pain and spasm in the stomach'* (Lancet Commission Report, undated). Wastage of food was noted amongst the old and toothless residents and for this reason their diet was *'uniformly insufficient'* (House of Commons, 1866). If the indoor paupers were certified sick by the medical officer it allowed the provision of a better diet: *'the number of sick is increased by fully one-third in most workhouses, simply in order to obtain for the aged and infirm a better dietary'* (House of Commons, 1866). A *'sick diet'* was prescribed for all patients except the *'undeserving'* by one medical officer and it was the medical officers themselves who could also order *'extras'* such as *'chops, fish and various delicacies'* (Sheen, 1875) including alcohol. Without the express recommendation of the medical officer, roasted food was rarely allowed to inmates (Abel-Smith, 1964). In one workhouse it was reported that unmarried, postnatal mothers suffered from extreme exhaustion because they were kept on a starvation diet for nine days after their confinement (Richardson & Hurwitz, 1989).

Investigators of this period criticised the prevailing systems of cooking and conveying food to the sick wards: in many workhouses kitchen apparatus was defective and very few employed skilled cooks. In London and the provinces *'the conveying of food is seldom effected with as much care to keep the food warm'* (House of Commons, 1866). In London, the transportation of food was necessary because there were *'no hospital kitchens in the detached infirmaries, nor separate kitchens attached to the sick wards of all the workhouses and invariably there are no day rooms'* (House of Commons, 1866).

2.3.2 Hospital food

2.3.2.1   1600 to 1800

The provision of food was not any better in hospitals (Box 2.1 shows the diet provided in St. Bartholomew's Hospital in 1687) with some patients likely to be

---

Box 2.1   The new diet table approved by the Governing Body of
St. Bartholomew's Hospital, April 1687.

DYETT APPOINTED

Sunday	10 ounces of Wheaten Bread, 6 ounces of Beefe boyled without bones, 1 pint and a halfe of Beef Broth, 1 pint of Ale Cawdell, 3 pints of 6 shilling Beere
Monday	10 ounces of Wheaten Bread, 1 pint of Milk Pottage, 6 ounces of Beefe, 1½ pints of Beefe Broth, 3 pints of beer
Tuesday	10 ounces of Bread, halfe a pound of Boyled Mutton, 3 pints of Mutton Broth, 3 pints of Bere
Wednesday	10 ounces of Bread, 4 ounces of cheese, 2 ounces of Butter, 1 pint of Milk Pottage, 3 pints of Beere
Thursday	The same allowance as Sunday, 1 pint of Rice Milk
Friday	10 ounces of bread, 1 pint of Sugar Soppes, 2 ounces of Cheese, 1 ounce of Butter, 1 pint of Water Gruell, 3 pints of Beere.
Saturday	The same allowance as Wednesday

Adapted from: Moore, N. (Sir) (1918) The History of St. Bartholomew's Hospital.

---

denied food for breaking rules such as Rule 5, established by the despotic governor of Guy's hospital:

> 'If any patient curse or swear or use any prophane or lewd talking, and it was prove on them by two witnesses, such patient shall, for the first offence, lose their next day's diet, for the second offence lose two days diet and third be discharged'.   (Weinreb & Hibbert, 1985)

However, the loss of diet was not thought to be a great punishment as in most large London hospitals the food consisted of a pint of water, gruel or porridge for breakfast, eight ounces of meat or six ounces of cheese for dinner and broth for supper (Abel-Smith, 1964). Patients might also receive up to a pound of bread each day and two to three pints of beer, twelve to fourteen ounces of bread but no fruit or vegetables (Abel-Smith, 1964).

By the middle to late 1800s the patients' diet had not significantly changed apart from the introduction of tea and in London hospitals, meat was more generously provided. For males in St Bartholomew's, the diets consisted of *'half a pound of potatoes, half a pound of meat, an ounce of butter, fourteen ounces of bread, two pints of tea and two pints of beer'* (Bristow & Holmes, 1864). The allowance of stimulants was *'becoming every year more liberal'* and it was generally viewed that *'alcohol was of medicinal value'* (Bristow & Holmes, 1864). Patients supplemented their diets with their own supplies, brought on admission and supplemented by gifts from relatives. Personal supplies of tea, sugar and butter were generally expected from the patients and it was noted that they included *'bacon, cheese, butter, bread, cakes, apples, slices of meat etc.'* (Gibson, 1926).

Then in 1859, Florence Nightingale in *Notes on Nursing* (Nightingale, 1859) commented on issues that were to become recurring themes throughout the history of catering in hospitals: patient observation, food standards and malnutrition.

2.3.2.2   Patient observation

'I would say to the nurse, have a rule of thought about your patients diet; consider, remember how much he has had, and how much he ought to have today ... incomparably the most important office of the nurse, after she has taken care of the patients air, is to take care to observe the effect of his food and report it to the medical attendant .... it is quite incalculable the good that would certainly come from such sound and close observation in this most neglected branch of nursing'.

2.3.2.3   Food standards

'Many a patient can eat, if you can only "tempt his appetite" The fault lies in your not having got him the thing he fancies. But many another patient does not care between grapes and turnips, – everything is quite distasteful to him. He would try to eat anything which would do him good; but everything "makes him worse". The fault here generally lies in the cooking. It is not his "appetite" which requires "tempting" it is his digestion which needs sparing'.

2.3.2.4   Malnutrition

'There may be four different causes, any one of which will produce the same result, viz., the patient slowly starving to death from want of nutrition:

(1)   Defect in cooking;
(2)   Defect in choice of diet;
(3)   Defect in choice of hours for taking diet;
(4)   Defect of appetite in patient'

Even though Florence Nightingale had raised the awareness of these important issues, progress in this area, as shown below, was slow to say the least:

2.3.2.5   1900–1930

Later, in the early twentieth century, food service in hospitals was a rather hit and miss affair and not regarded as warranting any degree of funding until the start of the Second World War (Wilson & Lecko, 2005). By the early 1900s ward sisters were responsible for housekeeping duties including food and dietetic services. As for the food, in 1922, *The Hospital* reported that *'bread was too thick and the mugs are too coarse and the like'* (The Hospital, 1924). The food was often made unappetising through 'want of care in serving it'. Hospitals responded to the criticism of poor food by complaining that they could not 'get good cooks: inefficient people were asking for exorbitant wages and having to be dismissed when their inefficiency became too patently obvious' (Abel-Smith, 1964). The Hospital believed that some of the difficulty was due to the 'post-war dislike of hard work, even when combined with good pay' (The Hospital, 1930) and it was suggested that the hospitals could band together to establish a hospital school of cookery. By the 1930s, following American practice, dietitians were being advocated (The Hospital, 1930), their role evolving to address the relatively new conception of special diets for certain illnesses, coupled with the fact that most of the vitamins had been discovered and shown to be therapeutically effective (Garrow, 1994).

At the time, there was discontent on the wards themselves with protests against the practice of early waking in hospitals being organised through the trade unions and the Labour Party. The Daily Herald reported that some patients were woken as early as 3 a.m. with a resolution submitted to the National Labour Party Women's Conference affirming that the practice of early awakening had 'grave results on the health of the patients', declaring that 'the first and main purpose of a hospital is the restoration to health of the patient, and feels therefore that no consideration of the convenience of doctors or nurses should be allowed to supersede the primary object' (The Hospital, 1930). It was subsequently revealed by the Central Bureau of Hospital Information that in two thirds of 63 hospitals investigated 'the work begins at 6 o'clock and the interval for breakfast is at any time between that hour and 8.30' (The Hospital, 1930). The Middlesex Hospital suggested that a solution might be a later hour for breakfast. In 1931, The King's Fund concluded that the difficulties in leaving the patients to sleep until 6.45 or 7 a.m. were 'insuperable' (King Edwards Hosptial Fund, 1931) and it was suggested that patients should be wakened at 6 a.m. at the earliest and should be given tea or breakfast before being washed. The real problem was to get everything done in time for the consultant's round or the start of operations. The Hospital commented that the argument looked 'suspiciously like making the patients' interests subservient to those of the staff' (The Hospital, 1931).

2.3.2.6   1940–1960

By the 1940s there was a need for the organisation of catering within hospitals. From this evolved two different modes of personnel: the catering officer with catering knowledge, but little or no nutritional background and the therapeutic dietician with specialist knowledge, but not much catering experience: they had separate training and therefore little in common (King Edwards Hospital Fund, 1986). There was more evidence of this 'rift' many years later when catering managers felt that dietitians became involved in catering issues with little understanding of the overall process of food provision, asked for too many extra food items for patients and that each team of dietitians made different demands on the catering service. The dietitians themselves felt marginalised from the process of developing hospital menus meaning that patients' nutritional needs were not met as well as they could be (Savage & Scott, 2005).

During the 1940s, hospitals had been accustomed to providing only one full meal a day, relying on provisions such as eggs, butter and fruit from patients' relatives. War time rationing stopped this source and a study of the nutritional value of food supplied in three hospitals, demonstrated serious inadequacies (King Edwards Hospital Fund, 1943). The newly formed NHS undertook to make full dietary provision for hospital patients, passing the management of catering in larger hospitals to catering managers. In addition professional chefs, largely recruited from the armed services, were appointed (Wilson & Lecko, 2005) and the National Trainee Scheme for Cooks was established (NHS, 1979). This initiative had its origins in the National Joint Apprenticeship Committee Scheme which started in 1954, initially aimed at school leavers who would eventually fill supervisory posts in hospital catering as cooks, head cooks or kitchen superintendents. The scheme established a valuable foundation, expanding to provide a comprehensive training scheme for the NHS with the objective of providing more uniform standards in catering. However, two standards of training were accepted in the NHS, one for those trained under the scheme and one for those who had not. This was reported to be 'anomalous' and therefore:

'both patients and staff are engaged in a lottery where their chances of receiving a uniformly good standard of meals are dependent upon a number of factors, often local, but in which the calibre of the cook is among the most important'. (NHS, 1979)

The 1950s also saw the start of the central tray system whereby food was served onto moulded insulated trays in the central kitchen using the patients menu to determine choice. More recently, this system was shown to use a conveyor belt assembling 500–700 trays in over 90 minutes. Eight trays per minute were assembled on the belt so that each operative had less than 10 seconds to determine what was required, select the items and place them on the patients' tray. The disadvantages were (Allison, 1999):

• Large variations in portion size and content unless rigorous control was exercised
• Plastic moulded trays might allow food to slop over from one section to another
• Plated food might move during transit
• Difficulty in maintaining food temperature, might be cold at point of service
• Food dried out in transit

Most hospitals were also using the bulk food service in which food was taken from the main kitchens to wards where it was plated and served (Wilson & Lecko, 2005). With the introduction of the cook-chill method, the food was distributed in insulated bulk food service trolleys to the wards where regeneration and heating took place before plating and service, preferably at the bedside. This system had several advantages (Allison, 1999):

- May obviate the need for a central menu system
- Patients got a better food choice
- Allowed patients to control portion size according to appetite and needs, thereby minimising food wastage at ward level

This system required careful management with the training and involvement of nursing and other ward staff increasing labour costs.

During the 1960s, there were rapid advances in nutrition knowledge and its application to the treatment of diseases which led to a growth in the number of dietetic departments in hospitals (NHS Estates, 2001a). Dietitians provided diets from a 'diet kitchen' usually separate from the main kitchen and advised hospital committees on nutritional and dietetic matters in general (Platt *et al.*, 1963). They were given considerable catering training and experience while catering officers had nutrition included in some of their courses (Royal Society of Health, 1966). The King Edwards Hospital Fund stressed the need for dietitians to be concerned with the nutrition of all patients in hospital, not just those on special diets. This point was reiterated in 1963 in the *Platt Report* (Platt *et al.*, 1963), which was a study of feeding arrangements and the nutritional value of meals in 152 hospitals, which noted that the dietician '*should be less exclusively interested in the provision of special diets and concerned with the everyday problems of hospital catering and with the requirements of all patients in hospital*'. Often dietitians' advice did 'not take sufficient account of practical difficulties' with one catering officer saying:

'*What is the use of telling me that watercress has more vitamins than lettuce, when nobody in this hospital will eat it?*'.   (Platt *et al.*, 1963)

It was observed that the role of the matron, acting as housekeeper in the 'Florence Nightingale' tradition, was diminishing and the increased numbers of patients from larger hospitals brought problems for the catering service in the timing of the cooking and the delivery of service which was becoming '*even more unwieldy and difficult*', hampered by the fact that problems were often dealt with *in situ* with no apparent planning (Platt *et al.*, 1963). There were also other problems:

- Hospitals did not estimate the nutritional requirements for patients with ordinary diets (i.e. how much food they both needed and were given), which was one of the reasons for the excessive waste. It also upset the balance of the diet as patients with the highest requirements brought in proportionally large amounts of their own provisions or they were provided by visitors.
- In general, the quality of the food was poor and lacking variety. The standard of the meal service in large hospitals was indifferent and compared unfavourably with small hospitals: 29% of larger hospitals described the meal service as bad and 34% described it as good. 52% of smaller hospitals described it as good.

- Approximately 65% of total calories were contributed by three main meals making the biggest contribution to protein, but this was reduced by food delivery issues and the patients own provisions.
- Food wastage was excessive: only 55–60% of the food was eaten by the patients. Approximately 10% of food served was left by the patients as plate waste, with the proportion of waste being higher in larger hospitals.
- The larger the hospital, the more inferior the administration and the quality of food served.

The reasons proffered for these defects in the catering service were:

- The division of responsibility between catering officers who organised cooking and preparation in the kitchen, nursing staff who served the meals, ward issues and dietitians who prepared special diet in kitchens
- Too little direct observation of the patient
- Too much concentration by medical staff and in the teaching of nursing staff upon the special dietary requirements of specific diseases to the exclusion of the requirements of general patients

The state of some of the kitchens themselves in larger hospitals were described as 'old' with one located in its original building built in 1933. It transpired that many of the hospital kitchens had been expanded without any pre-conceived plans resulting in the *'most complicated, sprawling and inconvenient layouts'*. In many kitchens the equipment and buildings were so inadequate that the *'most conscientious officer would be unable to maintain desirable standards'*. Issues of hygiene were also raised both on and off the wards:

'Men were seen with urinals on their bed tables, together with their meals'

'The kitchen was very cramped ... visibly dirty .... potato peeler and electric mincer both old and dirty. The whole place looked down at heels and dirty'

'The catering officer kept her pet dog in a dog bed in her office, adjacent to the kitchen'.   (Platt et al., 1963)

Indeed it was reported that *'conditions and practices in some kitchens might well have led to prosecution if they had been found in commercial catering premises'*. This was a referral to Crown Immunity whereby NHS authorities were theoretically servants of the Queen and could not be criminally liable for actions or failings connected with their work. This allowed them exemption from enforcement of public health standards (Deer, 1985).

However, it should be noted that it was not all doom and gloom, as suggested by the quotes below from the same survey:

'The kitchen was a pleasant place and well cared for'

'The kitchen was exceptionally clean and spotless .... a good deal of the equipment was old'

'*Very well managed* .... *clean and well cared for*'

'*Good kitchen run by a housekeeping sister in good, modern airy premises*'

As for the role of nurses, the 1966 *Salmon Report* (Salmon, 1966) on senior nursing staff structure gave the impression that the patient food service was a non-nursing duty: amongst other housekeeping duties, in the larger hospitals, '*control of catering can readily be exercised by people who are not nurses*'. This was not meant to imply that the nurses had no interest in its 'efficient functioning' with an acknowledgement that '*it is natural that nurses should feel dissatisfied with any role in which their contribution to nursing care seems diminished in the ordering of all things which go towards the well being of patients*'. However, the report is believed to have contributed towards the weakened importance of nutritional care as a key nursing role (Wilson & Lecko, 2005). Conversely, despite the considerable criticism of the Salmon nursing administrative structure, it has been purported that its introduction coincided with other changes which were occurring in the organisation of hospitals such as the appointment of group catering and domestic managers and the merging of hospital management committees. Therefore, it was deemed possible that some of the problems seen to have stemmed from nursing organisations, arose equally from other changes in hospital organisation and the social changes in the nursing profession as a whole.

At the time of the *Salmon Report*, nursing teams were still closely involved in day-to-day activities related to nutritional care, including helping patients to order meals, ordering special diets, making meals on trays for incapacitated patients, helping patients and monitoring what had been eaten (Savage & Scott, 2005). These tasks were viewed as time intensive by the Standing Nursing Advisory Committee (SNAC) (DHSS, 1968) with some tasks specified as taking more than four hours of nursing time per ward per week and occupying nearly 50% of the total average time spent by nursing staff, namely:

- Preparing of patients' food and drinks (except special diets)
- Distributing food and drinks including special diets at meal times
- Collecting and clearing meals

The SNAC recommended that new non-housekeeping teams should be introduced, but this package of measures was not widely implemented and nurses were left struggling to find time to cover all essential aspects of patient care (Savage & Scott, 2005).

2.3.2.7   1970s

The problems of hospital food were not confined to the UK: in 1974 it was suggested that in the US and Canada one of the largest pockets of unrecognised malnutrition was in the private rooms and wards of big city hospitals and not in rural slums or urban ghettos (Butterworth, 1974). Furthermore, a hospital stay was prolonged by:

> 'downright neglect of the patients' nutritional health ... iatrogenic malnutrition has become a significant factor in determining the outcome of illness for many patients. Since "iatrogenic" is merely a euphemism for "physician induced", perhaps it would be better to speak forthrightly and refer to the condition as "physician induced malnutrition".... when a person commits himself to the total unquestioning care of his doctor, his nutritional health at least, should be assured. Entering a hospital and placing oneself in the hands of doctors engenders a feeling of security akin to that experienced by a fugitive when he reached the sanctuary of the cathedral doors in legendary times. Certainly one doesn't expect to suffer because of the experience. Yet, there is evidence that many people do'.   (Butterworth, 1974)

The author suggested that just because a patient had reached 'sanctuary' it could not be assumed that the fulfilment of their basic nutritional needs could be regarded as 'divinely assured'.

In addition, it was reported that altogether, there were fourteen undesirable practices affecting the nutritional health of hospital patients including the lack of observation, failure to record weight and height and a lack of communication between the dietician and the physician. It was argued that malnutrition was the inevitable consequence of the neglect of nutrition education in medical schools and an examination of nutritional practices in hospitals would 'reveal a skeleton in the closet behind the first opened door' (Butterworth, 1974).

In a response it was suggested that subsequent surveys would show that many patients would:

> 'end up being little better off nutritionally than the poor natives of the drought ridden southern Sahara, there will be a hue and cry from the public; the media will churn up a medical Watergate and the malpractice lawyers will have a field day'.   (Enloe, 1974)

It was argued that although the owner of the 'skeleton in the closet' had to be found, the blame could not rest entirely with the surgeons, who although, it was believed, would realise the seriousness of the situation, would need help to rectify it. This help should come from the dietitians who were described as members of a respected essential profession who had emerged from the kitchen, having once been regarded as little more than nurses who could cook. As professionals they needed to assert themselves and not stand on the sidelines:

> 'Hopefully the day is coming soon when some pert little dietitian with fire in her eyes confronts a doctor, shakes her finger at him and asserting that she is just as much a professional as he is, declares she's not going to sit by while he orders parenteral[2] feedings that are nutritionally inadequate. I think surgeons

will welcome the stance. Certainly it heralds the dawn of "Dietitians" Lib!'. (Enloe, 1974)

This notion of how dietitians viewed themselves was also commented on in the UK, with it being noted that many were making the mistake of assuming that if their help was not requested they would probably have *'little to offer'* (Coubrough, 1978). It was also suggested that they should remember the *'deficiency in nutritional knowledge of many physicians and doctors and set about remedying the situation' but 'this is not an easy undertaking'.*

In 1975, back in the UK, the DHSS published *Nutrition Education* (DHSS, 1975a), which proposed that all caterers should have a relevant training qualification including a thorough grounding in the application of nutritional principles, nutrition should play a far more important part in the basic training of the healthcare professionals, more emphasis should be placed on nutrition as a component of health instruction and that there should be more reports on guidelines on nutritional matters by authoritative bodies.

But what was happening on the wards themselves? The 1976 report *The Organisation of the In-Patients Day* (DHSS & the Welsh Office) revealed that early morning tea was provided for patients but it was made by virtually anyone who was available and willing. In many instances the patients themselves were involved: some were happy to do this but for others it was viewed as a real strain. Early drinks were seen as an important part of the daily fluid intake and it was recommended that an alternative to tea should be available, seen as part of the regular meal and drink service for which appropriate staff arrangements should be made. In some wards there was no provision for an early morning drink, or they had to be specifically requested, which deterred some older patients. This was a concern as maintaining a sufficient fluid intake was viewed as a problem amongst elderly patients who also had difficulties with chewing and swallowing: a fair number had to be hand fed and it was essential that their food should be acceptably hot and appetising, with the quality of their diet needing to be just as high. This meant that there should be no significant differential between the food costs in general or geriatric wards. It was thought that the advised differential in food costs for different types of hospitals was minimal but it was apparent that there were places where food costs in geriatric hospitals were not as high as they were permitted to be, indicating a risk of unacceptably low catering standards.

On a practical level, the report considered and advised on the principles *'which should govern the organisation of the inpatients' day in hospitals, taking account of the medical and social needs of the patient and the efficient organisation of the work of doctors and nurses'.* It conceded that it was difficult to envisage a time *'when all the requirements of the hospital service would ever be satisfied'.* Finance was viewed as only part of the problem: the larger the organisation, the more difficult it was to provide a personal service. It advised that both doctors and nurses needed to be given a clearer understanding of their respective responsibilities and nursing staff should be encouraged to take a greater initiative in these matters. In addition, whatever method of food service used, it was recognised to be a fundamental duty of nurses to see that patients were offered the correct food in appropriate quantities and that they should be encouraged to actually eat it.

The earlier warnings about the nutritional health of patients and the resulting malnutrition, proved to be prophetic when in 1977, there were reported incidences of malnutrition amongst hospital patients in the US with a suggestion that it was largely unrecognised and untreated (Bistrian et al., 1976). As a result, a study was undertaken in 1977 in the UK to examine the nutritional state of patients in six general surgical wards at Leeds General Hospital during a 6-week period (Hill et al., 1977). The study concluded that the measures of protein-calorie malnutrition taken (body weight, arm muscle circumference and plasma albumin) showed abnormal but common values, corroborating the American studies. In addition there was an indication that abnormalities were particularly common more than a week after major surgery and that the changes were almost entirely unrecognised and untreated: few of the patients had even been weighed. It was generally agreed that treatment to improve nutrition in patients who were malnourished after major surgery was indicated *'particularly when the patient has sepsis as well'*.

In the same year, under Section 3 of the NHS Act, Health Authorities were obliged to provide 'comprehensive care' and to 'maintain' patients admitted for care and treatment. *'The provision of food and beverages to patients during their period of stay, is by inference, an inherent part of this care'* (South East Thames Regional Health Authority (SETHRA), 1983).

Part of this care was provided by dietitians. In 1978 their duties were divided into four main categories: advisory, educational, therapeutic and research and investigation (Coubrough, 1978). Their advisory role included:

- Planning of menus to ensure that nutritionally balanced meals are available for all patients and where there is a choice of meals that most diets can be selected from the range of food available
- Planning methods and timing of cooking to ensure retention of nutrients
- Assessing new food stuffs for example the potential and limitation of textured vegetable proteins in large-scale catering

As there was no formal training for diet cooks, apart from a two-week Scottish Health Service catering school, it was up to the dietitian to ensure that designated cooks and others involved in preparing special diets were taught what to do and to know why they were being asked to make some 'apparently strange dishes'. Dietitians were also expected to give tutorials to cooks to add to their basic diet therapy learnt at training college and trainee catering managers usually spent a few weeks in the dietetic department. In addition, student nurses were required to have six hours of applied dietetics in their training which should 'be given by a dietitian'. However, the lack of cohesion between the professions was all too apparent:

> *'We must all accept the fact that many young nurses are not in the least interested in food and find great difficulty relating their lectures, which they are given early in their training, to the care of patients'.* (Coubrough, 1978)

Even if special diets were available, there had been criticism about the fact that they were not given to patients because they were sometimes not delivered to wards or were forgotten by the ward staff (Evans, 1974). An example was given of a patient who had been moved to another ward and was given the normal hospital diet for two days before it was realised that he was on a special diet. However, it was also noted that disliked or unfavourable foods were often substituted by staff, thereby de-restricting their diets. It was suggested that this demonstrated the very low importance attached by nursing staff and patients to diet as a method of treatment and that their actions negated the expertise and work of the dietitian. Maybe nursing staff were actually duped by their patients. In reality, how many of us could refuse a hungry patient on a weighed diet an extra slice of bread or a bowl of soup, if we had not been properly trained ourselves in the importance of nutrition?

Perhaps it wasn't just nutritional care *per se* that was at fault, but something more fundamental – the kitchens themselves: a report on two hospitals in 1978 noted that their catering departments were '*designed on the Best Buy policy of reducing areas and scales of equipment to the minimum, consistent with efficient functioning*' (DHSS, 1980a). The kitchens had been developed ten years earlier and although based on sound advice, alterations based on both usage and developments should have taken place from time to time but design guidance for the kitchens and dining rooms had not been revised since 1962. Since the hospitals had been built, more comprehensive menus had been deployed requiring an even greater number of pre-portioned convenience foods, eating habits had changed and there was a greater awareness of costs related to both the food and the energy used in production. The report suggested that Area Health Authorities should invite Environmental Health Officers to report on the condition of their hospital kitchens which was 'long overdue'.

Hospital catering in general terms saw a decline in the bulk service with a focus on a centralised food service (discussed on page 123). Guidelines were produced on pre-cooked frozen foods (DH, 1989) and operational control of most diet kitchens was passed to newly appointed catering managers. In addition there was an integration of modified diets into the general menu through the issue of the DHSS catering manual in 1975,[3] *Nutrition and modified diets* (DHSS, 1975b) planned as a successor to *Therapeutic Diets in Hospitals*. Other Health Service Catering Manuals were available from the DHSS which contained standard recipes (DHSS, 1977).

2.3.2.8   1980s

Around this time the then Secretary of State, having learnt that patients in some hospitals in the Mersey region were provided with a 'continental breakfast' only, asked the DHSS to consider whether this policy should be commended nationally as a means of achieving economies in the £120 million catering bill. However, before there could be any change in hospital meal policy, it was felt that research was required to establish:

- The current pattern of breakfast provision in various hospital types and sizes
- The pattern of meals for the remainder of the day where continental breakfasts were the norm and the nutritional adequacy of this provision

---

Box 2.2 Types of breakfast.

A   *True continental* rolls, toast, butter and preserve and beverage only
B   *Light breakfast* fruit juice, cereal/porridge, rolls, toast, bread butter and preserve and beverage
C   *Light breakfast* and boiled egg, i.e. type B and boiled egg
D   *Full traditional*, i.e. type B and cooked dish
E   *Flexible choice*, i.e. patients choice of types A–D

Source: Department of Health & Social Security (DHSS) (1980c).

The resulting *Hospital Meal Survey* (DHSS, 1980c), which covered over 90% of all hospitals in England, involving 1863 patients showed that breakfasts were divided into five types (see Box 2.2) with 85% of patients in hospital receiving, or given the choice of having a full traditional cooked breakfast.

The highest proportion of these patients were, according to the author, 'as might be expected' in the mentally ill or mentally handicapped categories. The proportion receiving a true continental breakfast was negligible, while just over 14% were provided with a light breakfast (with or without an egg).

Breakfast and the midday meal were generally served at 'acceptable' times between 7.15 and 8.45 and noon and 12.30 respectively. There was considerable variation in the time at which the last meal was served, the earliest being at 3.45 p.m. and the latest at 7 p.m. The report recommended that the main meal should not be served before 6 p.m. but out of 33 observations only 11 showed the meal being at 6 p.m. or after. However, many people were accustomed to having their last main meal between 5 and 6 p.m. and this would be acceptable provided that a snack and hot beverage were available later in the evening. In the acute hospitals many of the patients expressed the view that two main meals a day would be adequate but opinion was divided as to whether breakfast or the evening meal should be lighter than the other two.

The majority of patients were satisfied with the quantity of food provided but many respondents said that they would have preferred smaller helpings with the opportunity of a second helping if they felt like it. Most patients thought the food was 'good' although there were several justifiable complaints about it being cold with 'all too familiar' reasons: failure to plug in heated trolleys, long distances from the central kitchen to the ward, slow service, and the transfer of food from the heated trolley to an ordinary one at the time of service. The availability of a menu and the freedom to make a personal selection was always greatly appreciated but there were instances, when with no good reason, the patient was not allowed to choose with the time lag between selection and service reported as often too great: 'illness produces rapid variations in appetite' and it was deemed pointless 'to ask patients to choose their meals four days in advance'.

The role of nurses was also discussed:

'The nurse is the person best equipped to observe the patient, recognise his needs and see that they are met: it is the caterers task to meet them ... anything

which affects the patient's care (and this must include feeding) is a nursing responsibility. To enable the nurse to direct her efforts to those things which require her special skills (discovering what the patient needs and what he eats; helping those who cannot eat unaided) various systems have been introduced to relieve her "of the actual service of the meal on the plate". It is disappointing therefore to notice that in some instances where assistance is provided it has resulted in the nurse taking less interest in assuming less responsibility for the patient's feeding. It seems that the nurse has yet to learn how to make use of the help offered without abdicating her responsibilities. There is a need to re-awaken the nurse's awareness and interest in patient feeding and equally to ensure that those who assist in the task recognise the nurse's role'. (DHSS, 1980c)

The report shows that the problems with hospital catering were not insurmountable and perhaps it would not have taken too much effort to maintain an efficient system, particularly as it was pointed out that the catering system was seen to be at its most efficient when it was operated by well-trained catering staff, working in collaboration with the nursing staff and at its worst when operated by a third party who had no direct responsibility to either catering or nursing management.

There were more calls for overall improvements in catering in 1981 when *Catering for Health in Hospitals* (South Manchester Health District Hospitals, 1981) claimed:

'While the health service has been in the forefront of developing and publicising new nutritional ideas it has not necessarily been the first to accept this advice and implement it'.

It recommended a health education campaign to include staff training, with the objective of involving staff and gaining their views on effecting change. In addition it stressed that attention should be paid to the presentation and the techniques of food serving and the importance of staff vigilance, noting what patients ate 'as a basis for patient counselling on diet'. It advised that attention should also be paid to long stay patients regarding the provision of fresh fruit and the 'requirement of their dentures to chew'.

It also reported that it didn't matter what combination of dishes were presented in a menu as it would not be necessarily what the patient would choose to eat. They envisaged that there were two ways to assist a patient to actually eat a healthy diet via the type of menu presented:

1. *The development of a system which guided choice whereby menu cards would have suggestions for healthy diets*

2. *The presentation of a choice of set menus, all of which would have been constructed to provide a healthy diet.*

It argued that although system 1 provided a high degree of choice, the evidence of a limited study commissioned by the group had shown that this was not associated with the majority of patients choosing and eating a healthy diet. They viewed system 2 as the most likely to be successful, based on existing knowledge that attitude change did not necessarily lead to behaviour change. However, changes in actions could lead to changes in attitude: information on the health benefits of fibre may lead to someone associating fibre with health but need not lead to them starting to eat wholemeal bread. On the other hand, wholemeal bread being presented on a plate, as part of a meal, could lead to a person trying it, getting used to it and learning to accept it as a normal part of their diet. Thus system 1 had the advantage of a compromise between peoples' desire for choice and the health services desire to provide an example. System 2 had the advantage of retaining some choice while maintaining a greater probability of setting an example which would actually be followed.

Meanwhile, the cost of catering for hospital patients in 1981/82 was reported to be around £250m with, on average, a District Health Authority (DHA) providing approximately 4000 meals a day in a dozen sites (SETHRA, 1983). Half the cost was attributed to the cost of food with the other half being virtually all labour costs.

Catering costs represented between 5% and 6% of hospitals' total revenue expenditure. Patient costs per patient day ranged from £2.13 to £3.28, amounting to an average of £2.40, excluding energy consumption and capital expenses (see Table 2.1). This variance in catering costs was explained by the classification of the hospital and the inconsistencies between hospital authorities as to what expenditures were included within the 'catering account': salaries for catering managers, the cost of general portering devoted to meal delivery, and special

Table 2.1   Patient costs per patient day.

Classification of categories for performance indicators	Number of hospitals	Cost per inpatient day		Average value
		Highest £	Lowest £	
Category A: comprising Types 1 (acute hospitals over 100 beds), 2 (mainly acute) & 3 (partly acute over 300 beds)	343	5.40	1.60	2.74
Category B: comprising Types 1, 2, & 3 hospitals (under 50 beds)	242	5.90	0.70	3.28
Category C: comprising other Types 1, 2, & 3 hospitals over 50 beds but under 100 beds (for Type 1) and under 50 but over 200 beds (as regards 2 & 3)	117	4.80	1.80	2.96
Long stay & geriatric: comprising Types 4 (mainly Long Stay), 5 (Long stay), and 5 (Geriatric) hospitals	377	4.50	1.20	2.36
Mental handicap	223	4.80	0.80	2.26
Mental illness	153	4.10	1.40	2.13

Source: SETHRA (1983).

dietary preparations could be charged to catering or general administration with a particular 'one off' expense such as the replacement of a set of crockery adding to the distortion. Other factors such as staff catering labour costs, the make up of the menu, food wastage and the 'generous views' of the management were also a consideration. The cost of catering for staff was about £114 million with over a third recovered through charges. The net cost to the NHS was £71 million which represented a notional annual subsidy to staff of around £90 per employee, per year.

The significance of costs were in the forefront of many minds because concern had been expressed for a number of years over the growing levels of public expenditure with increasing pressure being put on local governments, the civil service and the NHS to perform more efficiently. It was argued that competitive pressure would encourage more efficient operation and reduce costs in the management of these services, since failure to do so would result in the service being contracted out to a private firm (Kelliher, 1996). Thus in the 1980s, the majority of DHAs had determined that there was a need for a more commercial approach to the provision and management of catering services if they were to be seen to be providing high standards of service at the lowest possible cost: ministers asked all DHAs to draw up programmes to test the competitiveness of their domestic catering and laundry service by putting them out to competitive tender (CT) and in-house tender. Indeed, individual DHAs who developed catering service specifications reflecting viable business propositions, offering operational options and introducing greater cost effectiveness were advised to 'not delay in inviting CTs'. For other DHAs who may have been experiencing local problems in the development of an efficient catering service strategy or were intending to invite tenders for small units of catering on a one off basis, a two part tendering process was viewed as more 'advantageous' which would allow for the consideration of a range of service provision options in determining DHA policy. This two-stage tendering programme assumed that the DHAs had no preconceptions on the methods of production to be used and that they had two objectives, namely lowest possible unit costs and good standards of service provision (DHSS, 1985).

Despite these common objectives, it was acknowledged that there was no standard solution to the best form of catering and the methods of achieving the objectives would be influenced by differing local circumstances and needs: each DHA was unique and faced service development pressures from other departments which needed prioritising against the demands of a catering service. There were two service options incorporating four different methods of food preparation (see Table 2.2). Both the traditional and the new technology catering systems had advantages and disadvantages but '*in general terms new technology catering offers the greater opportunity in the longer term to secure cost reductions*' (DHSS, 1985). There was also an acknowledgement that new technology catering required much higher levels of capital investment which was justified by '*compensating reductions in manpower and operational costs*'.

Table 2.2 Catering services and methods of food preparation.

Method	Definition	Purpose
Traditional predominant within the health service Cook serve	Food is cooked as near to the time of service as possible and distributed hot or cold, as appropriate, for immediate consumption.	Allows: the use of freshly cooked foods, quick response to consumer demands, least number of processes and handling of food after cooking, all cooked foods of optimum quality with roast freshly sliced from the joint etc.
New technology Cook chill	Food is cooked, chilled to prolong its shelf life for up to 5 days, distributed chilled and reheated at the time of service.	Allows: off site production, economies of scale and manpower, minimal cooked product deterioration during distribution, flexible meal times with reheating as required.
New technology Cook freeze	Food is cooked, frozen to prolong its shelf life for a matter of months and reheated at the time of service.	Same as above.
Hybrid	Combination of production methods, designed to meet local needs in terms of quality, efficiency and flexibility.	Allows: availability of skilled chefs locally for emergencies and economies of manpower, flexibility to meet changing needs, ability to transfer from one system to another for public holidays, emergency cover or reduced manning levels at weekends and rest days. Good quality cooking results through integrating food production methods. Avoidance of palate fatigue from dishes tasting the same due to any flavour loss in chilling or freezing and avoids steaminess in reheating. Quick response to consumer demands for last minute meal adjustments

Adapted from: DHSS (1980d).

Box 2.3   Various assembly methods.

Bulk meals – individual menu items are placed in bulk containers directly from the cooking equipment, according to ward requirements

Portioned meals (plated individual marmites, salad bowls, vegetable dishes etc.) – individual consumer requirements are 'plated' centrally using purpose designed conveyor belts or table tops, supported by heated bain marie units and refrigerated units

Trayed meals – individual consumer requirements are plated centrally as described above and assembled on trays with cutlery, napkins, cruets etc.

Adapted from: DHSS (1980d).

The ward meal service itself involved various methods of assembly as shown in Box 2.3. Meals could be then transported to wards and serving points, via one or more of the following methods:

- Dual temperature bulk trolleys
- Dual temperature and regeneration tray trolleys with matching compartments for hot and cold foods
- Unheated tray trolleys with hot food being kept warm by preheated bases or insulated bowls for short delivery times

There was also the consideration of centralisation, of which there were three options (DHSS, 1980d):

Full centralisation. All meals are cooked at one point with little or no cooking at other locations. Requires a cook-chill or freeze system with centrally processed meals being assembled and reheated either in 'finishing kitchens' or in ward pantries and staff dining rooms.

Partial centralisation. Large hospitals provide a service to a smaller one or small ones linked together. Suggests a hybrid system, using a mix of chilled, frozen and freshly cooked foods. Meals are assembled and cooked (or reheated) in finishing kitchens for some meals and possibly reheated on wards for others.

Decentralisation. Each hospital produces it own meals, perhaps providing a cook-chill breakfast and evening meal but producing a freshly cooked midday meal or alternatively using the normal range of commercially processed foods to extend menus and provide staffing economies: may require a traditional cook-serve system if all food is to be cooked on site or a hybrid system if a mix of freshly cooked foods and processed items is to be used.

To add more confusion, authorities could start with a partial centralisation strategy and if it proved successful, move to full centralisation or decentralisation if the reverse applied. DHAs were also advised that:

> '*Care should be taken when planning Central Production Units to avoid over capitalising in anticipation of market growth. This is where investment and market appraisal must be carried out*'.

It was noted that the dietitian should be involved in the early stages of the planning and development of a new catering system to ensure that any changes in the catering system would not have a detrimental effect on the authorities' food and health policy.

Notwithstanding these complexities, Compulsory Competitive Tendering (CCT) was introduced in 1984 by the Conservative government. It has been suggested that the policy of 'contracting out' ensured that private contractors could compete on equal terms with in-house services, possibly in an attempt to reduce the power of the unions (Rivett, 1998). As a one off activity there were benefits to be gained from CCT but the cumulative benefits from successive exercises needed to be weighed against the costs incurred in staff morale and loyalty: as money was saved it meant that fewer staff were employed for fewer hours for the same workload with nurses often having to fill the gaps (Kellier, 1996): by 1987 they were leaving in droves (Rivett, 1998). More recently, it has also been proposed that NHS catering services have not benefited from major cost savings or the effect of reformed industrial relationships, with catering services developing policies that are poorly conceived (Hwang *et al.*, 1999). What is more, CCT was seen to limit the scope of nurses to influence nutritional standards (Savage & Scott, 2005).

CCT was not the only issue related to the catering service that needed to be addressed: as discussed earlier, the NHS was protected by Crown Immunity (CI) until a case of food poisoning had a dramatic effect on the way hospitals had been performing: on 26th August 1984 at the Stanley Royd psychiatric hospital in Wakefield, 350 patients and staff were affected by a salmonella outbreak, resulting in the death of 19 patients. There was speculation that the outbreak was the result of cooked beef being left un-refrigerated for ten hours on a warm day (Seton, 1984a). Later the kitchen was closed when traces of bacteria were discovered in the drainage system of the hospital kitchens (Staff Reporters). The Confederation of Health Service Employees were critical of the management and staff for refusing to isolate infected patients, adding to the death toll (Seton, 1984b), despite offers of help from outside experts which were duly shunned (Deer, 1985). During a public enquiry it was determined that the original source of the infection was 'virtually certain' chicken and beef which had been cross contaminated during preparation. The enquiry also learned of cockroaches and rats in the kitchen, with conditions described as a case of 'neglect and decay on a Dickensian scale' (Davenport 1985). It was reported that environmental health officers had been warning the hospital that both its kitchen and staff posed a threat to patients, advice that went unheeded and it was revealed that, surprisingly, Wakefield's health district budgets were under spent (Deer, 1985). The General, Municipal, Boilermakers and Allied Trades Union claimed that dirty kitchens, dangerous asbestos, unsafe laboratories and water supplies to disseminate Legionnaires disease were commonplace throughout British hospitals (Young, 1985). In addition the Institute of Environmental Health Officers cited 97 cases where prosecutions would have been instituted but for the protection of CI (McKie, 2000). Although an official enquiry found that the issue of CI was irrelevant, a campaign for the ending of CI was backed by MPs and health service unions. CI, in respect of food and health and safety regulations in the NHS, was finally lifted in 1986. This impacted financially on many hospitals with King's College Hospital particularly, having to spend nearly £2 million to bring its kitchen and catering facilities up to twentieth century standards: 'they were still in the 19th century'. This was at a time of severe financial restraint with a headline at the time suggesting 'NHS puts patients on sick list'. Many catering personnel lost their jobs with 'the emphasis very much on cost' (Wilson, 2005).

During the 1980s, guidance on hospital catering was presented through the publication of a raft of catering manuals which were, unsurprisingly, largely dominated by hygiene regulations. Others, pertinent to food itself included *Catering for Minority Groups* (DH, 1981), which stated that catering managers in the NHS had a responsibility to provide suitable food for all patients but the needs for some groups were not always easily identified: it was important that patients were provided with food which was suitable, familiar and acceptable. Guidance was given on Asians, Hindus, Muslims, Sikhs, Judaism, Vegetarians and Vegans.

In addition, due to the growing interest in the cook-chill system of catering the DH issued guidelines on cook-chill and cook-freeze methods saying that:

'Decisions to introduce cook-chill catering systems are taken by commercial or institutional managers in the light of local catering needs. The design of each system including its cost effectiveness must relate to those needs ... both systems can give increased flexibility in the preparation and service of meals'. (DH, 1981)

With more links between diet and disease being established (DH, 1984; DHSS, 1984), the *RecipeFile* (DHSS, 1988) was introduced which recognised that many preparation and cooking methods were based on traditional, out dated techniques which were not felt to be relevant or necessary. Many were seen to be wasteful, producing dishes which might not be as healthy as those using newer preparation techniques, particularly in relation to their fat content. Advice on alternatives to these redundant techniques was provided:

- The colour and flavour of vegetables was better if sautéing was eliminated
- Deep and shallow frying to be replaced by non-fat adding methods such as grilling and oven cooking
- Roux sauces to be discouraged as they required the addition of fat

Perhaps, more pertinent to the politics of the time, with the emphasis on cost cutting, *'forced air convection and steaming (ovens) were fast and needed less attention from staff'* with the simplified methods making food preparation easier for the staff, seen as a bonus when *'labour costs are high and trained staff a rarity'* (DHSS, 1988).

2.3.2.9   1990s

More on this subject of cost cutting was discussed in 1990 when it was suggested that the hospital catering service had been driven by costs, failing to keep pace with changing consumer needs and choices resulting in too many hospitals serving 1970s or even 1960s type of food to 1990s customers, seen as *'a recipe for disaster'* (Kipps & Middleton, 1990a). It was suggested that caterers should see menus less in terms of an operating system and more as an ideal opportunity to communicate messages (Kipps & Middleton, 1990b), perhaps no mean feat when at that time it was possible to obtain a degree in Hotel and Catering Management and become a Hotel Catering and Institutional Management Association professional with virtually no nutrition education. In addition, although the City and Guilds of London Institute which designed, moderated and examined catering courses intended to provide an understanding and expertise in professional cookery, there were few nutrition subjects in their examinations (Carlson & Kipps, 1990). At a Catering Teachers Association meeting it was noted that the public had high expectations of catering hygiene standards which would soon translate into high standards of nutrition and health: healthy food did not have to be less attractive or expensive but it required training and marketing (Robbins, 1990). However, as nutrition was often taught as a theoretical subject it was not integrated into all aspects of teaching catering students which meant that many students were ill-equipped to apply what they had learnt about nutrition into the work situation resulting in confusion: often healthy eating was envisaged as meatless meals and the 'healthy' meal often offered food such as quiche and chips. Salad bars were often presented as a solution to the problem of providing more healthy meals but then fatty foods such as pork pie, scotch egg and rich dressing were served with the salad:

'The healthy dish of the day mustn't imply that all the other food is unhealthy. It is better practice to modify the recipe of a well known and well liked dish'. (CTA, 1990)

However it was also pointed out that that it was impossible to contemplate the introduction of better choice and quality of meals without first appreciating the unnatural environment in which the bulk of hospital meals were chosen and consumed (Kipps & Middleton, 1990a). The patient 'constraints' included captive, 'unwilling' customers, meal times imposed by a dominant routine which included the inability to select food of choice when hungry and unnatural eating positions. The constraints of the caterers included budgets, standardisation and mass production, antiquated equipment, with the food service usually undertaken by untrained personnel.

On the wards themselves it was seen that achieving a 'positive sensation' about meal times could only be achieved with nursing staff co-operation and there was no convincing reason why medical routines could be avoided during mealtimes. There was limited evidence that most nursing staff positively welcomed the opportunity to spend time with patients at meal times, viewed as one of the few pleasant and unstressful interactions between them (Kipps & Middleton, 1990b).

Meanwhile, the nutritional standards of hospital food were seen to be declining to a point where they were unsustainable and in those circumstances it was impossible to provide adequate nutrition (Wilson, 2005). There were no minimum nutritional standards that hospitals had to deliver and no requirements for hospitals to feed anyone at all. Dietitians became more involved in clinical dietetics, particularly enteral[4] and parenteral[2] nutrition leaving menu development and the nutritional content of menus to catering staff (Savage & Scott, 2005).

Concern was also expressed about the drop in nutritional standards for older adults in hospitals, which resulted in the Royal College of Nursing (RCN) setting up a multi-disciplinary group to set nursing standards under the RCN Dynamic Quality Improvement Programme. These standards were published in 1993 and the project was extended to target hospitalised adults over 75 years of age: the resulting *Dietetic Standards of Care for the Older Adult in Hospital* (British Dietetic Association) were designed to be used by dietitians '*as they cover their unique role in nutrition care of this group of patients*'. The standards stated that the dietitian:

- Advises on nutritionally adequate food which is acceptable to patients and appropriate to patients needs
- Sets up a screening system with other professional staff whereby patients admitted to hospital are screened to identify those at risk nutritionally
- Advises on hospital policies that affect nutrition care of the older adult
- Assesses those patients identified as requiring nutritional intervention
- Manages the diet therapy for patients referred to the service
- Co-ordinates the provision of nutritional support
- Completes a written record for all patients seen for dietetic care
- Communicates dietetic treatment to the care team

However, in 1993, dietitians in the South East Thames Region (SETHRA) had other concerns regarding the results of an informal survey they had undertaken, which revealed the nutritional adequacy of hospital food. This resulted in a multi-disciplinary study day held at Guy's Hospital, where dietitians, caterers, nurses, general managers and medical staff agreed there was a pressing need for nutritional guidelines for hospital food services and that standards should be set for the delivery of food to patients in hospital. The subsequent *Nutritional Guidelines, Menu Planning* (SETHRA, 1993a), were aimed at those responsible for planning menus, that is catering managers in consultation with dietitians, ensuring '*that the content of the menu enables adequate nutrition of the patient group for whom it was designed*'. The complementary document, *Nutritional Guidelines, The Food Chain*

(SETHRA, 1993b) described the task of *'getting food from the provision suppliers' delivery van to the patients stomach'* as a:

> *'food chain – a complex task involving the coordinated efforts of a multidisciplinary team ... the chain is as strong as its weakest link and it is vital that every member of the multidisciplinary team fully understands where they fit into the food chain and exactly what their role and responsibilities are'.*

These observations were congruous with the 1994 publication, *Nutrition and Health* (DH, 1994), which suggested that the NHS could mobilise action through 'health alliances', with performance on effective action in directly purchased services and alliances with other agencies being monitored 'increasingly closely'. Advice was provided on how to become involved in developing a food and health strategy, setting nutritional standards, working in alliance with other agencies and the role of both providers and specialist training being explored. The handbook actually aimed to assist NHS organisations on what steps could be taken to help meet the coronary heart disease and stroke risk factors as detailed in the *Health of the Nation*, that is reducing peoples' average percentage of food energy derived from fat, particularly saturated fatty acids.

In the midst of the planning of these advisory documents on the NHS 'pulling together' to improve the nations' health, the issue of malnutrition had emerged again when a report by the King's Fund, *A Positive Approach to Nutrition as Treatment* (Lennard–Jones, 1992), declared that although it was 15 years since attention had been drawn to the high prevalence of malnutrition in hospitals, the problem remained with existing effective treatments not being utilised or being used inappropriately or badly. The report suggested that although the most cost-effective approach to overcoming malnutrition was to encourage patients to eat more normal food, this was not always possible and in these cases nutritional support via oral supplements, enteral tube feeding or parenteral nutrition, could radically improve recovery rates and quality of life. However, in over two thirds of UK hospitals there was an absence of formal nutrition teams who were responsible for organising the diagnosis, treatment and monitoring of malnutrition in at-risk patients. Hospitals, which already had a team, only covered parenteral nutrition and some functioned solely in specific specialities such as surgery. It was recommended that all patients in UK hospitals who were diagnosed as being malnourished or at risk of developing malnutrition should have access to a nutrition support team and all major UK hospitals or hospital groups should appoint a Nutrition Steering Committee (NSC), responsible for setting standards for and delivering catering services, dietary supplements and nutritional support. Additionally all NSCs should appoint at least one Nutrition Support Team (NST) to implement the standards of nutritional support laid down by the NSC. Perhaps more importantly the report estimated that the provision of nutritional support, based on a 5-day reduction in hospital stay for 10% of hospital inpatients could save £266 million annually, taking into account the cost of nutrients and increased nursing time for their administration.

As a direct result of this report, the British Association for Parenteral and Enteral Nutrition (BAPEN) was formed whose aim was to:

'Improve the nutritional treatment of all sufferers from illness who have become, or are likely to become, malnourished and who are unable to consume or absorb normal food in sufficient quantities to promote recovery'.   (BAPEN, 2007a)

In 1994 the BAPEN report, *Organisation of Nutritional Support in Hospitals*, stated that the nutritional care of patients throughout the UK was *'fragmentary and poorly organised'*, highlighting the requirement for NSCs (Silk, 1994). They commented that centralised hospital catering had made it difficult to provide pur-pose cooked meals or frequent snacks, further hampered by the demise of the ward kitchen. In addition some of the food handling legislation had had a significant and detrimental impact on what could be provided at ward level.

Perhaps then it came as no surprise that despite all the advice for the catering service and the realisation that things were not improving, the issue of malnutrition raised its head again when a study of 500 patients in the UK, concluded that 40% of patients were undernourished on admission to hospital, two thirds of all patients lost weight during their hospital stay, fewer than half had any nutritional infor-mation documented in their case notes and few had had their weight and height recorded (McWhirter & Pennington, 1994). The study stated that *'the continued lack of the awareness of clinical nutrition suggests the need for education on the subject of the incidence and recognition of malnutrition in hospital'* (some of the causes and effects of malnutrition are shown in Boxes 2.4 and 2.5).

Meanwhile there had been numerous calls for more education for all those involved in hospital catering, with SETHRA (1993b) advocating that medical schools introduce students to the hospital food chain during their clinical placement,

---

Box 2.4   Malnutrition can be the result of specific diseases which can prompt inherent nutritional problems.

- A high incidence of protein calorie malnutrition is associated with chronic obstructive airways disease
- Cancer may increase metabolic expenditure requiring an increased nutritional intake, yet the patient may be less able to eat due to pain, nausea or obstruction of the gastro-intestinal tract
- After a cerebral-vascular accident, patients with paralysis or weakness can be susceptible to nutritional problems due to difficulties with chewing food or handling cutlery
- Body fluid loss prompted by diarrhoea, wounds (blood loss), vomiting can deplete nutrients such as electrolytes or nitrogen
- Surgery or trauma can significantly affect body metabolism which can result in a proportionally increased metabolic rate and increased energy requirements

Source: Savage & Scott (2005).

Box 2.5 Effects of malnutrition.

- Malnutrition increases the rates of complications for medical and surgical patients
- The effects of malnutrition include reduced muscle power and motility with an increased likelihood of deep-vein thrombosis and pressure sores. Wound healing can be delayed and tolerance to therapies such as chemotherapy and radiotherapy may be reduced.

Source: Savage & Scott (2005).

---

all new medical staff to be familiarised with a hospitals' food service as part of their general induction on appointment, senior medical staff to ensure that they were in a position to give an informed opinion when influencing the allocation of resources to the food service and those who assisted in the task recognise the role of nurses: indeed the role of nursing staff and their perceived role in the food chain was recommended no less than eighteen times!

Then in 1995 the DH published a guidance document '*Nutrition Guidelines for Hospital Catering*' (DH, 1995), which placed an emphasis on the nutritional aspects of hospital catering while recognising the overwhelming importance of the caterers' role in addressing issues including: quality, taste and good preparation to ensure that food was actually eaten.

The subsequent '*Nutrition Guidelines for Hospital Catering, a Checklist for Audit*' (DH, 1996a) helped to measure the performance of a hospitals food service against the 1995 guidelines. There were no 'pass or fail' criteria but the aim was to raise standards by encouraging the use of the guidelines. It was intended to complement the document '*Delivering a Quality Service*' (NHS Executive), which advised that items under the heading 'meal and service quality' were mandatory, suggesting that a written menu must be produced, foods and cooking methods must be accurately described, menus must contain a sufficient range of meals to meet the dietary needs and preferences of care groups served for example vegetarians, ethnic minorities, and that catering managers must test the quality and temperature of cooked foods and replace sub-standard foods.

These mandatory points were, yet again, seen as guidelines and perhaps a member of the public entering hospital as an inpatient would have expected some of these seemingly simple ideas to already have been in place: with regard to the last two points, how many people at home would not cater to guests they were expecting at their table or indeed sample the food they were providing?

Delivering a Quality Service also included a questionnaire to enable Trusts to measure patient satisfaction and set performance targets stating that: 70% or more patients should give the service seven or more out of ten and that no more than 10% should give the service five or less out of ten. Would any of this help the catering service achieve higher standards:

In a nutrition audit at a community hospital using both the published guidelines and the audit checklist, the hospital menus appeared to be able to meet the national guidelines for intakes of vitamin C, fibre, iron and folate but in the elderly (65 years plus) the actual intakes of energy and several nutrients were inadequate. Additionally, patients on pureed diets had the poorest nutritional intakes and those on soft diets appeared to be disadvantaged (Mitchell, 1999).

Also in 1995, the *Patients Charter for England* (DH, 1996b) stated that, '*if you have to stay in hospital, you can expect to be given a written explanation of the hospital's patient food, nutrition and health policy and the catering services and standards you can expect during your stay*'. This assured that all patients had a choice of dishes including meals suitable for all dietary needs, had to order no more than the next 2 meals in advance, had a choice of the size of portion they wanted, were given the name of the catering manager, had help if needed, with menus printed in other languages and large print.

In 1996, education was on the agenda again at a workshop organised by the Stratford Executive Group, when representatives from medical schools involved in nutrition teaching and curriculum development agreed unanimously that human nutrition was well suited for medical undergraduate training, being of '*contemporary relevance to health and demonstrating a truly integrative theme throughout each year of the undergraduate curriculum*' (DH, 1996c).

But this knowledge would have to be applied in a practical sense because although the report *Hungry in Hospital?* (Association of Community Health Councils) acknowledged that the notion of patients being hungry in hospital was recognised by official guidance, the mere presence of official guidance itself, was not sufficient to solve the problem. It provided what, albeit retrospectively, could have been called, 'common sense' factors that contributed to patients not eating and drinking in hospital:

- Problems with ordering (dishes should be described accurately)
- Communication (lack of between catering and nursing staff)
- Quality (appearance, temperature and variety of food)
- Quantity (portion sizes)
- Inappropriate food (should be correctly prepared to patients needs)
- Choice (lack of options – set menu)
- Timing (inflexible meal times)
- Assumptions (regarding why meals are uneaten)
- Positioning (meals out of reach of patients)
- Utensils (inappropriate)
- Physical problems (difficulty opening pre-packed foods)
- Medication (affecting intake)
- Eating environment (patients comfort zones differ)
- Lack of assistance (some patients unable to eat unaided)

Of equal concern was the fact that in some hospitals nobody was taking responsibility for ensuring that patients were eating or investigating why some patients were not eating and drinking. This report prompted the Registrar of the then United Kingdom Central Council for Nurses (UKCC) to write to every hospital in the UK to remind them that *'nurses have a clear responsibility for ensuring that the nutritional needs of patients are met'*.

A response to this statement was provided in *Eating Matters* (Bond, 1997), which had been put together in response to requests from nurses for help in improving standards of dietary care:

'So it's official. Eating matters. As if we did not know'.

In the process of producing *Eating Matters*, the Chief Nursing Officer for England and her colleagues at the DH were concerned about ensuring that hospital patients received high standards in all aspects of care. A small number of people, who could contribute in different ways to raising the profile of the importance of patients eating, met at the DH and asked:

'Who is responsible for ensuring that hospital patients have enough to eat and drink?'

The simple answer was:

'The responsibility rests with nurses'

A letter, inserted into a nursing weekly publication to search for examples of initiatives that had improved patients eating, prompted only a 'single response' but this could be indicative of the nurses work-load and not their perhaps, perceived disinterest ... how many of the nurses even read a weekly publication? However, speculation aside, letters to the National Nurses Nutrition Group and the Nutrition Advisory Group for Elderly People of the British Dietetic Association together with leads from other sources were more effective in raising a wide variety of suggestions. The document stated that modern clinical practice meant the provision of food and drink for patients was a complex process involving a whole range of staff but whatever part other workers played in that process, it was ultimately the responsibility of nurses to ensure that the nutritional needs of patients were met. It was hoped that the contents would be stimulating and informative and that by using the document positively each practice would be enhanced, providing continuous and sustained improvements in the dietary care of patients. It also acknowledged that although nurses at the sharp end bore the responsibility for making sure patients ate, nutrition as part of a patients' treatment touched most hospital departments and personnel. However, without clear leadership from the top it was unlikely that patients' dietary care would receive the attention it deserved, including what was taught to professionals and support staff in their basic and continuing education and to the amount that was made available from hospital budgets to provide meals. It pointed out that ward staff needed to know why they did what they did and this demanded some sophisticated knowledge. Improving the dietary care of patients did not mean turning nurses into dietitians any more than they become, for example, occupational therapists. However, they did need to have sufficient knowledge of nutrition and to value its importance if they were to provide considerate and high-quality nursing and to play their part in an interdisciplinary team.

However, as suggested more recently, even armed with this 'knowledge of nutrition', nurses faced more frustrating, practical problems which had a direct impact on patients' food intake: in an ethnographic study of the role of nurses and patients' experience, there was considerable tension found between clinical and catering staff in a Trust due to health and safety policies (Savage & Scott, 2005). This resulted in a lack of meaningful flexibility making it difficult for individual patients to get something to eat when they felt like eating:

'You've got a patient who's dying who wants a particular meal and you have to stand there and say I'm sorry, we can't re-heat meals under regulation 460, paragraph 3'. (Ward Matron)

In addition, there was reportedly no access to a kitchen for visitors or patients. One of the reasons cited was hygiene, mainly whether visitors using the kitchen were sufficiently knowledgeable about food handling and safety. In addition the ward kitchen was small and food regulations did not allow public access. The nurses themselves could not perform tasks such as cooking light meals, for example, boiling eggs for patients, because kitchens on wards were designated food handling areas rather than food preparation areas: nurses are not generally trained in food handling! The 'bringing in of food' was not encouraged: following legal action over a case of food poisoning, the Trust did not allow patients or their visitors to bring in food to be reheated on the ward by visitors or staff for fear of breaching food handling regulations. Patients' food could not be stored in the ward refrigerators because of the risk of cross contamination, which could result in the Trust being fined by the Health & Safety Authority.

There was also concern that patients on a soft diet had little choice of food or a soft diet option was not even offered which resulted in patients being repeatedly offered mashed potato and gravy. Despite being aware of the consequences of the patients' nutritional status, nurses were not permitted to blend food from a trolley using a blender in the ward kitchen on health and safety grounds. Other, more complex reasons were offered: nurses might not appreciate the need for particular types of food consistency for certain patient groups such as those with swallowing difficulties. Additionally, it could take three or four attempts at ordering before the patient received the appropriate food and the supply could be intermittent with nurses either having to chase up the order or trying, often unsuccessfully, to find a suitable alternative from the menu. Indeed, the nutrition link nurse now telephoned the catering manager and asked him to come and explain what the problem was to the patients. The process for actually stopping a special order was also so erratic and it appeared that there was no established or commonly understood system for notifying the kitchen that a patient had gone home.

Despite these obstacles, on some wards there were high standards of nutritional care, with the nurses speaking highly of the dietitians and speech and language therapists but it did not reflect what happened in the rest of the hospital: many wards did not have a nutrition link nurse to help disseminate information about nutritional issues. This suggests the lack of uniformity, just from ward to ward, let alone amongst different Trusts.

And what of the patients' beliefs of the nurses role? There was an impression that patients had modest expectations of nurses and the nutritional care that they might offer with one patient suggesting that nurses might not be adept at nutritional care, viewing them as 'too young' to know about the nutritional value of food or that nurses from overseas would not necessarily understand what foods were healthy or unhealthy to eat in the British diet. Moreover, nurses seemed too busy to offer nutritional care and it was unrealistic to expect them to do anymore, with patients commenting:

'They already have enough to do'

'I do not expect nurses to be involved but I think perhaps they should be'.

There was no suggestion that patients thought nurses might have other, behind the scenes, less visible responsibilities such as influencing the choice or standard of food, which was difficult when the food was unappetising, with the main problems relating to the effects of regeneration, limited choice and the lack of fresh fruit and vegetables. The reported difficulties for nurses in tempting patients to eat could also have been influenced by the attitudes of some of the ward staff who were, on the whole, far more scathing about the hospitals' food, with one describing the quality as 'atrocious'.

Unsurprisingly, in 1999 a report by the Nuffield Trust, *Managing Nutrition in Hospital* (Davis & Bristow, 1999), concluded that there was a need for definitions of roles and responsibilities regarding nutritional care at ward level, for quality assurance and for coordination at a senior management level within each Trust, with food provision being managed as an integral component of clinical care rather than as a 'hotel function'. The BAPEN report, *Hospital food as treatment* (Allison, 1999), stated that it was unacceptable that catering should escape scrutiny, not only in terms of its costs but also in terms of its clinical effectiveness and before embarking on any charges, institutions should begin with an assessment of their current practices. It recommended regular audits to ensure continuing high standards. The nutrition audit, referred to earlier (page 131), concurred with the latter findings suggesting meetings every 4–8 weeks to set goals and monitor progress (Mitchell, 1999).

These recommendations seemed timely as in 2000, the problem of malnutrition was still shown to be in evidence when a study of 337 patients suggested that in acute hospitals it *'goes apparently unrecognised and unmanaged in 70% of cases'* (Kelly *et al.*, 2000). In addition, the incidence of undernourished patients admitted to hospital was documented in a comparison of studies from 1994 to 2000, shown in Table 2.3 (Stratton & Elia, 2000).

Table 2.3 Comparison of studies from 1994 to 2000 documenting the incidence of patients admitted to UK and Irish hospitals with a BMI <20 kg/m^2.

Study	Location and type of hospital	No. of patients	Type of patients	Patients with BMI <20 kg/m^2 (%)
Corish et al. (2000)	Dublin (teaching hospitals)	569	General medical, surgical, respiratory, care of the elderly and orthopaedic	13.5
McWhirter et al. (1994)	Dundee (teaching hospital)	500	General medical, surgical, respiratory, care of the elderly and orthopaedic	37.4
Kelly et al. (2000)	Glasgow (teaching hospital)	219	Acute medical and surgical	18
Strain et al. (1999)	Manchester (teaching hospital)	326	General medical, surgical and orthopaedic	≥24[a]
Vlaming et al. (1999)	London (teaching hospital)	423	General medical, surgical and orthopaedic (<65 years only)	15 (men) 18 (women)
Watson et al. (1999)	London (teaching hospital)	65	Care of the elderly	29.3
Weeks et al. (1999)	London (teaching hospital)	186	General medical	22
M. Ella[b]	Cambridge (teaching hospital)	57	General medical and surgical	21
J. Tharakan et al.[c]	Cambridge (teaching hospital)	100	Care of the elderly	21

[a] Additional anthropometric criteria were used in this calculation.
[b] M. Ella, unpublished results.
[c] J. Tharakan, R.J. Stratton and M. Ella, unpublished results.

Source: Stratton and Elia (2000).

2.4 Current decade

2.4.1 Audit Commission

So, with the issues of inadequate kitchens, CCT, centralisation, the confusing role of nurses, malnutrition, the patients' charter, guidance on nutritional guidelines and myriads of advice, just how did the catering service function in hospitals? The publication *Catering* resulting from a survey by the Audit Commission (AC) (Audit Commission, 2001), involving almost all NHS hospitals in England and Wales, based on data for 1999/2000, is significant because it provides an understanding of how the catering service is/was delivered in different Trusts:

- 71% of Trusts had in-house catering departments with the remainder having contracted-out catering
- 77% of Trusts had a nutritional screening protocol in place undertaken by nurses, but less than half of these Trusts reviewed patients' nutrition weekly to ensure their care was adjusted in line with their changing needs during their hospital stay. In the remaining 23 of the Trusts it was not clear how patient's nutritional needs were routinely identified.

The Trusts were asked to report patient satisfaction against the 1996 national targets as set out in *Delivering a Quality Service* (National Health Service Executive, 1996) (discussed on page 130): the average score on food quality and meal service was 7.6, which was seen as a positive endorsement of hospital food with the Commissions auditors finding many examples of high quality meals cooked to order, ethnic meals produced on site and appetising pureed foods. However it was also reported that more than one third of Trusts did not meet the DH targets.

The survey also reported on expenditure, non-patient costs, various cooking methods, cost and satisfaction, and meal service as detailed below.

2.4.1.1   *Expenditure*

The components of catering department costs comprised food and beverages, staff, consumables and overheads with food and beverages and staff typically accounting for 90% of the total cost.

Trusts received income from providing non-patient services such as meals served in the post graduate centre, staff restaurant or from providing a meals-on-wheels service for a local authority (see Figure 2.1).

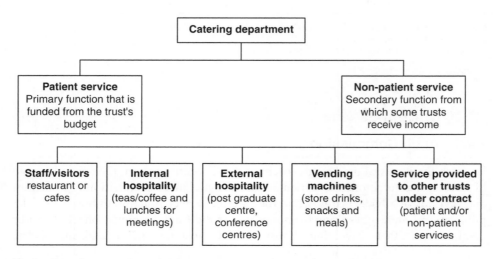

Figure 2.1   Sources of income for Trust. *Source*: Audit Commission (2001).

Within most Trusts, this income was retained within the catering department to offset the gross costs of providing patient and non-patient services. This meant that Trusts reduced the total catering budget by the predicted income, releasing the money for use in other areas of the hospital. Therefore, comparisons of catering expenditure are based on net expenditure with wide variations in the net expenditure per patient day, ranging from £2.80 to £20.00. Some of this was due to the level of income generated from non-patient services and the Trusts pricing policies. Some of the variation was explained by economies of scale: larger Trusts usually had lower average costs with the location and type of Trust also affecting costs.

There was no association between the net cost of catering and whether the service was provided externally or in-house, or with the type of cooking method used (methods of production and meal service are shown in Figures 2.2 and 2.3).

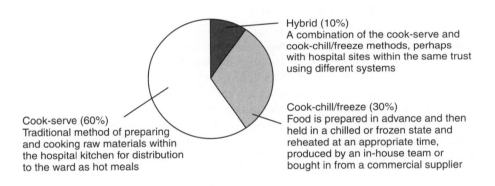

Figure 2.2 Percentage of Trusts using the different methods of production. *Source*: Audit Commission (2001).

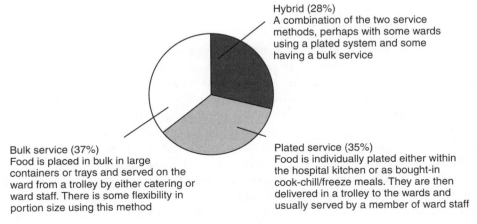

Figure 2.3 Percentage of Trusts using the different methods of meal service. *Source*: Audit Commission (2001).

Back in 1996, *Delivering a Quality Service* (National Health Service Executive, 1996) had recommended that each Trust set a daily food allowance and monitor whether they spent the full allowance and hence whether patients were receiving value for money from the service. The point of cost control was to establish the cost of ingredients for particular meals and then the average daily cost of food and beverages for each patient. By setting a daily food budget per patient day, three quarters of Trusts had made a conscious decision on their level of spending on patient food and beverages but only 66% of all Trusts monitored the actual costs to check that patients received the full allowance.

The average spending on food and beverages per patient was:

- £2.20 for a cook/serve production system
- £3.70 for cook-chill/freeze meals bought from a commercial supplier
- £2.40 for cook-chill/freeze meals made on site
- £2.70 for a hybrid production system

Within each method of production there was a considerable cost variation: for Trusts using a cook-serve production method the range was from £1.24 to £5.88. These variations in food costs did not reflect better or worse ingredients. They may have been due to differences in the effectiveness of purchasing or the control of raw ingredients in the production process. Therefore, it could be that some Trusts in the lower quartile provided the same range and quality of meals as Trusts in the upper quartile but at a lower cost. It was predicted that the future challenge for NHS Trusts would be to provide a 24-hour service incorporating a ward kitchen service and snack boxes within the current budget. This was a requirement of the NHS Plan – *A plan for investment. A plan for reform* (NHS 2000). It was also envisaged that the amount spent on patient food and beverages would need to increase, particularly for those who did not currently offer the recommended choices such as hot meals at night and those that did not use the high-quality fresh ingredients that were being advocated.

2.4.1.2   Non-patient costs

As discussed above, the income generated from non-patient catering costs was retained within the catering department, providing an incentive to the catering staff to improve performance and offer a high-quality service. However, this income did not always cover the cost of providing non-patient services: approximately three quarters of Trusts subsidised their non-patient services. Individual Trust boards decided whether non-patient services should be subsidised: almost a fifth of Trusts could not provide separate cost information for the different non-patient activities.

Only 35% of the Trusts in the survey monitored the actual contributions or subsidy achieved from providing non-patient services. Even fewer had established an appropriate level of subsidy and duly set a target. The average subsidy was approximately £153 000 per annum: equivalent to an additional 84 pence that could be spent daily on food and beverages for each patient. The reasons why one Trust might have a higher level of subsidy than another included:

- Longer opening hours in the staff restaurant, perhaps with a night service available for junior doctors to meet New Deal[5] requirements
- Discounts offered to staff to ease recruitment and retention problems
- Poor location of the staff restaurant or the facilities available to full-paying customers such as visitors

On average the staff/visitor restaurant at a Trust accounted for 69% of non-patient expenditure. In 1967 the Ancillary Staff Council established a pricing policy for staff meals, stating that the cost of food and beverages should account for 60% of the selling price which still seemed to be influencing pricing policy: the median distribution of food and beverage costs was nearing 60% of income. Clearly some Trusts had moved away from this policy, beginning to set prices based on local subsidy decisions.

Only a third of Trusts had a computerised catering information system aiding the setting of appropriate prices and monitoring the cost of catering activities. These systems were not always being used to their full potential: often there was insufficient investment in staff to maintain the information. There is a certain irony that back in 1983 SETHRA had welcomed the use of computers, regarded as a 'most valuable tool available to managers to aid them in controlling their service' (SETHRA, 1983). Ten years later SETHRA again commented that there were 'a number of very sophisticated software systems available to help with food service administration' (SETHRA, 1993a).

2.4.1.3 Various cooking methods

There were overall satisfaction levels which reflected a variety of aspects of the catering service including the extent of choice, whether meals were appetising and how they were served. Trusts used various methods for both cooking (production) and service (meal service) but there was no relationship between the type of method used and overall patient satisfaction.

2.4.1.4 Cost and satisfaction

As currently measured, patient satisfaction showed no relationship to the cost of providing a catering service. This was true whether costs were measured as net expenditure or as gross cost. It could have been that costs related solely to the catering department whereas, in reality, there were many stages and staff involved in the delivery of the catering service which could, again, affect the patients' satisfaction (see Figure 2.4).

This inverse correlation between cost and patient satisfaction had already been reported in 1980 in the *Hospital Meal Survey* (DHSS, 1980c), when economy and consumer satisfaction were seen to be incompatible and it was suggested that

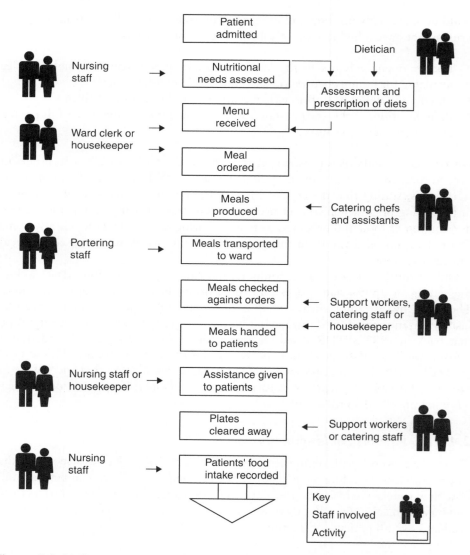

Figure 2.4 Various stages and staff involved in the catering service. *Source*: Audit Commission (2001).

most of the measures which should have been taken to improve standards might at the same time have yielded economies. In 1983 *The Cost of Catering in the NHS* showed that there was no correlation between costs and quality: patients in hospitals with low costs expressed high satisfaction with the meals provided whilst in high cost hospitals the patients were just as likely to express low levels of satisfaction (DHSS, 1983). Another possible consideration is the suggestion that patients' expectations exceed their perceptions for hospital meal services and in consequence the gaps that existed between their expectations and perceptions serve to lower their satisfaction levels (Hwang, 2003). This notion of patients' expectations and perceptions of hospital food was illustrated further in *Hungry in Hospital?* (Association of Community Health Councils) when a menu item 'chicken and potato' was perceived by patients as 'tender slices of easily digestible chicken and potato' and was presented as a 'chicken leg in a tough skin and a jacketed potato with a hard skin'.

2.4.1.5   Meal service

The report demonstrated that even if meals were of the highest quality, their value was lost if they were uneaten with the poor quality of service impacting on their presentation and delivery. They gave these examples:

- Hot food was served cold because the door to the trolley was left open as one member of staff struggled to deliver meals over 15 minutes
- Patients did not always receive the meal they ordered
- Patients were not able to eat their meals because they could not reach them, had inappropriate cutlery or needed help with lids or wrappers
- Elderly patients did not always receive assistance and were often not checked to see how much they had eaten
- Maternity patients often missed set meal times
- Meal times could be disturbed by doctors on ward rounds and nurses undertaking routine observations

Overall, it can be seen that there was a lack of homogeny amongst different Trusts: some of the disparities could be explained by the findings of another survey including all acute care NHS Trusts which investigated the hospital meal service process: many of the catering managers indicated a 'move to other catering policies' in the future which reflected the lack of agreement with regard to what constitutes 'an ideal catering set-up' (Hwang *et al.*, 1999). A lack of standardisation among hospital menus was also highlighted with the results, in general, across the hospitals being far from consistent or ideal. There was contention between the nurses and the catering staff about who should carry out distribution of the meals with the majority of Trusts using batch-cooking to prepare meals, with an indication that a number of Trusts intended to move to cook-chill, cook-freeze or bulk service methods. The mix between bulk and plated meal service was even with many Trusts deploying both methods. This switching between production and delivery methods was seen to create its own set of obstacles: each system had differing impacts on the flow of the catering system with different hospitals favouring different solutions, negating a consensus on the best way forward:

'... *so mixed between regions and lacking any discernable patterns that no region, nor any Trust, can adequately be labelled representative of the UK hospital catering environment as a whole*'.

It could be that the problem was compounded by the varying job descriptions and experiences of the catering management itself: more recently, from a survey 'under the auspices of the Catering Managers Association' it was reported that the diversity of job titles that catering managers embraced within the NHS service were said to be 'striking', with a total of 21 different position titles reported. These ranged from the highly functional kitchen manager to more strategic and corporate positions, for example, Director of Hotel Services, Director of Facilities, all pointing to a lack of professional cohesion and identity within the professional area (Baum, 2006). Their differing responsibilities were to manage on average:

- A direct catering budget of £2.07 million ranging from £0.6 million to £7.8 million
- An indirect budget of £3.25 million ranging from £0 to £11.45 million
- 78 staff of whom 10 were in supervisory roles ranging from 13 to 185
- The delivery of service to an average of 681 beds ranging from 175–2160.

It transpired that their core training did not necessarily equip them for the tasks they were expected to perform with the key features of their training and experience as follows:

- 35% had entered the profession as chefs via the professional cookery route (City & Guilds of London Institute)
- 61% had pursued the Hotel & Catering International Management Association qualifications (alternatively or in addition)
- 8% had no formal pre-entry qualifications
- The average time in current posts was 8.2 years
- There was overall a 'very long length' of service in the NHS, averaging 15.2 years
- There was very limited non-NHS career exposure except with early career work as commercial chefs and others who had pursued an armed forces/school meals route into healthcare
- There was reportedly very limited training external to the NHS (professional or academic)

The survey also indicated that there was an increasing focus on wider, non-catering responsibilities with some evidence that the respondents did not feel fully prepared for the challenge. Examples of some of these challenges were:

'Losing control after the food leaves the kitchen'. (Trust Catering Services Manager)

'Exposure to irate and stressed patients, customers and staff'. (Catering Manager)

'Delivering a quality service (both catering and domestic) with limited and diminishing budgets'. (Hotel Services Manager)

'Delivering nutritionally adequate patient meals for all patient groups, complying with national and local standards with poor resources'. (Head of Nutrition & Dietetic Services)

'Coping with unrealistic targets/expectations from senior management'. (Trust Catering Manager)

But despite their obvious challenges, difficulties and frustrations it is interesting to note that many of the employees did in fact show loyalty to the NHS as detailed in their length of employment. If there is that sort of commitment to a job, surely it is not beyond their employers to support this work force and somehow make their positions more tenable, even from an administrative point of view.

With all the many reports and noted trials and tribulations of feeding patients simmering away in the background, it suddenly seemed that changes to hospital catering were afoot when in the *NHS Plan 2000* it was reported to parliament that at a cost of £500 million, the NHS provided over 300 million meals each year, but the food was variable in quality, not provided in a way that was sufficiently responsive to patients and resulted in too much wastage (DH, 2000). These standards 'were not good enough' and subsequently it was announced that an extra £10 million a year was to be made available to deliver improvements in hospital food as part of a new NHS Plan, due in 2001, which would provide:

- A 24-hour NHS catering service with a new NHS menu
- A national franchise for NHS catering which would be subject to examination
- New Ward Housekeepers in half of all hospitals by 2004
- Dietitians to advise and check on nutritional values in hospital food.
- Patients' views measured as part of the Performance Assessment Framework
- Unannounced inspections of the quality of hospital food

2.4.2   Better Hospital Food Programme

As a result, in 2001 Chief Executives from NHS Trusts and Primary Care Trusts as well as Trust Catering Managers were requested to introduce the Better Hospital Food programme (BHF) (Wearmouth, 2001). This included the new National Health Service Menu and the NHS Recipe book, which in turn, incorporated Flexi Menu, Protected Mealtimes and 24-hour Catering. (NHS Estates, 2001a). It was designed to make country wide, effective changes to hospital food services.

The BHF programme acknowledged that some hospitals already provided modern, flexible catering services and that these should be maintained whilst others were raising standards. The three objectives in raising standards were:

- To ensure all hospitals at least met the required standards
- To bring all hospitals to existing levels of excellence
- To develop and introduce across the NHS, new catering systems, providing modern, highly efficient services which were responsive to the needs of patients

The minimum daily meals programme (The Mealtime Service) embodied the requirements set out in the NHS Pan and included:

- Early morning beverage
- Breakfast and beverage
- Mid morning (snack and) beverage

Box 2.6 The standard requirements for each meal under the BHF programme.

Breakfast
Fruit juice
Low fibre cereal
High fibre cereal
Porridge/Hot oat cereal
White roll/Toast/Bread
Wholemeal roll/Toast/Bread
Butter/Margarine/Portion
Preserve portion

Morning beverage and snack
Squash/Sugar-free squash
Drinking water
Tea
Coffee
Biscuits
Cake
Fruit
Additional sweet & savoury items

Light lunch
Fruit juice
Soup
Roll/bread and butter/Margarine portion
Light hot dish (meat/fish)
Light hot dish (vegetarian)
Sandwich (meat/fish)
Sandwich (vegetarian)
Fresh fruit
Energy/Protein-dense cold dessert

Afternoon beverage and snack
Squash/Sugar-free squash
Drinking water
Tea
Coffee
Biscuits
Cake
Fruit
Additional fruit & savoury items

Two course evening dinner
Main 1 (premium meat/fish item)
Main 2 (composite dish)
Vegetarian
Salad (meat/fish)
Salad (vegetarian)
Potato
Carbohydrate alternative
Fresh/chilled/frozen vegetable 2
Roll/Bread & Butter/Margarine portion
Hot dessert and custard

Evening beverage and snack
Squash/Sugar-free squash
Drinking water
Tea
Coffee
Hot milk-based drink
Biscuits
Cake
Fruit
Additional sweet & savoury items

Source: NHS Estates (2001a).

- Light lunch and beverage
- Afternoon (snack and) beverage
- Evening dinner and beverage
- Late evening (snack and) beverage

Standard requirements for each meal were also set as shown in Box 2.6.

A comparison of the Daily Meals Programme in 1975 and 2001 shows that they are very similar with the only differences being in 2001 when an early morning beverage and additional snacks were available (see Table 2.4), perhaps showing the acceptance of a more modern or realistic way of eating particularly with regard to 'snacking'.

Table 2.4 Comparison of Daily Meals Programme in 1975 and 2001.

1975	2001
	Early morning beverage
Breakfast and beverage	Breakfast and beverage
Mid morning beverage	Mid morning (snack and) beverage[a]
Lunch and beverage	Light lunch and beverage
Tea and beverage	Afternoon (snack and) beverage[a]
Supper and beverage	Early dinner and beverage
Bedtime beverage	Late evening (snack and) beverage[a]

[a] Snacks will be provided at least twice daily. The British Dental Association recommend that these are mid-afternoon and evening.

Adapted from: DHSS (1975b) & www.betterhospitalfood.

As well as standard requirements being in place, the NHS Purchase & Supply Agency (NHS PASA)[6] reviewed the specifications for raw ingredients in the National Dish Selector to ensure the use of value-for-money and good quality ingredients. This was to give patients greater confidence that their meals were made from wholesome ingredients.

To support the programme a Better Hospital Food Panel[7] was established, chaired by food critic and broadcaster, Loyd Grossman, who also headed a team of leading chefs[7] to develop a range of new recipes for use in NHS hospitals. In addition, leading chef, Shaun Hill, helped design a questionnaire asking patients to describe the consistencies and flavours of foods they preferred. The findings were subsequently incorporated into the dishes with a selection of the Leading Chefs' recipes published as the NHS Recipe Book. Further guidance was provided in the National Dish Selector, Nutritional Spreadsheets, Ingredient Specifications and Smaller Serving Recipes.[7] Trusts would be expected to conform to the specific guidance relating to the nutritional requirements (Nutritional Care), menu mix (Leading Chefs Dishes) and quality standards (Food Presentation) for each element of the menu.[7] They were also required to make appropriate arrangements to ensure that the specific needs of any patients from special groups were adequately met.

Trusts were requested to meet six requirements:

- Use the range of dishes created by the leading chef team (identified by the chef's hat logo)
- Redesign hospital printed menus to make them more accessible and easier to understand
- Implement a 24-hour food service comprising the Ward Kitchen Service, the NHS Snack Box and Light Bight
- Use the specially designed box for delivery of the Snack Box
- Move the main meal of the day to the evening
- Meet and exceed the standards

£401 334 was paid to outside organisations in connection with the BHF programme, covering design costs for the new menus, the implementation of the support pack, the establishment and testing of the full nutritional analysis of the NHS selector dish recipe and the development and management of the website. This equated to only slightly more than £1000 per Trust and was a fraction of the NHS budget for catering. In addition it was reported that central arrangement of much of this work would save the costs incurred in duplicating work across the NHS. Details of any payments made to outside consultants by individual hospitals were not available centrally (WrittenAnswers, 2001a). The costs for each component part of the programme varied from hospital to hospital, affected by a range of factors including current levels of investment in catering services, the type of catering service in use and the number of patients choosing dishes designed by the leading chefs. It was expected that an accurate forecast on additional costs for future improvements would be easier to ascertain when standards had been brought to a more equal level across the service (WrittenAnswers, 2001b).

Meanwhile, the panel of chefs were mocked by the press (Rayner, 2006) and the new menus, launched in a blaze of publicity, were criticised by managers for being too expensive and denounced by some nurses as 'slop' (BBC News, 2002a) with a suggestion that 'NHS caterers couldn't cook something like that' (Rayner, 2006). Among the items on offer were 'roast cod and garlic potato puree'; 'leek and mushroom sauce' and 'salad of spinach, tuna, egg and mung beans': patients said they would prefer more traditional dishes with some kitchen staff 'finding them difficult to prepare' (BBC News, 2002b). In Hungry to be Heard (Age Concern, 2006) Age Concern viewed the menu items as a challenge to older patients who may be confronted with 'navarin of lamb with couscous and grilled vegetables', when it could be their first time in hospital – feeling sick, frail, in a strange environment and just looking for something familiar to eat.

Notwithstanding the menu furore, 13 hospitals, known as Development Sites, worked with NHS Estates between May and December 2001, in bench-testing early implementation strategies of the BHF programme (NHS Estates, 2002). The Development Sites were hospitals which had introduced or developed examples of 'excellence' and hospitals which had implemented the Better Hospital Food Targets, initiating the Better Hospital Food Partnership Sites Club (BHFPSC). By January 2003, the membership stood at 51 NHS Trusts and almost 75 hospital sites. The purpose of the BHFPSC was to:

- Share ideas about the best ways of consistently providing high quality, patient-centred catering services in the NHS
- Act as reference sites for other hospitals
- Provide the NHS with free information about costs and performance associated with the BHF programme
- Encourage managers of different parts of the catering chain to develop and implement highly patient-centred practices and service standards

Their first 'interim' performance report was viewed as a benchmarking[8] exercise to act as a measure against which other hospitals could compare their own performance (NHS Estates, 2002). A total of 71 different performance indicators had been developed covering: the provision of 2 snacks per day; the use of snack boxes; the NHS Menu format; leading Chef Dishes; and the Ward Kitchen service.

The report came nearly a year after the BHF programme was launched and it was pointed out that *the detail in this paper is only the start – it has been put together in a very short space of time and serves only to place a foundation in the structure of what is to come*. The data were collected between 12th March and 12th April 2002, involving 37 hospital sites, representing 21 950 beds:

Catering services were provided in-house at 31 of the hospitals with 17 using bulk systems, 15 plated systems and 5 hybrid.

- 42% provided a housekeeping service to all wards
- 68% had introduced two snacks a day
- 81% had introduced the Snack Box service
- 61% had worked in collaboration from outside their own hospital in the design and printing of menus
- 73% had implemented 3 or more Leading Chefs' Dishes per day
- 90% provided a ward kitchen service
- 24% provided Light Bite meals

It was also revealed that 77% of the original Leading Chefs' Dishes had an average cost of 68.8p compared to an average cost of 56.2p for similar dishes which were not part of the Leading Chefs range. However, the total number of Leading Chefs Dishes increased to 116, including a significant range of 'Patient Favourites' said by the NHS to be very popular with patients which, after being reviewed had been added to the National Dish Selector. This had resulted in a decrease in the cost, to 63p. Twenty-two hospitals with a total of 14 000 beds had identified the most and least popular Leading Chef dishes as shown in Boxes 2.7 and 2.8.

Box 2.7   Most popular leading chef dishes (in order of popularity).

(1)   Cottage pie
(2)   Steak & kidney pie
(3)   Chicken pie

Source: NHS Estates (2002).

Box 2.8   Least popular leading chef dishes (in order of popularity).

(1)   Navarin of lamb with couscous & grilled vegetables
(2)   Seafood pasta with fresh dill & parmesan
(3)   Braised lamb with flagelot beans

Source: NHS Estates (2002).

Meal service at ward level: Environment, observation of staff involved, housekeepers, food delivery and presentation, monitoring nutrition for at risk patients

Menu content: Snack boxes, menu descriptions

Flexibility provided by the meal ordering and service systems: Negotiated meal service times, advance ordering, own meal selection, food upon admission if required, access to alternative food, snacks between meals

Customer awareness: Opportunity to talk with the catering manager, information prior to admission, opportunity for daily feedback, adapted cutlery, piloting patient catering satisfaction questionnaire, multi-disciplinary group to review patients needs

Organisation: Essence of care benchmarking

Eating environments: Different locations

Figure 2.5   BHFPSC Benchmarking focus. Adapted from: NHS Estates, 2003.

As discussed earlier, Age Concern viewed words such as 'navarin' and 'couscous' as a challenge to elderly patients but it could be argued that they would represent a trial to most individuals, hospitalised or not. The chefs undoubtedly understood what they meant but somebody at Trust level must have had to approve the descriptions and mistakenly believed that the general public had somehow developed a sixth sense in understanding 'fine dining' jargon.

The second benchmarking report was published in 2003 (NHS Estates, 2003), involving 31 Trusts for 42 hospital sites representing 19 746 beds with data collected between 9th August and 13th September 2002. It was said to focus on five key areas of the catering services (see Figure 2.5) although the heading '*Eating Environments*' was also included in the report:

- Meal service at ward level
- Menu contents
- Service flexibility
- Customer awareness
- Organisational issues

It was reported that catering services were provided in house at 29 of the 42 hospitals, a ratio which was said to accurately reflect the situation across the NHS, with 18 using bulk systems, 10 plated systems and 6 hybrids. This report was in a much more detailed format making comparisons to 2001 difficult but on housekeeping and snack boxes the results were as follows:

- 29% of hospitals provided a housekeeping service to all wards
- 81% provided snack boxes 24 hours per day

Table 2.5 Benchmarks for food and nutrition.

Factor	Benchmark of best practice
(1) Screening and assessment to identify patients nutritional needs	Nutritional screening progresses to **further assessment for all** patients/clients identified as 'at risk'
(2) Planning, implementation and evaluation of care for those patients who require a nutritional assesment	Plans of care based on **ongoing** nutritional assessments are devised, implemented and evaluated
(3) A conducive environment (acceptable sights, smells and sounds	The environment is **conducive** to enabling the **individual** patients/clients to eat
(4) Assistance to eat and drink	Patients/clients **receive the care and assistance** they require with eating and drinking
(5) Obtaining food	Patients/clients/ carers, **whatever their communication needs,** have sufficient information to enable them to obtain their food
(6) Food provided	Food that is **provided by the service** meets the needs of individual patients/clients
(7) Food availability	Patients/clients have set meal times, are **offered a replacement meal if a meal is missed and can access snacks at any time**
(8) Food presentation	Food is presented to patients/clients in a way that takes into account what **appeals to them as individuals**
(9) Monitoring	The amount of food patients actually eat is **monitored, recorded** and leads to action when cause for concern
(10) Eating to promote health	**All opportunities** are used to encourage patients/clients to **promote** their own **health**

Source: Department of Health (DH) (2001a).

It was also reported that 43% of hospitals had completed the DHs Essence of Care (DH, 2001a) Food & Nutrition Benchmark and of those 61% had included the Catering/Facilities team in the completion of the factors 4–8 (see Table 2.5). As discussed earlier these benchmarking reports were to serve as reference sites for hospitals to assist in the implementation of the BHF programme but there were/ are other parties involved in assessing the performance of the catering service as examined below.

2.4.3 Assessment

2.4.3.1 PEAT

Patient Environment Action Teams (PEATs) were established in 2000 to assess NHS hospitals. Under the programme, every inpatient healthcare facility in England with more than ten beds is assessed annually and given a rating. PEATs consist of NHS staff, including nurses, matrons, doctors, catering and domestic service managers, executive and non-executive directors, dietitians and estates directors. They also include patients, patient representatives and members of the public. Following the closure of NHS Estates responsibility for the day-to-day management of the programme transferred to the National Patient Safety Agency (NPSA) in 2006. In line with the approach taken by the Healthcare Commission (HC), PEAT is an entirely self-assessed system with validation carried out by independent teams (NPSA, 2007).

In 2002 food and food service was assessed for the first time by PEAT with a review of the six Better Hospital Food requirements. A traffic light system was used to represent the overall quality of food and food services:

- Green healthcare facilities were those providing high standards of food and food service which always, or almost always, met patient needs and generally exceeded expectations. They also met the requirements of the BHF programme. Rated as good.
- Yellow healthcare facilities were those providing standards of food and service that generally met patient needs. These facilities had room for improvement in some areas. Rated as acceptable.
- Red healthcare facilities were found to be providing generally poor standards of food and food service that did not meet patient needs, requiring urgent improvement. Rated as poor.

The results for 2002 and 2003 are shown in Table 2.6, but as the results represent overall quality it is difficult to judge where improvements could or have been made and therefore the reasons behind any changes in the percentage ratings, as discussed below.

In 2004 a new system was introduced whereby the facilities were rated as 5 excellent, 4 good, 3 acceptable, 2 poor, 1 unacceptable. The resulting assessment comprised of a review of nine components relating to meals and meals service and six BHF requirements. The results from 2004 to 2006 are shown in Table 2.7 which show an overall improvement.

Table 2.6   PEAT results from 2002 and 2003.

% Hospitals	Good	Acceptable	Poor
2002	17.0	81.0	2.0
2003	43.2	56.8	0.0

Source: BHF NHS Estates (2007).

Table 2.7   PEAT results from 2004 to 2006.

% Hospitals	Excellent	Good	Acceptable	Poor	Unacceptable
2004	8.1	50.3	35.2	5.9	0.6
2005	32.4	51.5	14.8	1.3	0.0
2006	33.8	57.8	8.3	0.08	0.0

Source: National Patient Safety Agency (NPSA) (2007).

Changes were introduced to PEAT for the 2007 assessment, which were said to reflect the comments received during the review of PEAT 'undertaken in the summer'.[9] The range of scores remain on a 0–5 scale but the definitions used as a guide are shown in Table 2.8. Questions were asked on issues such as the menu, availability, quality, portion sizes, temperature, presentation, service, beverages, protected meal times and nutritional care, for example the Malnutrition Universal Screening Tool (MUST) (see Box 2.9) but again the results only give an overall impression. The results for 2007 were: Excellent – 46.5%; Good – 48.5%; Acceptable – 4.5%; Poor – 0.5%; and Unacceptable – 0.0% (NPSA, 2007), showing an increase in the amount of hospitals reaching 'Excellent' with a downturn in the 'Poor' and 'Unacceptable' categories. Results for individual Trusts and hospitals are available online at: http://www.npsa.nhs.uk.

Table 2.8 PEAT Standards.

Standard	Definition
Excellent	Standards are consistently high, exceed expectations across all aspects of the element being measured. An occasional, obviously temporary incident can be overlooked if it is an isolated occurrence
Good	Standards almost always meet expectations and often exceed them
Acceptable	Standards usually meet expectations though there is room for improvement in some areas
Poor	Standards regularly fail to meet expectations and there is significant room for improvement
Unacceptable	Standards fail to meet expectations in most areas and improvements are required urgently

Adapted from: NPSA (2007) PEAT Assessments 2007.

Box 2.9 BAPEN Malnutrition Universal Screening Tool (MUST).

MUST is used to identify adults who are malnourished, at risk of malnutrition (undernutrition) or obese, involving five steps:

(1) Measure weight and height to obtain a BMI score using chart provided. If unable to obtain height and weight use alternative procedures
(2) Note percentage unplanned weight loss and score using tables provided
(3) Establish acute disease effect and score
(4) Add scores from steps 1 to 3 together to obtain overall risk of malnutrition
(5) Use management guideline and/or local policy to develop care plan

MUST is viewed as a multidisciplinary responsibility and most effective if deployed in a healthcare system that prioritised nutrition strategies, training and implementation. The development and dissemination of MUST was supported by the Dietetic Association, the Royal College of Nursing and the Registered Nursing Home Association.
   A comprehensive, free MUST guide is available to download from: http://www.bapen.org.uk/must_tool.htm

2.4.3.2 Benchmarking

In 2001 the DH introduced patient focused Benchmarking[10] (DH, 2001a) to support continuous improvement in the quality of fundamental aspects of health care, including nutrition (Ellis, 2006). In relation to food and nutrition, the agreed benchmark patient-focused outcome was 'patients are enabled to consume food orally which meets their individual need' (the 10 factors and the benchmarks of best practice are shown in Table 2.5).

The benchmarking tool-kit itself has been criticised as its use is inconsistent, with nursing managers struggling to have it recognised as an integral part of benchmarking activity (Ellis, 2006) with a suggestion that benchmarking raises expectations in highlighting areas for improvement but it can only work if the organisation is fully resourced, supporting planned changes and managing expectations of what can realistically be achieved (Matykiewicz *et al.*, 2005) Nevertheless, improvements are achievable as demonstrated by one group within the Central South Region (Chambers & Jolly, 2002), who reported changes of practice, directly attributable to the implementation of the *Essence of Care* benchmarks, for example:

- Mealtime activity – ensuring that staff are making it a priority to support patients with eating and drinking at mealtimes. This has meant rescheduling doctors' rounds and ward handovers
- Presentation of meals – implementing the privacy and dignity benchmark highlighted that patients felt rushed when presented with both main course and dessert on their trays and as a result did not finish their meals. Liaison with the catering department allowed for courses to be served individually and enabled patients to enjoy their food

In line with the previous comments, it was also noted that the success of this implementation relied heavily on the work of volunteers who undertook *Essence of Care* activities in addition to their full time jobs.

2.4.3.3 Inpatient surveys

These NHS patient survey programmes were designed to assess the quality of the patients' experience of care in acute Trusts. Prior to the surveys, a questionnaire was piloted to identify recently discharged patients' top priorities (Reeves *et al.*, 2002). Although questions on food had been included, it was one of the issues mentioned as not having been adequately covered with the researchers noting:

'Their concern was not only to receive appetising food but to get food appropriate for their dietary requirements and to receive adequate nutrition to promote their recovery from illness'.

'A number of interviewees commented that food was a particular problem in hospitals. Some interviewees thought there should be more questions to reflect the importance of this issue'.

Box 2.10   Questions that should have been included.

'Flexibility in obtaining food. It was not good'
'Should be appetising and attractively presented. Fish, peas and mash does not fill requirement. Rejected food not cost-effective. Bring back catering staff'
'When you are sitting around all day the highlight becomes the next meal, choice, size, hot'
'I think the food issue is quite important and inadequate diet does not aid a speedy recovery. Which is the common goal'
'Nurses were wonderful. Food is awful'
'Should have asked more questions on the food side'
'Dietary requirements'
'The food question. The standard of food and what could be done in future was not asked'
'Also a question about choice of food'
'Also more questions about the food (which was terrible)'
'Choice of diet, i.e. Coeliac + vegetarian'
'Choice of food and selection and distribution of food'
'Food was not mentioned'
'More time on the food to be talked about'
'Not enough on quality and quantity of food'

Source: Reeves *et al.* (2002).

The patients' actual comments on the questions that should have been included were as shown in Box 2.10.

Subsequently, the following questions were added to the questionnaire:

- Were you offered a choice of food?
- Did you get the food you ordered?

Inpatient surveys were carried out by the DH in 2001/2002 (Bullen & Reeves, 2003), and the HC in 2004 (Reeves *et al.*, 2005), 2005 (Boyd *et al.*, 2006) and 2006 (Boyd & Donovan, 2007). The results of the 2004 survey have been omitted as unlike the others, they sampled only patients aged 18 years and over, omitting those aged 16 years and above.

The results from the responses to the Inpatient Survey 'how would you rate the hospital food?' are shown in Table 2.9. In general, across England, there seems to be little change, although there are, of course, differences between individual Trusts.

The results from the responses to the question 'did you get enough help from staff to eat your meals?' are shown in Table 2.10,[11] which are perhaps more pertinent in light of the issues of malnutrition and might be deemed more factual rather than the subjective issue of rating hospital food. Alarmingly, in light of current policy, they show that assistance is not always available for patients who need assistance with eating.

Table 2.9 Responses to 'How did you rate the hospital food?'

	2001/2002 (%)	2005 (%)
Very good	18	18
Good	34.0	36
Fair	30	31
Poor	15	15

Adapted from: Acute Inpatient Survey 2001/2002 (Bullen & Reeves, 2003), Survey of Inpatients 2005 (Boyd *et al.*, 2006).

Table 2.10 Responses to 'Did you get enough help from staff to eat your meals?'

	Survey year (%)		
	2002	2005	2006
Yes, always	57.9[a]	61.8[a,c]	58.4[c]
Yes, sometimes	24.1[a,b]	20.6[a]	21.2[b]
No	17.9[b]	17.7[c]	20.4[b,c]
Total specific responses	**19 049**	**19 982**	**19 041**

Note: See note 11.

It should be remembered that the Inpatient Surveys use responses direct from the patients themselves which might well provide a more accurate appraisal than PEATs self-assessment system. In addition, the researchers and the HC set the core questions and the Trusts can 'top up' the questionnaires in order to 'allow for some flexibility and to enhance local ownership'.

Building on the 2002 questionnaire (Reeves *et al.*, 2002) the 2006 *Inpatients Importance Study* (Boyd, 2007) was undertaken to identify again, aspects of care that were most important to recent inpatients in England. This would directly influence the contents of the questionnaires for inpatient surveys from 2007 onwards. The question '*Did you have access to food whenever you were hungry (not just at mealtimes)?*' was rated as having relatively low importance by patients and therefore it was suggested that it might not be added to the core questionnaire unless other reasons could be provided for its inclusion. The question '*Did you get enough help from staff to eat your meal?*' was also rated as having low importance, but it was believed that there were good reasons to maintain it in the questionnaire. Despite these rulings, the patients' comments on 'food' seemed to provide more insight into what the patients thought about all aspects of the catering service (see Box 2.11).

These comments could be seen to reflect the true status of the quality of the food and its delivery but perhaps for short-stay patients the whole subject of

Box 2.11   Patients' comments on food.

'*Vegetarian food should be provided*'

'*When ill, food should be appetising*'

'*Having food saved for after an operation*'

'*While I have been an inpatient I have seen nurses serve food to elderly patients. These patients for whatever reason have been unable to feed themselves. At the end of meal time their trays have been collected and no-one has noticed it has been untouched*'

'*Being on (sic) special diet, it will be nice if one can contact a senior catering officer and explain fully ones choice and dislikes e.g. numerous allergies and taboo, and things one can or can't eat before a known admission and then pass this information to all concerned*'

'*I am 'coeliac' and my weight was very poor. [I ate] the same thing day after day and to top it all [I was] given a packet of build-up soup. I don't know what I was supposed to do with it as it was past its sell-by date and I couldn't make it up anyway*'

'*I was appalled at the lack of assistance given to elderly patients ... hot soup was just left. I got out of bed to help them myself*'

'*If admitted after the normal time for filling in a menu preference form, arrangements should be made by staff so that it can be filled in and acted upon. This should also happen when you are told to expect discharge on a certain day and this is changed after the time for filling in menu preference for lunch*'

'*A clean glass for water to each patient each day and covers for the water jugs*'

'*A mobile toaster – so fresh toast can be served for breakfast*'

Source: Boyd (2007).

food is seen as an understandably minor issue when a speedy admission would win every time over the expectations of the standard ofs food which are probably low to begin with. The results for the 2007 Inpatients Survey are due to be published in spring, 2008.

2.4.3.4   *Patient and public consultation*

Section 11 of the Health and Social Care Act 2001 placed a duty on NHS Trusts and PCTs to make arrangements to involve and consult patients and the public in the planning and development of health services and in how the services operate with the organisations below showing how this was achieved.

2.4.3.5   *Arms Length Bodies*

Since the NHS plan, a network of organisations was created to regulate the system, improve standards, support local services and protect public welfare. These organisations are referred to as Arms Length Bodies (ALBs).

2.4.3.6   CPPIH & PPI Forums

One of these ALBs was the Commission for Patient and Public Involvement in Health (CPPIH), which was established in January 2003 under the NHS Reform and Healthcare Professions Act 2002. Under the CPPIH, 572 Patient and Public Involvement (PPI) Forums were established involving almost 5000 volunteer members whose aim was to ensure an independent voice for patients and the public, not just in healthcare but in all decisions that could affect their health (CPPIH, 2006).

2.4.3.7   PPI Forums

In 2006, 2240 people in 97 hospitals in England were surveyed by PPI Forum members from 117 forums (CPPIH, 2006): some of the results and comments are shown in Box 2.12.

The Hospital Caterers Association (HCA) were disappointed by many of the findings from the PPI Forums Survey which again appeared to contradict the recent PEAT surveys which had indicated significant rises in patient satisfaction with hospital food. It would seem that this is similar to the situation with the Inpatient Surveys, discussed earlier, a paradox explained by the fact that one survey listens to Trusts and other surveys listen to the patients. The HCA also suggested that issues such as 'wrong meals' could be dramatically reduced by adopting practical measures such as ward house keepers or 'hostesses' being deployed (HCA, 2006).

2.4.3.8   LINks

Then in 2006, the Local Government and Public Involvement in Health Bill contained plans for the abolition of the CPPIH and the PPI forums which were to be replaced by Local Involvement Networks (LINks) covering an area rather than being tied to a specific organisation (DH, 2006). This decision was in line with the emphasis of the NHS Improvement Plan, namely, that the balance of power in the NHS should shift towards the frontline (DH, 2002). This was further strengthened by the fact that strategic Health Authorities now held Primary Care Trusts accountable for the services they commissioned (DH, 2005b). In the context of devolution, the wider network of ALBs was deemed too cumbersome and, therefore, streamlining would 'increase efficiency in the public sector' (Gershon, 2004) and conducive with the principle of the Lyons Review that public sector jobs should be relocated away from London and the South East (Lyons, 2004). The DH commented that the reasons for the changes were because:

'Although there are many examples of good practice found across the NHS, there are inconsistencies with the NHS still having much to learn about the more localised social care approach to involvement'.   (DH, 2006)

The establishment of the LINks system is still being determined by legislation, with a date for Royal Assent on the Local Government and Public Involvement

Box 2.12   Results of PPI Foodwatch Survey.

96% responded that they were given sufficient time to eat their meal.

85% responded that the menu was easy to understand but a quarter of patients in specialist hospitals had difficulty in reading the menu:

'Patients do not get to see a menu, it is read by the housekeeper. When the food trolley comes – if you're at the end of the ward – you do not get your choice.'

'I am nearly blind and cannot see the menus easily and do not receive help'

85% responded that the menu suited dietary requirements but how they accessed this information is unknown.

82% responded that all items were available but nearly a fifth of the respondents stated that not all items were available once they had ordered them and this was seen as a particular concern in Mental Health and Elderly Care Centres where over a quarter had experienced this problem.

81% responded that there was a choice of meals in advance but the figures were much lower in Specialist and Other health facilities. Some patients were disappointed with the quality of the choice they received:

'Menu needs to include more vegetarian choice. Have to go to Asda for more variation in diet'

'My family need to bring me fresh orange juice as this is not readily available'

'From a diabetic point of view, fruit salad choice and quality could be better'

78% responded that the temperature of 'hot' meals was just right but there were compounding factors:

'Only problem, all courses served simultaneously'

'Meals covered with metal lids causes condensation and leaves food swimming in water'

74% responded that help was available with eating if required. Over a quarter of respondents had not received any help with the highest figure recorded in General Hospitals and 'other' health facilities:

'Sometimes not enough staff for amount of patients who need help'

'Family members help more than nursing staff with the meal'

'I do not require assistance but saw patients who did and the help was not always forthcoming'

58% responded that snacks were available between meals. 17% said they didn't know about them which could intimate a lack of information.

40% responded that their diet was supplemented by food brought in by family/friends with this occurring most frequently in Specialist Units and least in Community hospitals.

37% responded that they had left a meal because it looked/smelt/tasted unappetising. There were notable differences in different types of health facilities with the biggest response from Specialist Units and other health facilities such as Mental Health Units and Elderly Care Centres:

'Food smelt awful and tasted worse – caused me to vomit on three occasions'

'The quality is ok although things would be better if they were fresh e.g. vegetables'

'Disgusting, vile, nasty, sloppy, piggish'

Source: CPPIH (2006).

in Health Bill anticipated for October 2007 after the summer recess (private email from PPI Mailbox). Based on this assumption the timescale for implementation is as follows:

- LINks will begin procuring for Host organisations soon after Royal Assent
- The abolition of PPI Forums will take place at the end of March 2008
- The work of the CPPIH will cease operationally in March 2008
- LINks should begin to emerge by 2008 with the appointment of Host organisations
- LINks will begin to carry out functions from April 2008

LINks will be funded by local authorities and has the power to defer matters to Overview and Scrutiny Committees (OSCs): the OSC's will be encouraged to focus their attention on the work of the commissioners of health and social care services, being ideally placed to ask commissioners about the decisions they have made thereby 'ensuring they reflect the health needs of the local populations and reflecting public priorities in the communities' (DH, 2006).

2.4.3.9   Core Standards

In November 2005 the Healthcare Commission (HC) announced that it was starting visits and spot checks at almost 120 (20%) NHS Trusts to ensure compliance with the government's core standards (Health and Social Care (Community Health and Standards) Act 2003), as outlined in *Standards for Better Health* (DH, 2004a). This process was to form part of the new annual health check, replacing star ratings (HC, 2005) which did not include hospital catering. The HC also cross-checked Trusts' declarations, using other sources of information such as patient surveys, clinical audits and data from other organisations (HC, 2005). The HC itself is responsible for determining how it assesses core performance, taking account of the targets that the department had set and assumed to be achievable. This enables the public to identify progress against the standards by individual organisations and determine which Trusts are to be considered for Foundation Trust status. If 'exceptionally', a Trust fails to satisfy the HC that it meets the core standards, consideration will need to be given on how performance should be improved. In these cases, the Trust would have to develop proposals for improvement, negotiating with its Strategic Health Authority. In addition, the legislation gives powers to the HC to recommend to the Secretary of State, or in the case of Foundation Trusts the Independent Regulator, that they take special measures in relation to any significant failings (HC, 2006).

Within the NHS there are 24 core standards which are based upon:

'A number of standards or requirements ... serve as a platform or bottom rung for progress against the developmental ladder, providing a marker to show where service is now and to assure the public that all services, wherever provided, will be safe and of an acceptable quality'.   (HC, 2006)

The core standards are split into seven domains. The fourth domain, patient focus, contains core standards C15a and C15b which are directly related to food provision in hospitals.

Core Standard C15a: where food is provided, healthcare organisations have systems in place to ensure that patients are provided with a choice and that it is prepared safely and provides a balanced diet (excluding ambulance services).

Core Standard C15b: where food is provided, healthcare organisations have systems in place to ensure that patients' individual nutritional, personal and clinical dietary requirements are met, including any necessary help with feeding and access to food 24 hours a day.

For 2005/2006, Trusts self-assessments showed there was 98.4% compliance for Core Standard C15a and 97.6% compliance in 2006/2007. For Core Standard C15b there was 98.4% and 96.9% compliance consecutively.

These self-assessment methods used have been criticised by Age Concern (Age Concern, 2006) as details on specific measures to comply with the standards, or any statement to justify how the Trust came to view their own compliance, were not included – are tick boxes enough? They also viewed the core standards as having a direct link to the issues of malnutrition and despite their presence along with a raft of other regulations,

'*Malnutrition in hospitals continues to be all too prevalent: policy is not being put into practice*'.

2.4.3.10   Independent assessment by Which?

In 2006 Which? (Which?, 2006) carried out an online survey of 833 of their members who had stayed in hospital during the past twelve months – 70% had been NHS patients in NHS hospitals, 25% private patients in a private hospital and 5% private patients in an NHS hospital. A comparison of NHS and private patients' experience of the food service are shown in Table 2.11. With regards to the quality of the food itself, a comparison is shown in Table 2.12.

The Which? results indicate more patient satisfaction within the private sector and Which? reported that the reason for this was due to the fact that private hospitals spend more money on food, nearer £10 per day, and cook using fresh ingredients. It has to be said that with the amount of money generated by private health care subscriptions it would be almost impossible for them not to provide decent food, but this is only a discussion on food and not other services provided by the private sector.

As has been illustrated, the assessments of the catering service are wide ranging, but despite their presence, yet another report on malnutrition in hospitals, *Hungry to be Heard* (Age Concern) was published in 2006 which depicted the plight of the elderly in hospitals:

'*It is a national scandal that six out of ten older people are at risk of becoming malnourished, or their situation getting worse, in hospital. Malnourished*

Table 2.11 Comparison of NHS and private patients' experience of the food service.

Food service	NHS (%)	Private (%)
Meals at fixed times	88	64
Always shown a menu	59	86
Portion size correct	66	91
Received food ordered	53	88
Sufficient variety	13	43
Access to hot and cold drinks 24 hours	15	47
Had to order food the day before	53	18
Still hungry after meals	29	4
Restaurant standard	15	62

Source: Which? (2006).

Table 2.12 Comparison of NHS and private patients opinions on the quality of the food.

Food	NHS (%)	Private (%)
Tasty	35	76
Healthy	42	72
Appetising	29	76

Source: Which? (2006).

patients stay in hospital for longer, are three times as likely to develop complications during surgery and have a higher mortality rate than well-fed patients. Ending the scandal of malnourished older people in hospitals will save lives'.

Their findings underlined the gravity of the situation:

- Up to 14% of people aged over 65 years in the UK are malnourished
- Four out of ten older people admitted to hospital are malnourished on arrival
- Patients over the age of 80 have a five times higher prevalence of malnutrition than those under the age of 50
- Whether their condition goes untreated, unnoticed or worsens during, their hospital stay is a lottery, with patients and relatives concerned about appropriate food and the absence of help with eating or drinking
- Up to 50% of older people in general hospitals have mental health needs
- Six out of ten older people are at risk of becoming malnourished or their situation becoming worse in hospitals
- The cost of malnutrition on health and health care systems is estimated to exceed £7.3 billion per year with over half the cost expended on people aged 65 and above

2.4.3.11   NICE

The same year, following the Age Concern report, the National Institute for Health and Clinical Excellence (NICE) with the National Collaborating Centre for Acute Care, launched a clinical guideline, *Nutrition Support in Adults,* to assist the NHS in identifying patients who were malnourished or at risk of malnutrition (NICE, 2006):

- All hospital patients and outpatients should be screened and at their first clinic appointment
- Nutrition support should be considered in people who are malnourished
- Nutrition support should be considered in people at risk of malnutrition
- All acute hospital Trusts should employ at least one specialist nutrition support nurse and establish a nutrition steering committee (NSC)
- All healthcare professionals directly involved in patient care should receive relevant education and training on the importance of providing adequate care
- All acute hospital Trusts should employ at least one specialist nutrition support nurse
- All hospital Trusts should have an NSC

Dr Mike Stroud of the Institute of Human Nutrition, Southampton General Hospital and Chair of the Guideline Development Group said that the guidelines contained one obvious and simple message:

'Do not let our patients starve and when you offer them nutrition support, do so by the safest, simplest, most effective route' (NICE, 2006).

However, it was reported that eight months later, hospitals were not acting quickly enough in setting up NSCs and challenged all Trusts to ensure that both NSCs and Nutrition Support Teams were in place by February 2007, the first anniversary of the publication of the NICE guidance (Elia, 2006).

Moreover, it was also suggested that the raft of guidelines and standards might produce a different set of problems for Trusts, namely in the form of 'guideline fatigue' and 'conflicting' guidelines. For example, during this time, NICE published 20 guideline appraisals each year, which meant that they would have to be fully implemented every 2–3 weeks to keep up with publication. In addition an independent survey revealed that out of 28 NICE guidelines, 12 were considered to be under-implemented and 4 over implemented: more than half did not meet the target. This might have been because NICE guidelines do not have the status of core or mandatory standards thereby undermining the motivation to implement them (Elia, 2006).

2.4.4   Better Hospital Food Panel disbanded

Problems with guidelines aside, in 2006, 5 years after its launch, the BHF panel was formally disbanded: in a radio 4 programme (BBC, 2006) it was revealed that the Health Minister, Jane Kennedy, had written to each member of the BHF panel:

'The time for strong central directive and targets has now passed … accordingly I am now standing down the panel and for the moment don't intend replacing it with any formal group … it's local action that matters to patients and it's local action that we are now looking to see'.   (BBC, 2006)

Loyd Grossman's response to the 'local' issue was:

'Delivering of power locally is incredibly important but there must be certain policies that have a national direction … I don't see how you can individually convince every Trust that they must adopt certain food standards and it seems to me unfortunate that something of national importance can't be directed from the centre as a compulsory national programme … anything that is going to allow hospital food to slip off the agenda is not desirable because it is going to have a very bad affect on a lot of patients'.   (Grossman, 2006)

Dr. Gill Morgan from the NHS confederation had a different view:

'I think it's really important that over time we take all these important central initiatives, of which there are large numbers and do put them into the responsibility of local boards. The reason I think that's important is that you can't from the centre monitor everything that is going on and we have to get boards to take that type of responsibility … . at the end of the day things are going to be improved when every clinician, every board puts this high on their agenda. Certainly in the confederation we think the panel has done a fantastic job over the last years but now is the time to get the responsibility into every organisation'.   (Morgan, 2006)

Loyd Grossman responded:

'I still feel that whilst I believe in devolution of power, I still feel that in terms of driving the programme forward, keeping it high up in the minds of ministers, keeping it in the public eye, keeping it in the minds of funders, it does require a national focus and I am very, very concerned that national focus is going to be lost now'.   (Grossman, 2006)

These comments seem to encapsulate the findings of a study in 2005 (Savage & Scott, 2005) undertaken in a general medical ward, committed to improving nutritional care with a large proportion of its patients being long stay, dependent and/or at risk of poor nutritional status: whether or not nutrition was seen to be high on the Trusts' agenda was dependent on whom the researchers spoke to their place in the organisation and whether they thought of nutrition as a form of therapy or as the delivery of food and fluids. In addition, nutrition tended to be subordinated to other priorities: distinctions between 'bottom up' initiatives such as the nutrition strategy which were seen as important in improving the therapeutic impact of nutrition and 'top down' initiatives such as protected meal times that tended to treat nutrition with a broad brush and emphasise the aesthetic aspects of food. This particular Trust tended to focus on top-down initiatives at the expense of more life-and-death aspects of nutrition and resources for specialist staff. It came as no surprise to read that 'clinical equipment was given priority over catering equipment with repair or replacement of catering equipment always going on the back burner as it was difficult to see the impact of investment in this area' (Savage & Scott, 2005).

2.5 Other initiatives

Following the disbanding of the BHF programme what had happened to other initiatives relating to hospital food as determined by the NHS Plan? They included protected meal times, the promise of the presence of ward housekeepers in half of all hospitals by 2004, the introduction of modern matrons, a reduction in food wastage, with healthcare catering services and other NHS organisations being encouraged to develop sustainable food procurement policies. These initiatives are explored below.

2.5.1 Protected mealtimes

Protected Mealtimes were introduced in 2004, whereby hospitals were encouraged to stop all non-urgent clinical activity during mealtimes so that patients could eat their meals without interruptions with nurses being available to offer assistance to those who needed it. This initiative received the full support of the Royal College of Nursing and the British Dietetic Association.

Implementation of the initiative involved negotiations between medical staff and health care professionals such as radiographers who could then structure their visits to patients accordingly (Hospital Caterers Association, 2004) although one Trust reported that this was not always possible: for many surgeons racing between theatre lists and clinics, the hours of lunch and supper were often the only ones free to visit patients (Savage & Scott, 2005). However, the Protected Mealtimes scheme was widely accepted as a useful initiative but in a few areas it seemed to have introduced tensions between nursing staff who endeavoured to make sure it worked and medical colleagues who were not convinced of its value. It was seen by some staff as a reminder to take their own meal break and for nursing staff it tended to extend the period that they could work without a break. Although it could be seen as a 'top down' project, like other nutritional initiatives it tended to be destabilised and given less priority by Trusts who had other items on their agenda such as meeting targets associated with star ratings (Savage & Scott, 2005).

2.5.2 Ward housekeepers

The funding and implementation of the housekeeping process was the devolved responsibility of local NHS Trusts (May & Smith, 2003) who were encouraged to establish contact with each other to allow, amongst others, rapid problem solving of any housekeeping issues (NHS Estates, 2001b).

Housekeeping was published in 2001 which was a first guide to the new, modern and dependable ward housekeeping services in the NHS (NHS Estates, 2001b). Ward housekeepers themselves, were described as ward based and non-clinical, coordinating a range of ward services including catering, cleaning and maintaining the environment and equipment. They might also coordinate the clerical, transport and linen services, working closely within the Trusts' support service departments to ensure that national standards in key areas (hygiene, catering, maintenance, receiving visitors and handling complaints) were met (NHS Estates, 2001b). To be employed as a ward housekeeper there are no set minimum entry requirements although previous experience in the hotel service either within healthcare or the private sector is usually required. National Vocational Qualifications (NVQs or SVQs in Scotland) were being introduced in 2001 with units that supported the development of ward housekeepers, namely Cleaning, Science, Customer Service, Food & Beverage Service and Health & Social Care (NHS Estates, 2001b). As described above, the ward housekeepers role is diverse but for the purposes of this chapter the main focus will be on their contributions to catering.

In 2001 it was acknowledged that the ward housekeepers role would vary depending on the type of ward: in an elderly care ward providing food and cleaning may take a similar amount of time, in A & E departments more time might be spent cleaning and in ICU where patients are artificially fed providing food would only form a small part of the job (NHS Estates, 2001b). *Housekeeping* provided model examples of the ward housekeepers relationships with other staff members and how they might work with others to provide food services. Therefore, it would appear that there were to be systems in place for food distribution but improving the quality of the food itself, yet again, had not been addressed.

The role of these ward housekeepers was not a new concept as some Trusts already had successful housekeeping teams on site (see Box 2.13). Hospitals that did not have housekeeping services were advised that they should make sure that everyone on the ward understood how important food was, both clinically and socially and to make sure that wards had basic food supplies available at all times. In addition, the ward housekeeper should always be able to tempt patients with a choice of hot and cold drinks and snacks, as well as choices from the new NHS menu (NHS Estates, 2001).

In evaluating the various approaches that had been adopted in developing, implementing and funding the ward housekeeper role, including its value, one study documenting a series of six case studies within different NHS Trusts, noted that with regard to catering some of the ward housekeepers were responsible for the patient meal service in terms of menu completion, ordering the meals, regenerating and serving the food to patients while in other hospitals members of the catering teams performed these roles (May & Smith, 2003) (see Table 2.13).

This glaring disparity is not conducive to establishing continuity for the patients themselves. The importance of this continuity in patient care was demonstrated

Box 2.13   Examples of successful ward housekeepers.

'The housekeeping team is responsible for the ordering, storage, delivery, preparation, regeneration and service of food....such services have greater flexibility where new technology cook-freeze/chill meat systems are used and there is a need for specialist and user-sensitive services'.
(South West London and St Georges Mental Health Trust)

'The trust has introduced a 24 hour food service for patients, with different snack boxes for patients with specific dietary needs, for example low fat, diabetic diet, vegetarian. Catering staff prepare the snack boxes which are delivered by ward housekeeping teams to refrigerators located around the trust. Snacks for maternity and paediatric areas are available from the ward kitchen. The trust has a hospital restaurant which is staffed 24 hours a day and is open to patients and relatives as well as staff'.
(Walsall Hospital NHS Trust)

'Sylvia Smith, an assistant catering manager, recognised the special needs of certain patients who have problems maintaining their food intake, for example terminally ill or elderly patients. Sylvia set up a special care scheme to provide these patients with food of their choice – called 'Sylvia's Specials. Patients can only access this service through referral from their dietician or nurse in charge. Nurses inform the catering department of any patients who are not eating. Catering staff then visit those patients every morning to discus the menu and offer suitable alternatives. Kitchen staff cook the patient's chosen menu to order. If patients require very small portions, they are served on a small plate to make them look more attractive. On one occasion the catering department prepared a candlelit dinner for two for a terminally-ill patient's wedding anniversary. The service has been extended to all wards in the hospital. It works well because the hospital has a traditional kitchen offering a plated meal service. At any one time there can be between two and twenty patients receiving this dedicated service. It means patients get what they want to eat, less food is wasted and nursing staff do not have the worry of patients refusing to eat. As well as boosting the patients nutritional intake, the service lifts their moral and relatives appreciate the service'.
(Central Sheffield University Hospitals NHS Trust, Royal Hallamshire Hospital).

'Each floor has a kitchen that supports four wards. Each kitchen provides regeneration facilities, while vegetable and potatoes are cooked from fresh. Sandwiches and salads can also be plated to improve presentation. Nursing and catering staff work together to meet patient's needs'.
(Royal Group of Hospitals and Dental Hospitals Health & Social Services Trust)

Source: NHS Estates (2001b).

in some hospitals by the presence of a 'dedicated and permanent housekeeper' allowing the WH to familiarise themselves with the patients' particular needs, for example, diet. Another issue raised was the fact that only one Trust included the WH at a supervisory level, as recommended in *Housekeeping*. They had chosen to do so as they felt that:

'It would help raise the profile of the housekeeper and assist in their responsibility of overseeing non-clinical duties in the absence of the ward manager'.

Table 2.13 Summary of the main characteristics of the housekeepers in different hospitals.

Hospital type	
General	*Case study 1*: Mainly catering relating work but also responsible for the laundry cupboard, replenishing stores and general tidiness
Acute	*Case study 2*: Purely catering work, i.e. ordering and serving patient meals and the cleaning of the crockery and cutlery afterwards
Acute	*Case study 3*: Supervisory role, responsible for overseeing all non-clinical work on the ward
District	*Case study 4*: Serving meals, cleaning and tidying the ward, making beds
Community	*Case study 5*: Mainly catering-related duties such as ordering and serving patient meals. Some general work such as bed making and checking linen trolleys
Acute	*Case study 6*: Mainly focused on cleaning the ward, however they are responsible for serving hot drinks

Source: May & Smith (2003).

There was also a suggestion that the role being only at a supervisory level was down to funding and one of the problems in the recruitment of housekeepers was due to the levels of pay: In 2001 there was no national pay and reward structure for ward housekeepers but they were to be included in the new National NHS pay scheme. As the new scheme had been designed to facilitate career development, Trusts were required to use existing reward mechanisms to remunerate the post locally at relevant salary levels. In 2005, one Trust admitted that its slow deployment of ward housekeepers was mainly because the ward managers were expected to employ them out of the nursing budget (Savage & Scott, 2005). Their duties included cleaning and porterage – a domestic service which, if paid for out of the nursing budget, would have to be balanced by a reduction in nursing staff. As it was, it was argued that too many things were already coming out of the nursing budget for each ward, including £188 per month to cover all cereals, biscuits, condiments, crockery, cutlery, paper towels and so on, an amount that was often overspent. Under the Private Finance Initiative (PFI), it was anticipated that in a new hospital building, ward housekeepers would be funded via the facilities budget with all facilities services being provide by a non-NHS contractor. The intention was for ward managers to be involved in the interviewing and management of housekeepers so they could see whoever was to be appointed as part of their team. How this arrangement, with joint management across NHS and non-NHS sectors would work in practice, remained unclear. Overall it was reported that the ward housekeepers who had been employed, received positive comments from a number of sources with the catering manager remarking that wards with housekeepers gave him no catering problems at all. From the patients' perspective these wards were reportedly, the best run in the hospital (Savage & Scott, 2005).

In 2004, the Health Minister, Lord Warner, announced that the NHS had ward housekeepers in 53% of all hospitals, rising to 70% in larger hospitals where the majority of patients received treatment. This meant that two thirds of Trusts (66%) had introduced ward housekeepers effectively meeting government targets (DH, 2004b).

In 2007, the Heart of England NHS Foundation Trust provided a further example of the positive effects of WHs who had already been employed in some ward areas for nine years. However, over a period of two years there had been a concerted effort to employ housekeepers to comply with the requirements of the NHS plan (Richmond, 2007). All wards had a budget for a housekeeper, who had been funded by 'nursing monies'. This had been agreed by the directorates as the housekeepers were taking on tasks which had been traditionally carried out by nursing staff. The housekeepers were employed by the senior nursing sister and integrated into the ward team as advised by NHS Estates. Within the Trust it had been observed that some areas of good practice, in particular, nutrition, were not being exploited to improve care Trust-wide. By developing the service to ensure sufficient training, support and opportunity to share best practice for the housekeepers there was a demonstrable improvement in the way patients' nutritional requirements were met. This service included:

- A mandatory, corporate induction day with guidance issued to all ward sisters regarding the setting up of their housekeeper induction programme, downloadable from the Trust's Essence of Care intranet site
- Each clinical area having different requirements for its housekeeper
- A Monthly newsletter sent to each housekeeper via internal mail
- A six point plan developed containing a six point checklist before the serving of meals to those who needed assistance
- A Top Tips for Protected Mealtimes leaflet was developed
- A corporate Key Performance Indicator (KPI) agreed that every ward should score 90% or more in quarterly nutrition audits as their end of year target

The resulting successes are shown in Box 2.14.

The Trust has shown that the development of the housekeeper role within a multidisciplinary framework has had a beneficial effect on patients' nutrition, demonstrated by improved audit results and reduction in Patient Advice and Liaison Services (PALS) complaints. For 2007, additional data was to be collected

---

Box 2.14   Nutrition successes.

Year on year improvements in audits
Sharing of best practice trust wide
Introduction of cooked breakfasts to the elderly directorate
Serving of soups and desserts separate to the main meal service
Halal picture menu available on all wards
Introduction of healthy drinks and snacks and monitoring of usage by catering staff
Red trays given to patients identified as those in need of assistance/monitoring
Mealtimes changed to enable nurses to assist with the meal service

Source: Richmond (2007).

about the use and accuracy of the Nutrition Screening Tool and there were plans to develop pathways to respond to patients' nutrition risk score.

Another positive example of how a co-ordinated approach to addressing nutrition at ward level was shown during a successful pilot study on two medical wards over a period of 6 months (Hayward, 2003) when a multidisciplinary team was formed to share their specific nutritional concerns, devising a new role of nutrition coordinator: after a week's intensive multidisciplinary induction an existing health-care assistant was given the role whose main focus was to facilitate rather than undertake the nutritional care of patients throughout their stay. After 6 months, the role demonstrated a significant impact on nutritional screening, nutritional service, patients' perceptions of their nutritional care and staff satisfaction:

- The accuracy of food ordering increased on the pilot ward, resulting in less catering wastage with a projected saving on this one ward of £500 annually
- 76% of staff thought the nutrition coordinator role greatly improved patients nutrition (18 respondents)
- 67% of staff felt their jobs had been made easier
- 82% of staff thought that all wards ought to have a nutrition coordinator
- Twice as many patients awarded 'good' or 'excellent' on the pilot ward (28 respondents) when asked about meals and service related to eating and drinking in comparison with the other wards (39 respondents) and there were no reports of poor service in any of the areas of nutritional care on the pilot ward
- Giving nutritional supplements to patients who had missed a meal was achieved 86–100% of the time compared to 8% of patients Trust wide
- Enhanced communication between the ward and the catering manager via the nutrition co-ordinator meant that patients with special needs were catered for appropriately. Traditionally, the catering department offered a service whereby any patient with specific needs could be referred to them for a one-on-one visit. This is still available but rarely used on the pilot ward as the coordinator managed nutritional problems, allowing the catering department to use its resources elsewhere
- On admission to the pilot ward nutritional screening was undertaken on 75% of the patients compared with 57% of patients across the whole Trust. This was an overall improvement of 24% when compared to the findings from 2000
- 82% of patients were weighed weekly compared with 36% in 2000. Height recordings were 82% vs 34%
- For patients on the pilot ward for longer than 2 weeks nutritional screening was achieved 100% of the time
- Appropriated referral rate to the dietetic department was 100% compared to 14% hospital wide
- Monitoring with a nutritional intake chart was achieved 75–100% of the time (where required)

So all this seems to show that this kind of undertaking is not insurmountable, it just requires determined application and, of course, funding.

2.5.3   Modern matrons

By 2002, NHS Trusts and Primary Care Trusts with wards were required to have identified matrons (senior sisters or charge nurses) each accountable for a group of wards, whose presence would be highly visible, identifiable and accessible to patients (DH, 2001b). They were seen as performing a modern and more important role than that of the matron who had disappeared in the late 1960s and would help 'get the basics right' (Richmond, 2007) including good food: number 6 of their ten key responsibilities, was to ensure that patients' nutritional needs were met. In 2003, *Modern Matrons – improving the patient experience* (DH, 2003) provided examples of good practice:

> 'Our core philosophy is that eating should be a pleasurable experience. Recently a lot have resources have been concentrated on waiting lists. But I have been able to demonstrate that if we get nutrition right then we can discharge patients promptly to a more appropriate setting'.   (Royal Berkshire and Battle Hospital Trust)

> 'We are also encouraging relatives to come in and help with the patients' nutrition. They eat at the same time and so encourage patients to eat'.   (Birmingham Heartlands & Solihull NHS Trust)

In 2004, *The Evaluation of the modern matron role in a sample of NHS Trusts* (Savage & Scott, 2005) reported on how NHS Trusts, including Primary Care Trusts, established modern matron posts, the experiences of nurses in these posts and the impact of their activities on patient care. With regard to key responsibility 6, ensuring patients nutritional needs are met, there appeared to be a limited involvement of matrons in the improvement of nutritional standards. The contracting out of catering services, coupled with the lack of influence matrons had over the allocation of contracts or the auditing of contracted services, meant that matrons were restricted in the extent to which they could improve patients' food. This was viewed as one of the most surprising findings of the study. However, in some Trusts, matrons as a group were becoming more effective in influencing the contracting service which highlighted the benefits of collective action more generally. The researchers had also not expected to find so few matrons mention their responsibility for patients' nutrition in the 'matron survey or during interview'. Furthermore, in the patient survey most patients failed to identify hospital food as a responsibility of the matron which contrasted with a widespread understanding about matrons' responsibility for cleanliness and standards of nursing care. It also seemed that operational activities such as bed management seemed to have precedence over key roles, which included the nutritional needs of patients. The research demonstrated that across the Trusts there were differences in how many matrons had been appointed, significant variations in their salaries, only 19% of Trusts had made new money available to support their introduction, and the title of 'matron' or 'modern matron' was not widely used with 113 different job titles in use.

Following an audit at a South Essex Partnership Trust to provide an accurate picture of the impact of modern matrons it was found that matrons accessibility and visibility was affected by the amount of meetings they had to attend and that they had no formal direct management responsibilities (Shanley, 2004). On a more positive note, matrons worked closely with ward housekeepers and received all copies of monitoring sheets on, amongst others, the quality of the food. They worked collaboratively to respond to all housekeepers in addressing any problem areas. Overall it was felt that modern matrons were definitely raising standards but further improvements could be made. Many of the findings illustrated by the latter studies were also found in another study which audited the impact of implementing the modern matron but it concluded that overall, although the role was challenging, matrons had been shown to be vital to service delivery and quality of care (Dealey *et al.*, 2007).

2.5.4 Food wastage

The significance of food wastage was realised in 2001 when it was reported that the annual cost to the NHS from 'unserved meals' was £18 million or an average of £55 000 per Trust. If all hospitals achieved the lower quartile level for Trusts of their type, the NHS could save a total of £8 million or the equivalent of an additional 25 pence that could be spent on food for patients each day (AC, 2001). Wastage rates varied dependent on the type of service method used with Trusts using the bulk service methods experiencing considerably higher wastage rates. This was because food was served in trays of a set size and if the tray contained eight portions then eight portions were produced even though only 6 might have been ordered. On any level, this seems to be an obvious, unnecessary waste of both money and food and the kind of issue that needs addressing at a local level.

The subject of food wastage in the NHS has been a recurring theme: In 1983 it was reported that food was wasted at the point of consumption with three underlying causes: too much food was ordered, the food was unsuitable and the food was of poor quality (DHSS, 1983). In 1999 (Edwards & Nash) a study undertaken in elderly, medical and surgical wards across four hospitals showed that in general:

- Food wastage was lower at the breakfast meal
- Female food wastage was higher than male food wastage
- Wastage was higher where food was plated in wards rather than in the kitchen
- Wastage was higher where food was purchased-in ready prepared, rather than prime cooked in the hospital kitchen

On looking at these findings, perhaps breakfast is the most important meal of the day and maybe the one that should be the focus of future attention for its nutritional content. It would also seem that patients preferred 'home cooked food' which was served to them *in situ* … not much of a surprise really.

The publication *Managing Food Waste in the NHS* (NHS Estates Hospitality, 2005) identified the reasons why food wastage occurs in the ordering, distribution and service of food at ward level, suggesting how this waste may be effectively managed in a cost-effective way. It was intended as a best practice guide for modern matrons, doctors, dietitians, catering managers, Ward Housekeepers and ward-based teams. It recommended that a management checklist was completed at least once a year, with an operational checklist completed on a monthly basis with both being completed if there were any changes to the catering service. In addition it included a daily ward food waste record and summary sheet for plated food service, a ward food waste daily record sheet for bulk food service, a ward food waste summary sheet for bulk food service, a healthcare facility food waste summary sheet, an observational audit of plate waste, an observational audit of meal service and a sheet to record either the total number of patients who received support when required and/or which groups of staff participated in the recording. All these checklists could be adapted for use at local level to be used in audits as follows:

- At least two wards should be audited during breakfast, lunch and dinner as arrangements can differ significantly
- Preparation and service should be observed at each mealtime as arrangements can differ significantly
- Staff on each ward should be interviewed regarding roles and responsibilities for catering, meal service and nutrition
- Findings should be summarised and discussed with catering staff, Ward Housekeepers, nursing and support staff and dietitians

It is a very comprehensive publication but begs the question as to how much time these audits would take and what extra demands would be put on the staff required for such an undertaking. Indeed, this could explain why it has been suggested that:

> *'The behaviour of the medical, catering and allied professionals have not changed significantly to ameliorate the problems of extensive food waste and inadequate dietary intakes within the hospital setting'.* (Marson *et al.*, 2003)

2.5.5   Procurement and sustainable food

The Sustainable Development Commission (SDC) was set up in 2000 to provide independent advice to the government on sustainable development (Cole, 2008). Under the BHF programme, it was hoped that sustainable food procurement policies would result in the production of food that would do as little harm to the environment as possible (NHS Estates, 2001a). Stakeholders were advised that sustainable food procurement included sourcing fruit and vegetables locally to avoid transport pollution and composting peeling and other preparation waste to keep landfill to a minimum. Other sustainable measures could include using 'fairly traded' or organic goods, energy efficiency and reducing food preparation waste.

But can this be achieved? In *Getting more sustainable food into London's hospitals* (Hockridge & Longfield, 2005), Sustain, the alliance for better food and farming reported on a two-year Hospital Food Project, run in partnership with the Soil Association, whose aim was to tackle these problems, focusing on four London hospitals, namely Ealing General, Royal Bethlem, Beckenham and Lambeth, Royal Brompton and St. George's (not necessarily concentrating on patients' food but some focusing on staff restaurants). Their goal was to increase the proportion of sustainable food in the hospitals to 10% of their routine catering. The project acted as a 'dating agency' to find suitable suppliers to match different hospitals' particular needs and solved problems such as transport, distribution and continuity when they arose. The new supplies arranged by the project include a range of vegetables, apples, eggs, milk and beef. To 'sell the idea to everybody involved' – the catering team, patients and their visitors and hospital staff, the project provided a wide range of training events and promotional activities such as celebratory food events and visits to suppliers.

Once a new system was in place it was felt that extra assistance for the funding of the practical help offered by the project would not be required indefinitely but progress would be hindered by conflicting policy signals which extolled the virtues of sustainable food but insisted on budget cuts. In addition the lack of equipment and staff enabling food to be cooked from scratch did not allow for any flexibility needed for the gradual increase in the proportion of sustainable food and more people needed to be convinced to help those already engaged in the promotion of sustainable food, which required vigorous marketing. Also, to ensure that a wide variety of sustainable food was available everywhere, supported by an adequate transport and distribution infrastructure, investment was required.

However, early indications, resulting from independent evaluations of the health and economic effects of the project, showed that although it was not feasible to expect any physical health changes, there had been improvements in knowledge about and support for more healthy and sustainable food with an improvement in food quality and variety, service levels, and staff and customer satisfaction. All this, with some sustainable food suppliers in London and the South East having increased their businesses, without increasing hospital food budgets (some food products had increased but had been offset by savings elsewhere and/or by increasing the prices in the restaurants).

In 2004, the BHF programme commissioned the King's Fund to identify opportunities for managing food procurement, sustainability and promoting healthy eating in acute hospitals. The resulting project considered activities in three acute care Trusts involving cook-chill food manufacturer's drawn from the top five suppliers to the NHS and the Purchasing and Supplies Agency (PASA). A framework was developed for organisations to assess and change their own procurement and catering practices, policy recommendations, menu designs and contract specifications.

In their subsequent report, *Sustainable food and the NHS* (Jochelson, 2005), it was revealed that Trusts had limited knowledge about food sustainability policies and that their menus and sourcing policies were cost driven. This resulted in a food system that favoured standardised meals with ingredients that were '*sourced internationally with little awareness of the potential economic, social and environmental and health impacts*'.

The report also said that over two thirds of all food procured by the NHS was via NHS Purchase & Supply Agency (NHS PASA) contracts with the remainder independently sourced by individual Trusts. This meant that was a gatekeeper for much of the purchasing for the NHS, potentially influential in changing specifications for food contracts to ensure better quality and more sustainable food. For potential suppliers tendering for NHS contracts, PASA has produced a guide to try to make the health market more accessible to smaller, local companies which also reduced their documentation costs. It had also developed a 'patchwork' approach to sandwich, meat, fruit and vegetable contracts in order to open up a public sector market for smaller contractors. Regarding its meat and poultry contract, PASA found that national and regional companies bid for tenders with national companies who were not always equally responsive to local conditions. PASA could not confirm if the patchwork approach had increased the number of contractors but believed that opening up the bidding field made the tendering process fairer. PASA also offered a few organic and fairly traded options where they met value-for-money criteria. The report said that critics from local food organisations argued that PASA could do a lot more, suggesting that they should be more explicit about their commitment to sustainability in their contracts and should include sustainability in their evaluation criteria. It was also pointed out that other countries, particularly Italy and France did not see EC procurement rules as an obstacle to local sourcing by the public sector.[12]

Hopefully the sourcing of better food will become easier as in 2005 it was reported that PASA have provided a tool, developed for all food items which allowed all NHS Trusts to compare the nutritional content of products by brand so that Trusts could make informed decisions on the make up of their recipes and menus. The tool will also aid PASA to award contracts based on Trust requirements and track changes in producer levels of salt, sugar and fats. They were also hoping to work with suppliers to reduce products with high levels of these items and to increase the consumption of dietary fibres and fruit and vegetables (Tiddy, 2004).

According to the National Audit Office (NAO) savings were achieved by PASA by tendering for all types of NHS food requirements in one go (with the exceptions of baby milk, fruit and vegetables and 'ready meals'), a market worth, in total, about £130 million (NAO, 2006). The agency achieved more competitive bids and achieved further reductions by holding e-auctions[13] to decide the final value of successful bids. Overall they achieved savings of 9% (just under £12 million).

There were three other bodies holding significant responsibilities for hospital food at a national level:

- NHS Logistics Authority: buys certain food items in bulk which Trusts may in turn buy. Orders are delivered from its network of regional warehouses

Table 2.14　Variations in prices obtained by the public sector procurers.

	Milk (1 pint whole milk) (Pence)	Bread (800 g wholemeal) (Pence)	Specified brand of cola (330 ml can) (Pence)
NHS Trust (range)	18–27	32–84	20–29
NHS Trust (average)	20.9	55.4	25.3

Source: NAO (2006).

- Department of Health: The Chief Nursing Officer has overall responsibility for patient experience including the user experience of hospital food
- NPSA: In April 2005 NPSA acquired responsibility for some operational aspects of hospital food delivery from NHS Estates. The focus of this work has been on improving nutrition whilst maintaining close attention to food quality and delivery

The NAO also reported that at a local level, NHS Trusts were free to buy from suppliers through the framework contracts negotiated by PASA, to buy direct from NHS Logistics or to negotiate their own deals with suppliers. In practice, many Trusts employed a mixture of these, often mixing and matching, depending on where they could find the best prices for different items. However, the majority of spending goes through PASA frameworks (NAO, 2006).

With regard to pricing, there were variations reported in the prices paid for goods with the lowest prices being genuinely competitive, but many were comparatively expensive (see Table 2.14). The variations could be explained by the different sizes of organisation as well as their differing standards of nutritional quality and the ease with which smaller suppliers were aware of opportunities and thus able to compete for contracts. Also reflected were the differences in the professionalism of the food purchasing. There was an indication that there was considerable scope for many organisations to purchase the same quality of items for significantly cheaper prices. The NAO pointed out that food procurement objectives were often not integrated into the wider objectives of organisations: the catering service should be designed around the needs and policies of the organisation as a whole.

An example of where food procurement performance has progressed is at Southampton University Hospitals Trust, which contracted out its catering management while still directly employing its own kitchen staff. As a result the Trust had expert catering managers, focused on running an efficient service and maximising sales. The retention of in-house catering staff removed any incentive for the contractor to save money by reducing the level of service with all savings being retained by the Trust. Food wastage rates were far below the national average while the staff and visitors' restaurants operated without any subsidy, making a small profit for the Trust. In addition, it moved from buying items from several different suppliers to sourcing all its food items through one supplier, reducing the prices paid by an average of around 10% and reducing the number of deliveries.

In addition, in 2004, the Nottingham University Hospitals NHS Trust, one of the largest in the country, whose City Hospital Campus caters for a 1100 bed capacity, adopted the Public Sector Food Procurement Initiative (PSFPI). In realigning their catering plan with the PSFPI, the campus opened the entire catering menu to local and regional suppliers as well as drawing employees from the community. Some of the resulting changes are highlighted below (Sustainable Development Commission (SDC), 2007):[14]

- Nearly 1000 pints of milk per day come from a farm 11 miles from the hospital
- The campus gets 95% of its meat from a local supplier, guaranteeing traceability
- The site is working with local suppliers to use seasonal surpluses of fruit and vegetable to feed patients
- The campus is using larger containers from the milk supplier, reusable food containers in the canteen and biodegradable sandwich boxes in the retail shops

The catering manager admitted that he was very cynical when he began the search for alternative, local suppliers, but he was proved wrong. In addition he said that 'the principal selling point is that heres something operated by the NHS, that's developed by the NHS and all the profits go back into the NHS' (Cole, 2008).

Other examples of good practice are:

- The catering department at the Northern General Hospital was accredited with ISO 9001:2000, which gives a rigorous programme of procedures and commits to its continuous improvement. For instance, every delivery problem with a supplier is recorded and automatically compiled into a quarterly report which is used in future negotiations with suppliers.
- The Cornish Food Consortium, a collaboration of the five NHS Trusts in Cornwall who worked with a local supplier to reduce the cost of packaging, thereby making their products cost effective.

Despite being one of the most economically deprived areas of Europe, the Cornish Food Consortium has created a model, some might say a blueprint, to enable Trusts throughout the UK to provide tasty and nutritious meals, boosting the local economy and aiding environmental sustainability by switching to local and organic suppliers. The success of these Cornish Trusts, has been well documented in a report by the Soil Association, *A Fresh Approach to Hospital Food* (Russell, 2007).

This success began in 2001 when a hospital patient complained that the sandwiches were from a national supplier in Oxford: why give the contract to a national caterer when local ingredients could be used, boosting the local economy? A new source was located and the feasibility of sourcing more food locally was examined.

At the time there were five healthcare Trusts in Cornwall covering twenty hospitals, of which the largest, the Royal Cornwall Hospitals Trust (RCHT), was providing food for 1035 beds. It operated a cook-serve system for 80% of these beds, with the rest being provided with cook-freeze meals produced in their own kitchens. This service delivered 1500 main meals daily. The combined Trusts had an annual food budget of £1.5 million, of which 60% was spent out of the county. It was decided that the best long-term option would be a new Cornwall Food Production Unit (CFPU) supplying a cluster of hospitals, a decision which took into account the expanding demand for food across the county and the size and age of the existing RCHT kitchens. The unit is scheduled to open in 2008.

The Soil Association became a partner of the Cornish hospital food project via its regional arm, Organic South West (OSW), supporting the key role of sustainable food development manager through the EU Objective One (EUOO) programme, matched by SA funding, all working towards achieving Food for Life[15] targets in Cornish hospitals.

Meanwhile, the first locally produced sandwiches provided positive feedback from patients with the head of hotel services realising that this new initiative required specialist staff who were duly appointed. Critical to the success of the project was the support of the NHS chief executives in Cornwall. It was initially hosted by the Cornwall Partnership Trust but in the second phase the capital project was taken over by the RCHT. All five NHS Trusts made a financial commitment to the project, confirming that they would use the CFPU as a provider of some of their meals in the future.[16] With the support of the Trusts in place, further assistance from a host of stakeholders was sought, advice was gained on what was locally available, meetings were held with policy makers, together with a wider group of NHS contacts and media, attracting considerable interest and encouragement.

By 2003, the political climate had changed with an interest at national policy level in sustainable procurement, with PASA looking for opportunities to increase local sourcing. The Cornish project was recognised as a positive pilot scheme, 'an exemplar of sustainable principles'. The ensuing stream of awards included a *Health Service Journal* accolade in 2004, *Local Food Initiative of the Year* 2006 in the SAs Organic Food Awards and a silver award at Hotelympia 2006 for a menu designed around local and organic ingredients.

By specifying exactly what the Cornish project wanted from its supply contracts, some of the improvements felt by patients included the use of:

* Clotted ice cream which is higher in calories and less likely to melt before patients eat it. This has cut the amount spent on expensive, powdered drink supplements previously given to elderly patients to maintain their calorie intake
* The new fish cake whose fish content has increased from 30% frozen fish to 40% fresh fish

With patients commenting:

'The food at Treliske is the best hospital food I have ever come across'

'The food was exceptionally good, healthy and attractively cooked and presented, which hastened recovery'

'The quality of the food and the menu options were good, arriving as ordered and hot where necessary'

Box 2.15   Sample menu, main meals in Cornish hospitals.

Cornish fish pie – fresh local fish in a white sauce with mushrooms,
topped with potato
Chicken in mustard, leek and coriander sauce
Creamy cauliflower and broccoli pasta
Vegetable balti

Source: Russell (2007).

Box 2.16   Sample menus, puddings.

Bread & butter pudding
Stewed plums
Cornish soft cheese and biscuits
Seasonal fresh fruit
Cornish ice cream

Source: Russell (2007).

Sample menus of food on offer in Cornwall's hospitals are shown in Boxes 2.15 and 2.16.

An example of how savings had been achieved and waste reduced was the switch from buying 115 g pots of long-life yogurt to custom-sized 80 g pots of fresh yogurt. The Cornwall Food Programme has achieved these improvements without increasing costs and within its budget of £2.50 per patient per day.

In 2006 the total spent by the Cornwall Food programme on food produced in Cornwall was around £402 000 which was 41% of the £975 000 budget. This figure rose to 83% of the budget, £812 000 when produce ordered through Cornish companies (though not necessarily produced in Cornwall) was included.

The environmental effect of the programme has also been noted with a reported 110 000 road miles being cut from deliveries annually.

The Soil Association says that Cornwall's emphasis on supporting local suppliers and sustainability might appear to be at odds with the government's Gershon Efficiency Review which placed an emphasis on public sector bodies achieving efficiency savings in their procurement purchasing. The Soil Association have received reassurance in this matter from the agency responsible for improving the efficiency and effectiveness of procurement in the public sector, the Office of Government Commerce, who said that efficiency did mean a return to the lowest price as a basis for decision making, pointing out that a sustainable solution might offer better value for money when issues such as energy savings and recycling were considered. The Soil Association saw this as a positive clarification but argued that there is still confusion among public sector procurers because the government is trying to get two messages across: all buyers must comply with European procurement regulations and that these regulations should not be used as any form of barrier to sourcing more sustainable, environmentally friendly products.

In the awarding of contracts, the inclusion of external costs are not permitted but the government suggests that they are included in the specification criteria. In the majority of cases where contracts have been awarded locally in the UK, careful specification of what was required had been followed up. The smaller or local companies often have the advantage where clear criteria such as nutritional quality and freshness are included in the contracts. In the Cornwall Food Programme's tendering document for their fish contact, potential advantages that local companies might be able to exploit were highlighted but by including suppliers from further afield the public procurement regulations were not contravened. It was suggested that any supplier could adhere to the arrangements as specified in the tender document and although local companies would have to compete for business, 'fresh fish suggested a local source who might have lower transport costs too'.

In 2006, the NHS Supply Chain, took over the procurement of some categories from PASA, including food. The SA say that they expect that there will be changes to working practices but are hoping that there will still be a mix of local and national contracts in NHS procurement.

The Sustainable Development Commission (SDC)[17] has developed a good corporate citizenship toolkit that enables Trusts to check their performance on a whole range of issues related to sustainability (Cole, 2008). However, the SDC know that their powers are limited:

> 'There is no co-ordinating body compelling trusts to develop sustainability and the SDC do not have any "clout" ... it might be that the only way to do this is through compulsion. The bottom line is that this really must be done. We just can't afford not to'.   (Cole, 2008)

Issues around procurement were discussed at a Westminster Diet & Health Forum seminar on *Food in Hospitals*[18] when the 'prohibiting of the movement for quality food' was blamed on Compulsive Competitive Tendering by a representative from the UK's leading foodservice distributor: If an NHS tender suggests the use of a well-known brand of baked beans then the catering supplier does not have the ability to suggest the low salt version. The same applied to bakery products with regard to their fat, sugar and salt content:

> 'Any supplier of food into the NHS needs to have a range portfolio that meets the aim. And interestingly, in food distribution all carry between 12,000 and 15,000 wide ranging products and these products are as wide ranging as supplying someone like Buckingham Palace down to a greasy food café on the A2'.   (Kemp, 2005)

This must be achievable, but as *'food is seen as a cost and so immediately it's an add on ... catering departments need to be specific about what they want'* (Jochelson, 2005). It has also been suggested that standards should be built into catering contracts so it actually becomes a contractual requirement to meet expected standards (Morgan, 2006). Although the organisations are not comparable in the service they provide it has also been said that:

'... the MoD are superb at ensuring that all of our forces when they're eating abroad are eating nutritionally balanced food and I think this is a lesson that we should start to learn within the NHS'.   (Kemp, 2005)

2.6   Alternative hospital catering facilities

2.6.1   Vending machines

It must be remembered that there are other sources of food in hospitals such as vending machines and restaurants to which the publication *Choosing a Better Diet* (DH, 2005a) apply. This document was seen as a food and health action plan presenting the actions that the Government would take across a wide range of areas including ensuring that the NHS promoted healthy eating in all aspects of its work, promoted opportunities for healthy eating in the workplace and ensuring that the public sector led by example: the public sector including the NHS had a corporate social responsibility to offer healthy nutritious food in its institutions and to lead by example in improving the diets of its staff and patients. As has been observed, 'if you want to improve food in a hospital you have to improve the food of the whole hospital (Kitson, 2005).

Timely advice when *Sustainable Food and the NHS* (Jochelson *et al.*, 2005) reported that hospitals provide vending machines selling anything from canned soft drinks, chocolate and crisps to hot meals such as chicken rolls, cheeseburgers, meat kebabs or chicken nuggets with fries. A nutritional analysis of these commonly available foods showed that they were energy dense, high in sugar and saturated fats and low in protein. At the time, catering managers believed that a 'healthy' vending machine would be unprofitable. The hospitals were tied into contracts with companies that owned or managed the vending machines, filling them for a percentage of the profit, making efforts to change the vending content more difficult. This, arguably, boils down to funding, with the Trusts having to decide on profit over health. As the chairman of the HCA has said:

'It has to be recognised that market testing and the privatisation of catering services leads to food being driven by price over value and quantity over quality. We need to turn this situation on its head as value and quality need to become the key drivers'.   (McCree, 2005)

It could be argued that the vending machine food provided is driven by demand, from patients, visitors and staff but as the latest *Consumer Attitudes to Food Standards* (Food Standards Agency, 2007a), shows that healthy eating is a key issue for consumers, perhaps a good example should be set at a time when there is this heightened awareness. However, with obesity levels at an all time high, what consumers admit to being concerned about and what they are actually prepared to do about it is probably another issue.

2.7   Events in 2007

In 2007 there has been a veritable hive of activity regarding patient nutrition with some of the organisations involved detailed below.

2.7.1   Royal College of Nursing (RCN)

The RCN has launched the campaign, *Nutrition Now* (RCN, 2007a) to improve patient nutrition in hospitals and the community. The campaign built on work that the RCN had undertaken in collaboration with the Government and other stakeholders. To launch the campaign a set of RCN *Principles for Nutrition and Hydration* (RCN, 2007a) were published, providing nurses with a set of basic guiding principles to be used to push forward and improve patient nutrition, stating that nutritional care should be prioritised at board level with systems in place for support. An online *Hospital Hydration Best Practice Toolkit* (RCN, 2007b) was also developed via partnerships involving nurses, patient groups and key stakeholders – including the RCN, the National Patient Safety Agency (NPSA), and Water UK, to improve water consumption by patients.

2.7.2   National Patient Safety Agency (NPSA)

NPSA released new data on patient safety incidents relating to nutrition and hydration in hospitals. This was based on a systematic review of 423 incidents relating to nutritional care as reported by healthcare staff: although 90% of incidents resulted in low or no harm to patients, 3 incidents resulted in death while a further 8 resulted in severe harm. Most reported deaths and incidences of severe harm related to patients receiving inappropriate meals or fluids (e.g. a glass of water being given to a patient with dysphagia[19]) or to poor intravenous fluid administration. Some of the cases involved patients' existing conditions being exacerbated and complicated by poor nutritional care (NPSA, 2007). Although NPSA acknowledged that approximately 400 000[20] meals are served safely across the NHS daily, *'poor nutrition and hydration are patient safety issues and it is vital that they are recognised as such'*.

The NPSA is currently building on an existing programme of work on dysphagia and working with speech and language therapists, nurses and catering providers in order to identify factors that contribute to patients choking. In association with NPSA and BAPEN, the RCN is also holding a programme of Nutrition workshops across England and Wales for nurses and other health professionals.

2.7.3   The Council of Europe Alliance (UK)

This Council represents Government and non-Government organisations across the UK who have an interest in nutritional care, including organisations such as NPSA, BDA, RCN, BAPEN, the British Medical Association (BMA), and the Hospital Caterers Association (HCA). They have produced *The 10 Key Characteristics for good nutritional care in hospitals* (NPSA, 2007), which was launched in October 2007, containing the following recommendations:

- All patients are screened on admission to identify the patients who are malnourished or at risk of becoming malnourished. All patients are re-screened weekly.
- All patients have a nutritional care plan which identifies their nutritional care needs and how they are to be met.
- The hospital includes specific guidance on food services and nutritional care in its Clinical Governance arrangements.
- Patients are involved in the planning and monitoring arrangements for food service provision.
- The ward implements Protected Mealtimes to provide an environment conducive to patients enjoying and being able to eat their food.
- All staff have the skills and competencies needed to ensure that patient's nutritional needs are met. All staff should receive regular training on nutritional care and management.
- Hospital facilities are designed to be flexible and patient centred with the aim of providing and delivering an excellent experience of food service and nutritional care 24 hours a day, every day.
- The hospital has a policy for food service and nutritional care which is patient centred and performance managed in line with home country governance frameworks.
- Food service and nutritional care are delivered to the patient safely.
- The hospital supports a multi-disciplinary approach to nutritional care and values the contribution of all staff groups working in partnership with patients and users.

The Chair of the Council of Europe Alliance (UK), Rick Wilson, said:

'All patients have a right to expect that their nutrition and hydration needs will be met when they are in hospital. For the first time we have broad agreement across all the caring professions and the relevant Government bodies on how this can be best achieved, this can only improve nutritional care for vulnerable patients in all our hospitals and caring institutions'. (NPSA, 2007)

2.7.4 British Association for Parenteral and Enteral Nutrition (BAPEN)

With reference to this 10 point 'Mission Statement', BAPEN welcomed the particular emphasis on the involvement of senior hospital management, the multi-disciplinary approach to and responsibility for malnutrition, screening for malnutrition for all on admission to hospital and the importance of sustainable and regular training for all staff in nutritional care, including screening (BAPEN, 2007b).

BAPEN have recently published *Organisation of Food and Nutritional Support in* Hospitals (OFNoSH)[21] (BAPEN, 2007c) whose purpose is to:

- Collate existing initiatives and drivers which are easily accessible
- Provide a framework for their implementation
- Consider where further advances can be made
- Provide an aspirational model for progressive improvements in the delivery of nutritional care in hospitals

From 25th to 27th September 2007, BAPEN undertook the first prospective national nutrition screening survey in the UK across both hospitals and community care settings (BAPEN, 2007d). Christine Russell, the BAPEN lead for Nutrition Screening Week, explained that it was not known how many people at risk of malnutrition were being admitted to hospital or care homes, with current data being over 10 years old and having used different criteria to define malnutrition. Based on MUST assessments (see Box 2.9, page 151) the resulting data would provide evidence for hospitals and care homes on the scale of the problems that need addressing, that is the number of patients and residents for whom a nutritional care plan should be provided (BAPEN, 2007d). Professor Marinos Elia, chair of BAPEN, commented:

'Malnutrition is preventable in the long run and if treated early can improve outcomes for patients ... treatment saves the NHS and social care systems money as the cost of treatment is small compared with the potential benefits to be gained'.   (BAPEN, 2007d)

National Screening Week (NSW) was undertaken in collaboration with the BDA and the RCN with support from the NPSA, DH, Welsh Assembly Government, Scottish Government and the Chief Nursing Officer in Northern Ireland. The results of the NSW were announced at the BAPEN conference, *Nutrition Matters* in November 2007 (BAPEN, 2007e) showing that the percentage of patients on different wards at risk of malnutrition were:

- 41% on oncology wards, 33% of those on care of the elderly wards, 31% on medical wards, 27% on surgical wards and 15% on orthopaedic wards

Patients at risk of malnutrition from various diagnosed conditions were:

- 42% patients with GI disease, 34% of those with disorders of the central nervous system, 33% of those with respiratory conditions, 24% of those with genito/renal disease, 22% of those with cardio-vascular disease, and 18% of those with musculo/skeletal conditions.

Age also had a bearing on the risk of malnutrition:

- 47% patients <65 years of age. In the age range <20–59 years malnutrition risk ranged from 22% to 30%
- 53% patients >65 years of age. In the age range 60–>90 years malnutrition risk ranged from 26% to 38%

BAPEN concluded that patients of all ages in hospital were at risk but there was a significant increase in risk with age.

2.7.5   Food Standards Agency (FSA)

The Food Standards Agency have published *Guidance on Food Served to Adults in Major Institutions* (FSA, 2007b), including hospitals. Example menus were provided for 'adult men aged to 19–74', which seems a rather extreme age range, but as the FSA point out:

'The guidance is not intended for those who may have different nutritional requirements due to illness or disease and are undernourished or at risk of under nutrition'.

This would seem to negate many of the hospitalised elderly population included in this age range and are probably the 'group' that the FSA describe as those 'outside the scope of this guidance'.

2.8   Hospital food Scotland

2.8.1   Audit Scotland

In its first review on hospital catering, Audit Scotland published *Catering for Patients* (Audit Scotland, 2003) which was based on data for 2001/02. It reported that each year, NHS Scotland (NHSS) provides approximately 28 million patient meals costing £55 million. Since 2000 the cost of total spending had increased by around 8% each year but spending on catering services had been reducing slightly each year with the catering services becoming a smaller proportion of overall NHSS spending. As with the England and Wales audit in 2001 (AC, 2001) this audit provided a valuable insight into how the catering service in Scotland operated.

2.8.1.1   *Total costs*

Budgets were set for the catering service as a whole, thereby including the patient service, staff meals and visitors' meals (non-patient catering).[22] This allowed any income generated from non-patient catering to be used to reduce the overall cost of the catering service. The largest proportion of the catering departments based their catering service budget on historical information, which generally meant increasing the cost element each year for inflation. This took account of pay rises and increases in the costs of food and beverages but not the variation in the number of meals produced or other changes such as revisions to the menu. To offset these increased costs, income generated targets were likely to be increased each year and may be set even higher to reduce the overall catering budget. Other catering departments based their budgets on target patient cost per patient week, daily food allowance and contract price.

2.8.1.2   Total gross cost

This included the cost of food and beverages, staffing, other indirect costs such as cleaning materials and a proportion of Trust overheads. Food and beverages and staff accounted to just over 90% of total gross profit.

2.8.1.3   Net costs per patient day

Net costs per patient day[23] ranged from £3.50 to £7.50 with the average cost being £5.50. Some of this variation was due to the level of income generated by non-patient catering services and the hospitals pricing policies. No relationship was found between cost and production type or patient satisfaction.

2.8.1.4   Patient catering services

The lack of control over the costs of the catering service was highlighted by the fact that only a third of the hospitals were able to split the costs of the catering service between patient and non-patient activities. For example, if a daily food allowance was set most hospitals would be unable to calculate whether they were meeting this allowance. Around 40% of hospitals had set a daily food allowance but did not appear to be using it properly, for example, only half were using this to calculate the budget required for the catering service.

The cost of patients' food and beverages varied significantly ranging from around £1.25 to over £3.00 per patient day. These variations did not necessarily mean better or worse ingredients which were purchased through national contracts meaning that costs varied only marginally. The variations in costs could be as a result of the quantity of ingredients used in production, poor portion control or food waste.

2.8.1.5   Non-patient catering services

Most hospitals provided non-patient catering services for staff and visitors via dining rooms and vending machines, and hospitality for meeting and events. Some had extended the service by operating shops and cafes and providing catering for external functions such as parties and supplying meals to non-NHS bodies, for example, police stations and local care homes. The income from non-patient services was generally used to offset the cost to the catering service: 84% of catering departments had set income generation targets allowing catering managers to manage their budgets effectively. It was noted that income from non-patient services should at least cover the costs of non-patient catering and where possible should contribute to the cost of the patient service unless a Trust had a clear written policy on subsidising staff meals. In this situation a target level of subsidy would be set and monitored. It was normal to have a separate pricing policy for staff and visitors with the latter being charged higher prices. All the hospitals had pricing policies in place but in the main they were following a pricing policy that was originally set in 1978 which stated that staff prices should be set at provisions cost, plus 50%, plus VAT: this was unlikely to recover all of the costs associated with providing a non-patient catering service. Thus the income generated from non-patient catering rarely covered the costs of the service. Approximately three-quarters were subsidising their non-patient catering services, most unknowingly, with the level of contribution or subsidy achieved ranging from an annual contribution of £118 000 to a subsidy of £266 000. The average hospital subsidy was around £110 000 per annum and the cost to NHS Scotland was approximately £4.2 million per year.

2.8.1.6 Service providers

Eighty per cent of catering service providers were in-house teams. As a result of a Private Finance initiative/Public Private Partnership deal or as a direct result of market testing of the service, the remaining 20% of the hospitals provided catering services through the use of private contractors.

2.8.1.7 Production methods

The production methods used are shown in Figure 2.6.

2.8.1.8 Meal delivery service

The different methods of meal delivery service were hybrid 29%, bulk 34% and plated 37%.

2.8.1.9 Menus and choice

The majority of Trusts undertook a formal menu-planning process but compliance with the principles of menu planning varied. In addition, 86% of Trusts

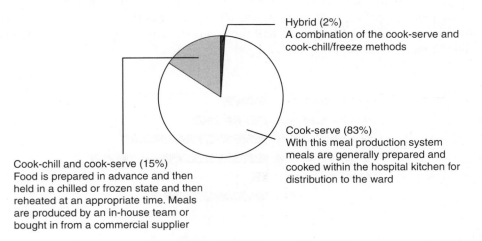

Figure 2.6 Percentage of hospitals using the different methods of production. *Source*: Audit Scotland (2003).

had nutritionally analysed menus but the extent of the analysis varied considerably with one in five Trusts not having standard recipes in place, viewed as fundamental to the whole process of providing nutritionally analysed food to patients. Around three in five catering specifications did not fully comply with the model nutritional guidelines for catering specifications in the public sector in Scotland as recommended in *Eating for Health – a Diet Action Plan for Scotland* (Scottish Office, 1996).

All long-stay hospitals had at least a three-week menu cycle in line with recommended good practice. Three quarters of acute hospitals were operating at least a three-week menu cycle with the remaining acute hospitals operating a two-week cycle.

Ninety-eight per cent of hospitals had at least two main meal choices from the menu at each mealtime with many offering alternatives such as salads and sandwiches. There was a limited choice for vegetarians, patients on therapeutic diets and for patients with eating or swallowing difficulties: in some cases there was only one choice available for these types of diets and in others these meals were not available on the menu but had to be requested by patients and ward staff. All the hospitals had arrangements in place to offer meals to minority ethnic patients but often staff were not aware of this provision. Nearly all the menus provided an accurate, easily understandable description of dishes with the majority providing a range of portion sizes. Eighty-three per cent of menus were coded for special dietary needs, allowing some patients to choose a suitable meal.

2.8.1.10   *Ordering and delivery of patient meals*

Only 43% of hospitals were operating a system that allowed patients to order their meals no more than two meals in advance with 17% operating an 'other' ordering system (see Figure 2.7). It was often dictated by the patient group itself: acute patients ordered 48 hours in advance whilst elderly patients' meals were ordered one week in advance. In half the hospitals, 10% or more of the patients did not receive the meal they had ordered.

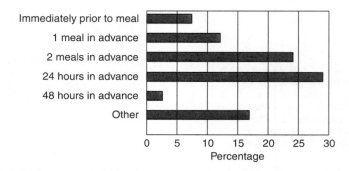

Figure 2.7   Advance ordering of patient meals. *Source*: Audit Scotland (2003).

2.8.1.11   Out of hours service

Most hospitals operated fixed meal times. All the hospitals had kitchens at ward level where snacks could be prepared for patients. Three quarters were able to provide snacks from hospital kitchens outside meal times.

2.8.1.12   Patient satisfaction

Sixty-nine per cent of Trusts carried out patient-satisfaction surveys, with the frequency varying considerably from one month to every two years. The remaining Trusts obtained patients' views from other sources such as comment cards, informing staff or via the formal complaints procedure. Patient satisfaction levels were generally high ranging from 74% to 100% with an average satisfaction level of 92%. All of the private contractors undertook their own regular monitoring of the catering service with around half of the Trusts using patient groups or the local health council to obtain the views of patients and give an independent view on the quality of the service.

2.8.1.13   Quality of meals

An independent survey on the quality of patient meals in each hospital scored against taste, texture, aroma, temperature, appearance, portion size and correct item being delivered, supported the high satisfaction scores from the patient survey with the results ranging from 81% to 99%.

As with other studies discussed earlier, no relationship was found between patient satisfaction levels and the cost of the service or the service provider.

2.8.1.14   Nutritional screening

Around 70% of Trusts had a validated nutritional screening tool in place. A further 10% were screening patients for risk of undernutrition but were using a screening tool that had not been validated for the patient group, meaning that 20% of Trusts did not have an effective nutritional screening tool.

2.8.2   Standards and assessment

In 2003 NHS Quality Improvement Scotland (NHS QIS) published *Clinical Standards for Food, Fluid and Nutritional Care in Hospitals* (NHSQIS, 2003).
There are six standards:[24]

- Standard 1. Policy & Strategy: Each NHS Board has a policy and a strategic and co-ordinated approach, to ensure that all patients in hospitals have food and fluid delivered effectively and receive a high quality of nutritional care.
- Standard 2. Assessment, Screening and Care Planning: When a person is admitted to hospital an assessment is carried out. Screening for risk of undernutrition is undertaken both on admission and on an ongoing basis. A care plan is developed, implemented and evaluated.

- Standard 3. Planning and Delivery of Food and Fluid: These are formalised structures and processes in place to plan the provision and delivery of food and fluid.
- Standard 4. Provision of Food and Fluid to Patients: Food and fluid are provided in a way that is acceptable to patients.
- Standard 5. Patient Information and Communication: Patients have the opportunity to discuss and are given information about their nutritional care, food and fluid. Patient views are sought and inform decisions made about the nutritional care, food and fluid provided.
- Standard 6. Education and Training for Staff: Staff are given appropriate education and training about nutritional care, food and fluid.

Between June 2005 and February 2006 performance assessment reviews were undertaken (NHSQIS, 2006). It was agreed that three of the standards (1, 2 and 6) would be assessed during the first round based on the fact that the complete six standards 'represented a formidable challenge to implement' with the chosen three representing 'the bedrock on which the other standards rest' (McKinley, 2006):

- Standard 1 provided the strategic direction for the implementation and achievement of the national standards
- Standard 2 was critical in terms of frontline patient care
- Standard 6 needed to be in place to ensure staff were provided with the appropriate education and training to effectively carry out assessment, screening and care planning

The results of the resulting review were varied:

Standard 1

- All the NHS boards had started work on a nutritional care policy but their objectives had not been implemented.
- Many of the NHS boards were using complex feeding techniques but did not have access to a clinical nutritional support team.

Standard 2

- Most NHS boards were actively developing assessment, screening and care planning.
- The current wording of the standard did not fully reflect the local dimension of identifying malnutrition.

Standard 6

- At a local level (ward/department) training and education had been in place for some time.

- There was little evidence that additional training and education in nutritional care was a priority within national undergraduate and postgraduate medical training, notable in relation to complex nutritional techniques.

In conclusion it was stated:

'What we do not have yet is a co-ordinated approach that is risk-assessed and proportionate across whole organisations and, as a result, we are not making the best use of what we have. Nor are we getting the best outcome for patients, particularly for the increasing number of older people admitted to hospital as well as for those with complex nutritional needs'.

At a public meeting there was criticism of progress to date, concluding that as better nutritional care was part of the patients' basic care, 'a system that tolerates poor quality meals or provides insufficient staff to allow patients to receive help at mealtimes' was not understood (McKinley, 2006).

Overall, it seems that the standards themselves focus on the issues of malnutrition with the actual quality of food not in evidence with a follow up report in 2006 on *Catering for Patients* (Audit Scotland) stating:

'catering services are offering patients an inproved level of choice but boards still need to do more to ensure patients' nutritional care'

Currently, a programme of work on food, fluid and nutrition is being prepared in conjunction with other agencies. It is too early to say what it will encompass but it is anticipated that a further round of reviews against the standard in 2008/09 will form part of the work (private email NHS QIS).

2.9   Hospital food – Wales

2.9.1   Reports

In 2001 in *Improving Health in Wales* (National Assembly), it was stated that specifications for hospital catering would be established and monitored on a regular basis. Patient satisfaction surveys would include questions on hospital food for Trust Boards to evaluate with prospectuses, including results of annual catering reviews. In addition, hospital nutrition teams would report on the adequacy of food and the quality of service and develop a nutritional study to develop policy and practice.

In the same year, 106 (of 126) hospitals in Wales were involved in a study – *Food and catering policies in NHS hospitals in Wales* (Paisley & Tudor-Smith, 2001) which investigated food provision, with respect to the DH 1995 *Nutrition Guidelines for Hospital Catering* (DH, 1995) and the 1997 *National Standard for Hospital Caterers* (Health Promotion Wales) The results are summarised below.

2.9.1.1 Policy production

Of the 96 hospitals for which a catering manager questionnaire was completed, 96% had a food and catering policy, of which 92% were written. Responsibility for developing policies was said to lie mainly with Trusts (77%) but in practice 92% of policies were developed by the hospital without a representative from the Trust or Health Authority management. Responsibility for monitoring the implementation of policies lay mainly within the Trusts (76%) with two thirds (68%) of policies being formally approved by Trust Boards.

This high percentage of Trusts with a food and catering policy was seen to reflect recommendations but the lack of approval from Trust boards was something that needed to be addressed to ensure that policies met the requirements of the patients as stated in the guidelines (Health Promotion Wales, 1997).

2.9.1.2 Catering arrangements

In all, 70% of hospitals carried out their own catering with 35% also catering for other hospitals. Almost half used the cook-freeze method. On average hospitals catered for 117 patients and 170 staff per day (ranging from 12 to 920 patients and 4 to 800 staff). All policies covered meals for patients while most covered meals supplied to staff (91%). Other sources of available food such as cafes, food trolley services, sandwich person and vending machines were not present in less than half the hospitals. These outlets were generally well covered by the food and catering policy with the exception of cafes run by outside organisations. There was concern that there was no information available on the usage of these outlets by patients which impacted on their food intake.

2.9.1.3 Food production

All policies included the monitoring of food production – food stock management, food hygiene standards, storage of food, cooking methods, temperature of food, delivery of food to hospital and wards and quality control procedures. With the exception of food stock management, monitoring occurred in most hospitals daily.

2.9.1.4 Menu planning

The different aspects of menu planning included in policies varied only slightly from 99% of policies including menu planning involving a State Registered Dietitian to 89% including menu planning to provide required daily energy intake for patients. In practice, these different aspects of menu planning most frequently took place 'always' or 'often', rather than 'sometimes', 'rarely' or 'never'.

2.9.1.5   Monitoring of patients

Monitoring of patients' food and fluids intake was included in policy in less than half of hospitals. Although, in practice, the extent of monitoring appeared to be greater than half indicated by policy content, on most aspects, daily monitoring took place in less than half of hospitals. Nurses were responsible for keeping records of patients' food and fluid intake in all cases, being solely responsible in approximately three quarters of hospitals. In less than 20% of hospitals, a State Registered Dietitian was responsible for keeping records. This lack of monitoring of patients' food and fluids intake both in policy documents and practice was seen as a main area of concern and seemed to be on par with other findings related to malnutrition in hospitals.

2.9.1.6   Meals and repetition

The monitoring of repetition of main meals was part of the policy in 82% of hospitals. In practice, 59% monitored practice with 21% doing so daily. The average length of the menu cycle was 15–21 days (45% of hospitals) with 36% having a cycle of 8–14 days. Overall, 37% repeated main course dishes every 15–21 days with 52% repeating main dishes every 8–14 days. This latter point was not in line with the recommendations that main dishes should not be repeated within 14 days but it was also unclear how close meal repetition was to the 14-day recommendation due to the grouped nature of the findings. Meal repetition could also have been related to the average length of patient stay, for which further information was required.

On average, menu choices were made three meals in advance (44%). This again, was not in line with recommendations which suggested no more than two meals in advance. In 67% of hospitals, new patients were given the menu choice of a previous patient and if a patient who ordered food missed their mealtime they would always or often be given a snack (63%), an alternative meal (60%) the ordered meal when they were ready (24%) or no meal or snack (19%). On average breakfast was served at 8 a.m., lunch at 12.10 p.m., the evening meal at 5.30 p.m. and a bedtime meal or snack at 8.30 p.m. The timing of meals showed that many patients experienced a gap of more than twelve hours between the evening meal and breakfast which concurred with other research findings.

2.9.1.7   Staff training

The provision of training in food serving and food preparation for catering staff and assessment of patients' nutritional requirements for nurses, either annually or at some stage during their employment was lower in practice for nursing than for catering staff, which reflected policy. The researchers pointed out that this lack of training was not conducive to the key role of a nurse which is to 'ensure that patients' nutritional needs are met'. In addition, their perceived inability or willingness to carry out this assessment and monitoring could also be affected by their time constraints and perceptions of this role. It was recommended that other ward staff could support the nurses in this area.

2.9.1.8 Health promotion

Over 95% of catering managers stated that their policies promoted healthy eating or eating for health,[25] the consumption of five portions of fruit and vegetables a day and a low fat intake: 73% of hospitals offered patients a daily low fat option (48% labelling the option as low fat) and 71% a daily healthy option (42% labelled). This was seen as 'encouraging'. The caterers' use of low fat options was lower than the use of other healthy options. Over 95% of hospitals made the following items available for patients 'every day or most days':

- A vegetarian option at lunch or evening meal
- A cold meal or salad option at lunch or evening meal
- Low fat milk
- Five portions of fruit and vegetables per day

The following options 'were always' available to patients:

- Wholemeal or brown bread rather than white
- Polyunsaturated spread rather than butter or margarine
- Jacket or boiled potatoes rather than chips
- Brown rather than white rice or pasta

The study concluded that efforts towards improvement in hospital catering appeared to focus on production systems rather than food choices and patients' intake.

In 2002 the Audit Commission report *Food for Thought in hospital catering in Wales* (AC, 2002) revealed that:

- 80% of the hospitals surveyed had developed tools to assess patients dietary needs
- Dietitians were commonly involved in menu planning
- There were encouraging examples of flexible, ward-based careering services being introduced

However the report also said that best practice needed to be more widely applied, with more scope for improvement required in several important areas:

- Three quarters of Welsh hospitals did not systematically screen patients on admission to identify their nutritional needs
- Waste food from unserved meals cost the NHS in Wales almost £1 million a year with a significant number wasting 10% or more of the meals they produced
- Patients missed out on meals by, for example, not being given assistance, or arriving on wards outside set meal times

- Only one third of hospitals were routinely using standard costed recipes to ensure consistency of quality and cost
- Nearly three quarters were subsidising the catering service provided to staff and visitors, but only 1 in 5 had set a target for contributions from non-patient services

At the time of the report, NHS in Wales spent over £20 million a year on hospital catering, producing in excess of 16 million meals.

2.9.2 Standards

In 2005, a total of thirty-two Healthcare Standards for Wales, with four domains were published by the Welsh Assembly Government (WAG, 2005a). Under the umbrella of the First Domain – The Patient Experience, is Standard 9 which states that: Where food is provided there are systems in place to ensure that:

(a) patients and service users are provided with a choice of food which is prepared safely and provides a balanced diet
(b) patients and service users' individual nutritional, personal, cultural and clinical dietary requirements are met, including any necessary help with feeding and having access to food 24 hours a day.

In 2007 every Local Health Board, NHS Trust and Health Commission Wales completed a self-assessment against the standards, together with an annual public declaration of how they had performed, which were submitted to the Health Inspectorate Wales (HIW) for testing and validation. In the publication *How Good is the NHS in Wales?* (HIW, 2007) key issues were addressed: in relation to food, the question to be answered was: *Is the food good, readily available and appropriate assistance given when needed?* The results were as follows:

- The quality and choice of meals was not consistent across all NHS organisations
- Protected meal times had been introduced on many wards but in some cases this has been applied too rigorously, for example, speech and language therapists who needed to review the swallowing reflexes of some patients were not allowed on the wards at meal times.
- Some Trusts had introduced a colour-coded tray system, which easily identified those patients who needed assistance to help them to eat. Again, these practices were not consistent across all organisations.
- Dieticians were attached to some wards and provided individual advice on what patients could and should not eat, with good instances of innovative approaches to encourage patients to eat
- 24-hour access to food was limited, although most wards were able to provide snacks such as toast, bread and spreads

- For those patients with specific dietary or cultural needs, choice was even more limited. Some Trusts were tackling this, for example by introducing menus for specific ethnic groups
- As part of their self-assessment, the majority of Local Health Boards, indicated that they considered Standard 9 only appropriate to provider organisations

This latter point was a concern to the HIW because they felt that Commissioners should be ensuring that provider organisations had arrangements in place to meet the dietary and nutritional requirements of their patient population, thereby ensuring that that the whole patient experience was a good one.

By the end of November 2007, every NHS organisation in Wales was also required to publish a Healthcare Standards Improvement Plan.

2.9.3   Sustainability

With regards to sustainability, in 2005 it was announced that Welsh hospitals would be 'dishing up Welsh beef' thanks to a deal worth around £750 000, supported by the Welsh Assembly Government's Procurement Initiative, Hybu Cig Cymru (Meat Promotion Wales) working closely with NHS Trusts. It was reported that one of the Welsh Assembly Government's top priorities was to encourage hospitals to purchase more Welsh produce, thereby reducing food miles, cutting carbon emissions and ensuring that patients were served high-quality meat (WAG, 2005b).

2.10   Hospital food – Northern Ireland

2.10.1   Assessment

In 2001/2002, the Department of Health, Social Services and Public Safety commissioned auditors to carry out a value for money study of catering services. The study was based on the Acute Hospital Portfolio developed by the Audit Commission. Data were collected for 2000/2001 from fifteen catering departments in eleven Trusts providing acute services (DHSSP, 2003). The results were as below.

2.10.1.1   Total costs

These included provisions and beverages, staff costs and other indirect costs such as uniforms, cutlery and central overheads. Portering and transport costs had been excluded. The net cost was obtained by deducting the income received from the non-patient catering services from the total cost. The total net cost per patient day ranged from £4.21 to £10.56 with the variations explained by:

- Economies of scale, with larger departments potentially able to achieve lower costs
- The level of income generated from non-patient services
- The Trusts' pricing policy

Costs could also be increased by the provision of specialist services catering for patients with more complex needs, often requiring more flexible meals and greater supplements.

2.10.1.2 Patient provision costs

These included all food and beverages provided to patients, which varied from £1.26 to £2.75, the variations arising from the quality of ingredients, effective purchasing or good control of raw materials in the production process. A comparatively low spend may have indicated that a department was unlikely to provide the range of meals and snacks to meet the needs of patients. The departments that had low patient provision costs were still able to provide sufficient menu choice.

2.10.1.3 Non-patient services

Generally, income generated from providing meals for non-patients was retained within the catering department and used to offset the cost of the service. Any shortfall had to be subsidised and any excess income could make a contribution to the cost of providing the patient meal service. Having considered its overall priorities, it was up to the Trust to decide whether non-patient services should make a contribution or be subsidised. Many Trusts could not reliably split costs between patient and non-patient services.

2.10.1.4 Quality

This was assessed by reviewing if patients were satisfied by the service received and the number of complaints received by the department on catering. The benchmark for performance was as in *Delivering a Quality Service* (National Health Service Executive) (discussed on page 130). The average score on food quality and service from the satisfaction survey was 8.0 with only two departments not meeting the 70% target.

2.10.1.5 Nutrition

* 40% of departments had a ward nutritional screening tool in place, with five departments actually carrying out ward nutritional screening and four performing the task on a weekly basis.
* At five sites dietitians were unable to see all referred patients
* At all but five sites audits were conducted on the meal service and nutrition
* Dietitians at eight departments considered that there was sufficient menu choice
* At twelve sites dietitians checked the menus for nutritional adequacy

2.10.1.6 Daily food allowance

Ninety-three per cent had set a daily food budget per patient day with thirteen sites actively monitoring the daily food expenditure, 67% fully and 20% partially.

2.10.1.7   Non-patient subsidy/contribution

Eleven of the sites had set a non-patient catering contribution/subsidy and 40% monitored the actual level achieved.

2.10.1.8   Standard costed recipes

Forty-seven per cent had standard costed recipes in place.

2.10.1.9   Computerised catering system

There were computerised catering systems in use in nine of the sites with a further three sites having systems partially in place.

2.10.1.10   Wastage

Seventy-three per cent monitored ward wastage, 60% fully and 13% partially. 87% monitored dining room wastage but only 33% performed this fully. The bulk service method tended to produce more waste but conclusions could not be drawn about the effective method of service delivery based on wastage results alone as cost and quality of the service also had to be considered. Where waste levels were high, poor performance could be the result of either over-production or over-ordering. It could also result from providing a greater choice of meals for patients.

2.10.2   Future plans

In 2007, it was announced in the House of Lords, that a review on the DHPSS[26] catering operations would be completed by November 2007 taking forward the development of the DHPSS catering strategy by March 2008. In addition an assessment of the DHPSS position against 'essence of care' with regard to the Council of Europe (discussed below) statement on hospital food and nutrition would be completed by 30th November 2007 and lead to the exploration of appropriate initiatives to improve nutritional standards by 31st March 2008 (Written Answers, 2007a).

2.11   Hospital food – Europe

2.11.1   Council of Europe

The Council of Europe determined to collect information regarding nutrition programmes in hospitals via a European network established in 1999, consisting of national experts from Austria, Belgium, Cyprus, Denmark, Finland, France, Germany, Ireland, Italy, Luxembourg, the Netherlands, Norway, Portugal,

Table 2.15   Specific non-prioritised problems in European hospitals.

Country	Main problems with regard to food service and nutritional care and support
Denmark	Low priority, inflexible food service systems, unsatisfactory eating conditions and environments
Finland	No systematic arrangement, information, follow-up and evaluation
France	Lack of dieticians, lack of national guidelines, lack of interest and low priority
Germany	No adequate recognition of the problem. Lack of dieticians and nutritional support teams
Italy	Inadequate recognition of the problem, low priority, unsatisfactory eating conditions and environments, lack of national guidelines, lack of expertise, and lack of nutritional support teams in most hospitals
Netherlands	Inadequate recognition of the problem, lack of interest and low (financial) priority
Norway	Lack of dieticians, lack of implementation of national guidelines, low priority and lack of time
Portugal	Inflexible food service systems, lack of expertise, organisational and staff constraints, lack of national guidelines and perceived low quality of hospital food
Slovenia	Low priority, lack of interest and time
Sweden	Lack of staff, reduced length of stay and lack of expertise (including the primary health care sector)
Switzerland	Lack of dieticians and nutritional support teams, lack of national guidelines
UK	Inadequate recognition of the problem, inflexible food service systems and perceived low quality of hospital food

Source: Beck *et al.* (2003) The European View of Hospital Undernutrition.

Slovenia, Spain, Sweden, Switzerland and the UK, chaired by Denmark. Their aim was to:

- Review the current practice in Europe regarding hospital food provision to patients prone to develop, or suffering from disease-related undernutrition and highlight deficiencies in the current food service systems.
- Issue recommendations which ensure that assessment of nutritional status and requirements, hospital food and nutrition support and monitoring are regarded as important and necessary components of patient care.
- To consider how national authorities of food service representatives, healthcare personnel and hospital managers might work together to improve the nutritional care and support of hospitalised patients

Each participating European country was asked to indicate the main (non-prioritised) problem with respect to undernutrition in hospitals (see Table 2.15). Five of these problems were common in most/all countries (Beck *et al.*, 2001):

- Lack of clearly defined responsibilities in planning and managing nutritional care
- Lack of sufficient education level with regard to nutrition among all staff groups
- Lack of influence and knowledge of the patients

- Lack of co-operation between different staff groups
- Lack of involvement from the hospital management

In November 2003, the Council of Europe's resolution on food and nutritional care in hospitals made over 100 recommendations for improvement contained within the following headings:

- Nutritional assessment and treatment in hospitals e.g., easy to use screening method, evidence based.
- Nutritional care providers e.g., distribution of responsibilities, communication, education and nutrition knowledge at all levels.
- Food service practices e.g., food policy, guidelines and standards for out sourcing, eating environment.
- Hospital food e.g., monitoring of food intake, nutrient content, portion sizes and food wastage audited annually.
- Health economics e.g., cost effectiveness and cost–benefit considerations, food service and food wastage costs.
- Definitions e.g., artificial nutritional support, nutritional steering committee, food service and hospital food.

It was recommended that the governments of the member states should:

- Draw up and implement national recommendations on food and nutritional care in hospitals based on the principles and measures of the resolution.
- Promote the implementation and take steps towards the application of the principles and measures contained in the resolution in fields where these are not the direct responsibility of governments but where public authorities have a certain power or play a role.
- Ensure the widest possible dissemination of this resolution among all parties concerned, particularly public authorities, hospital staff, primary health care sector, patients, researchers and non-governmental organisations active in this field.

Discussions took place with stakeholder groups, including the British Dietetic Association, and the Health Caterers Association to establish the most effective strategies regarding the Council of Europe's recommendations (private email DH).

2.11.2   European Nutrition for Health Alliance (ENHA)

With reference to the Council of Europe's declaration, the project *Nutrition Day* (ENHA, 2008), was launched in Europe in 2007, to 'move the political declaration to reality'. It was organised by ENHA and was the first project whereby patients and caregivers in hospitals, amongst other settings, were interviewed in more than 30 countries. The results of *Nutrition Day* showed that:

- 47% of the patients had been hospitalised with signs of disease-related malnutrition. Only one out of three patients (38%) eat all that they have been served with the consequence that the length of stay is increased by six days.

- One in five patients ate less than a quarter of their food or nothing. Only 11% of those eating very little indicated that they did not like the food. The majority (47%) had no appetite with some suffering from nausea (14%). This was reportedly due to illness or just being in hospital.

The next Nutrition Day was held in January 2008.

Also in 2007, it was reported that although a few countries and institutions had made some progress in establishing systems and policies to prevent malnutrition, 'this is still a complex issue that remains poorly understood and considered of little relevance to most European countries' (ENHA, 2007). In addition, although solutions did exist which would reduce healthcare expenditures and most importantly improve the quality of care and clinical outcomes, they were not currently being implemented even though they were part of the Council of Europe declaration.

2.11.3   The Prague Declaration

'Against this background', the European Society for Clinical Nutrition and Metabolism (ESPEN), the Medical Nutrition International Industries (MNI) the European Nutrition for Health Alliance (ENHA) and the members and partners of these organisations joined forces to fight malnutrition in Europe. In the Prague Declaration (ENHA, 2007), they called upon EU institutions – the European Parliament, the European Commission and the European Council of Ministers, and national governments, providers of health services and other relevant bodies to:

- Acknowledge that malnutrition and obesity are both results of poor nutrition with significant consequences for health outcomes and healthcare expenditures.
- Recognise malnutrition as a distinct pathology and its nutritional support as an integral part of each medical treatment.
- Affirm that access to proper nutritional care and support is a fundamental human right.
- Offer political direction and support for all stakeholders involved in the fight against malnutrition.
- Provide coherent reimbursement policy for nutritional support across health and social care systems.
- Develop nutrition care plans for all healthcare settings and promote the implementation of existing solutions to fight malnutrition for the benefit of patients, healthcare systems and society.

As has been reported the issues around malnutrition are not confined to the UK. With these problems being recognised at an international level, policy will hopefully move forward, providing the myriad of red tape and yet more reports aren't allowed to cloud the issues.

2.12   Conclusion

This chapter has attempted to unravel the maze of events that have made hospital food what it is today. Currently, from procurement to delivery it is a complex system involving a 'food chain' (SETHRA, 1993b) of many individuals whose objective should be 'better hospital food'.

The procurement process is often restricted by funding constraints with complex rules and regulations that in themselves can be daunting (NAO, 2006) with pressure on Trusts to develop sustainable food procurement programmes. Therefore, hospitals that have made a success story of this issue should be congratulated on their performance as it takes dedication from a team of people who actually think it matters:

> *'there are many instances of very good practices that can be replicated, it's very easy to focus on the negative, but we have to look to the likes of the Royal Brompton, Royal Cornwall, Nottingham – islands of best practice in a sea of mediocrity'.*   (Email Rosie Blackburn, Sustain)

In many cases, it requires expertise from trained individuals and funding to employ them, as demonstrated in the example set in Cornwall (Russell, 2007). Whether or not this example is transferable is debatable. However, the London-based Hospital Food Project has shown that a hospital's location need not be a barrier but, again, without assistance it might not have been possible: the London Project was funded by the Department for the Environment, Food and Rural Affairs (Defra) under the England Rural Development Programme and European Guidance Fund. It is co-ordinated by Sustain in partnership with the Soil Association. The King's Fund also provided a grant and has been 'generous with its expertise' (Hockridge & Longfield, 2005).

There is also the issue of new hospitals being built without kitchens and as the Catering Services Manager for the Royal Brompton Hospital said, this means that:

> *'somebody in South Wales, for instance, is producing the food for patients in London. That may save money short term but in the long run I don't think we're doing anything for peoples health'.*   (Cole, 2008)

Therefore, presuming the procurement has been successful and the menus are available on the wards, the patients now actually have to select their food: what individuals choose to eat in normal circumstances is a complex matter, influenced by the food's appearance, aroma, taste and texture but will be determined by the actual 'liking of the food'. Other factors include the consumer's own attitudes, seen as far more important than perceived social pressure, for example, concerns about the nutritional benefits of food with habits often over-riding other aspects (Shepherd, 1990). In addition there is the link between food and mood, when, for example, a cup of coffee can provide a boost or be associated with a positive social event such as meeting a friend or items such as chocolate which are often associated with feelings of pleasure (Geary, 2004). Other contributing factors for food choices are the external and social environment in which the choice is made (Shepherd, 1990) and this could be where the choosing of hospital food is so problematic: it is unnatural to have to choose all one's meals for the next day or beyond, anticipate appetite requirements – 'I could do with a snack' – and perhaps be bored enough to be deliberating about mealtimes which become important markers throughout a long day, making food an exaggerated focus with exaggerated expectations. As noted back in 1990:

> 'There is much emphasis on pre production and production systems of patient feeding but this is probably because they can honed and quantified whilst patients suffer all the vagaries and contradictions which are common to the human condition'.   (Kipps & Middleton, 1990a)

Thus, the NHS is trying to provide food to a diverse population who are in these unfamiliar surroundings and eating in this unnatural environment. It must be a logistical nightmare. It would be impossible to please all of the people all of the time but even if the food is not the food of natural choice it should conform to a certain standard, served with quality ingredients: if patients are judging food by its appearance, that is very different to what they will or won't eat, despite having made their choice. As one patient recently commented:

> 'At lunchtime the chicken soup was yellow with orange dots, lukewarm and served in a polystyrene cup ... why do they do that? ... wouldn't do it at home'.   (Interview with former inpatient, November 2007)

The quality of the food, coupled with its efficient delivery, is paramount if the food is to benefit patients holistically. The efficiency of this delivery is the link in the hospital food chain which, in many instances, could be the link that is sometimes broken: even if the food is suitably tempting and, hopefully nutritious, this can be lost in the actual food service. Who is to 'blame' here? A 2005 survey (Savage & Scott, 2005) reported that in some hospitals domestic staff played a central role in food regeneration and service and although ostensibly part of the ward team they were only marginally responsible to ward managers as they were employed by an external contractor. This could lead to a fragmentation of the service as it was difficult to get service level agreements which spelled out staff responsibilities in detail regarding for example, how food should be served. This meant that domestic workers might know which supplies like condiments or cutlery were running low but it was not in the service agreement for domestics to ensure that supplies were available – this was a nursing responsibility because these supplies come out of the nursing budget. Furthermore, in some instances, there was a high turnover of domestic staff which impacted on the quality of the food service.

As one patient recently noted:

'The nursing staff were exemplary in their attitude, unlike the catering staff. The one in charge of the ward kitchen could barely look anyone in the face and grunted when spoken to, not at all welcoming. She also sat eating something out of a plastic bag ... is that allowed? ... I wouldn't have dared asked a question ... in the afternoon she would bang down the water jugs as if doing us all a favour and rolled her eyes when somebody asked for more ice on a very warm afternoon'.   (Interview with former inpatient, November 2007)

There surely is no excuse for this kind of attitude and it should not be taken as the norm: the 2005 survey also reported that in other 'parts of the Trust' domestics were employed by the NHS and were well integrated into ward teams, taking pride in their work even though they were paid less for the same work with poorer conditions of work (Savage & Scott, 2005).

Any negative attitudes, no matter how unacceptable, could be fuelled by the fact that 'HCA members feel undervalued, underpaid and under-resourced' (Kemp, 2005), with the reasoning behind this outlined further:

'... and I can honestly tell you that there are people out there thirsting to come into our industry provided they get the right money. And if you've got staff employed on minimum wages using archaic kit then we're not going to attract the right people into the industry particularly in the NHS area and we're not going to keep our employees working there. So it is about cash. It is about investing inpatient care and hospital care and a holistic approach'.   (Kemp, 2005)

This might explain why, with the high cost of living, it has been suggested that the delivery of food and food services in London hospitals is different because one of the difficulties is recruiting and retaining an experienced well trained workforce (DH, 2004c).

The food chain could have been strengthened by the introduction of ward housekeepers and modern matrons who were supposed to address catering and nutritional issues but the quality of food and/or its delivery has not necessarily improved. This is mainly due to the disparities in how their roles are viewed (May & Smith, 2003; Read & Ashman, 2004) and the differing funding priorities amongst the Trusts (Read & Ashman, 2004; Savage & Scott, 2005). However, in some hospitals there are single wards making a difference to issues of catering and nutrition, yet again due to a determination to make that difference, with examples of sterling work by some Ward Housekeepers (Richmond, 2007), modern matrons (DH, 2003), and one particular multidisciplinary team, formed to share specific nutritional concerns, creating a new role to address the problem (Hayward, 2003).

Dietitians also have their part to play in the food chain with approximately two thirds of the British Dietetic Association membership employed in the NHS. Their role is often seen as science-based, being 'uniquely qualified to translate scientific information about food into practical dietary advice' (BDA, 2007).

However, since the 1960s there have been reported tensions between dietitians and caterers which were still found to be evident in a study in 2000 (Donelan, 2000) when it was recognised that although both groups were clearly very different they both demonstrated attributes of professionalism: in being considered 'professional' by both peer and lay groups, dietetics had achieved more success than catering maybe because of their regulated qualifications compared to the caterers 'diverse routes of training' within the umbrella of the service industry:

'Why we never placed caterers, new assistants, supervisors, etc., to shadow dietitians in the same way as they did with catering, I'll never know. Of course, with dietitians as students, they have to do it and be assessed on it. But no damn reason why we shouldn't have done it unofficially ourselves. Perhaps and induction, two to three days'. (Caterer)

It was also suggested that there were 'constraints and barriers' because both dietitians and caterers worked within different working environments, worked with a 'divergent calibre of staff and colleagues' and had different status within health care. As has been noted:

'... I think this is now a habit ... the expectation that dietitians and caterers are not going to get on and therefore they fulfil that expectation ...' (Dietitian)

'... I do think we are poles apart I must admit ... they [dietitians] come from an ideal world, 18g of protein and all that. As a caterer, I think that, as long as the patient eats something, that's important ...' (Caterer)

However, although this apparent gulf should not be taken as the norm, there was clearly an indication that problems of attitude do exist. It was expected that these attitudes could impact on the 'path to optimal patient feeding' which could only be realised through 'mutual aspirations'.

From a scientific viewpoint, dietitians involvement in menu planning should assure the nutritional content of the food in the planning stages but what happens to that nutritional content during the subsequent cooking and delivery is not assured. Let it be hoped that, as anticipated, the effective implementation of their toolkit as demonstrated in *Delivering Nutritional Care Through Food and Beverage Services* 'has the potential to really make a difference to the nutritional status of our patients in hospital' (BDA, 2006).

Another link in the food chain are nurses, with their role in hospital food being the subject of much debate. On one hand they are restricted by safety standards, time constraints and low staffing levels but also maligned for their lack of education and therefore presumed lack of interest in the importance of food (DHSS, 1990c).

However, in 2007, a survey of 2193 nurses from different care settings across the UK undertaken by the RCN revealed that 95% of the nurses rated patient nutrition as important or extremely important with more than half of those involved actively in patient care saying that they did not have enough time to devote to it. In addition, a quarter of the nurses said that guidelines from NICE, regarding screening patients on admission, were not being met. Barriers to achieving good patient nutrition were seen as the lack of availability of food outside mealtimes (49%) not enough staff to ensure patients got the help needed to eat (46%), the choice of food (42%) not enough staff to monitor patients' intake of food and water (38%) the quality and presentation of food (36%), and staff concerned with other priorities such as medical rounds (34%) (Waters, 2007).

Therefore, the awareness is in evidence but if it is the nurses' responsibility to ensure that patients eat their food, then they should officially be made accountable instead of being judged on a role that in some instances is confusingly supposed to be the responsibility of others such as ward housekeepers and modern matrons. As the chairman of the National Nurses Nutrition Group said:

'If a nurse had failed to give a patient their intravenous drugs that would be considered a very serious incident. However, if they don't ensure that their patients have had a meal that just seems to be 'well ok they didn't bother eating their dinner, does it really matter?' And of course it does, foods a treatment equally as much as drug therapies are'.   (Colagiovanni, 2006)

And somebody does have to take responsibility with issues of malnutrition at stake. The role of nurses has again been in the forefront of these malnutrition issues, mainly for their lack of observation around mealtimes which again suggests a lack of cohesion in perceived roles. If malnutrition occurs during a hospital stay, it is the food chain which is at fault. However, one of the reasons for the high prevalence of malnutrition is the amount of patients' already malnourished when they are admitted to hospital (Elia, 2005), a situation which will hopefully be more controllable with the guidance from MUST (see Box 2.9, page 151) The seriousness of being malnourished on admission is that it would be compounded by a patient eating poorly prior to surgery with an expected poor appetite post surgery:

'And if at this point you don't act you've only got about ten days before the patient dies of malnutrition'.   (Stroud, 2004)

As many of the malnutrition issues are relative to the elderly, it was disturbing to read that, back in 2001, the Nursing and Midwifery Advisory Committee had expressed concern about the persistent negative attitudes towards nursing older patients, saying that there were deficits in core nursing skills with many nurses regarding fundamental skills, such as assisting patients with feeding, as tasks to be delegated to health care assistants, often without supervision (DH, 2001c).

But there is another aspect to consider in the area of malnutrition: arguably, most people would associate malnutrition with individuals who look undernourished, usually thin and of course for these physical signs to go unnoticed is not acceptable. But let us consider the overweight individual who may be overfed but malnourished. With obesity levels out of control this paradox may be the 'unnoticed' norm. For these patients nutritious food could be viewed as doubly important as any perceived weight loss might be viewed as 'healthy' but actually adding to their general malnourishment.

An alternative to food for patients such as those with malnutrition is artificial feeding, which has its place, but as the Council of Europe advises:

> 'Ordinary food by the oral route should be the first choice to correct or prevent undernutrition in hospitals ... artificial nutritional support should only be started when the use of ordinary food fails or is inappropriate'. (Council of Europe, 2003)

It has also been suggested that there are times when patients are given more expensive alternatives to food when this should be the 'last resort' (DH, 2004d). However, if the 'ordinary' food is not up to standard either nutritionally or even visually, artificial feeding might well be the only 'appropriate' course of action or indeed the 'last resort'.

The lack of education amongst those involved in the food chain has also been well documented. It has been suggested that there is an assumption in policy documents that all health professionals should be giving dietary advice but research amongst doctors and nurses in primary care has indicated disappointing nutritional knowledge (Barratt, 2001). But is this surprising? How many people actually know anything about the nitty gritty of nutrition? It is a specialised subject, as any dietician or nutritional therapist will testify. Somehow, for those involved in the food chain, there just needs to be a way of making everybody aware of how important food and nutrition are. Whether this is via emails, a poster campaign or any other form of simple communication that the Trust sees fit, is it that difficult to impart a simple message without the threat of 'education' hanging over people, who are in the main, overworked with time already being at a premium? Yes, there are instances when staff need more specialised knowledge, but leave it to the specialists: a surgeon performs an emergency operation without having to know finer details such as the patients shoe size, this does not make him less effective as a surgeon. A domestic help uses a cleaning product, unaware of what the actual ingredients are but knows it has to be used. They are both specialists in their own right but don't require the entire minutia to perform effectively. A simple message about the importance of nutrition is all that is required in the majority of cases. The question 'is the patient eating and drinking?' is a simple question of which everybody should be made aware. It is the responses, 'yes' and/or 'no' that then become somebody's responsibility. Again, as long as the food is nutritionally appetising and appealing, these questions and their answers too should be noted and acted upon, with the responsibility properly assigned:

> 'I don't like milk and for breakfast that was all that was on offer with rice krispies ... what sort of diet is that ... not even any bread, mind you the toaster was broken anyway'. (Interview with former inpatient, November 2007)

Inevitably, this patient did not have any breakfast, just a cup of tea. Nobody noticed.

What seems to be required is a more comprehensive education process aimed at the people in the food chain who can make a difference to the quality of food. Even then best intentions can go awry: an example of this was seen when *Catering for Health* was launched jointly by the Food Standards Agency and the DH, which was a guide for teaching healthier catering practices (FSA/DH, 2001). It was aimed at lecturers and assessors of City & Guild NVQ catering courses, seen as the most popular catering course amongst students who go on to work in a wide range of environments including nursing homes, schools and hospitals. The guide set out the 'fundamentals of nutrition without the baffling science and terminology often associated with such a subject'. However, an evaluation of this guide revealed that it had not reached its target audience due to a lack of funding and the fact that the key awarding bodies had not identified demand for training in nutrition by the catering colleges or the catering industry (FSA, 2003).

The lack of funding in all areas of the food chain is often quoted but this does not explain the paradox that there is no relationship between cost and the quality of food provided (DHSS, 1983; AC, 2001) with the Cornwall project demonstrating that by buying high-quality meat there was less shrinkage so they needed to buy less, high-quality bread was more filling so patients ate less and when they started to make their own soup they made a profit (Jochelson, 2005). As has been noted by the catering manager from the Nottingham Trust:

> *'Unfortunately a lot of Trusts have not understood that things like the hospital site and facilities are big assets and can be huge generators of profit. The continual outsourcing of these assets shows a real lack of vision ...'*

This whole issue of funding has perhaps been put into perspective as narrated at the Westminster Diet & Health Forum seminar on *Food in Hospitals*:[18] in 2005, the food bill at the King's College Hospital for staff and patients was around £3 million a year with virtually zero inflation for the last five or six years. This figure was not increasing so 'we're having to do more of the same for the same amount of money'. However, the drugs bill was £26 million with inflation on drugs running between 10% and 15%. Moreover, a lot of these drugs might have been avoided if patients were fed or hydrated better – a fair chunk of the £26 million was spent on laxatives. At the time, a day spent in a hospital bed cost £270, with a high dependency unit costing nearer £1900 or £2000. When a young fit man was admitted, paralysed from the neck down, he not only had an enormous appetite but needed help and assistance with eating and there was 'all sorts of trouble trying to get adequate amounts of food for him ... its too much, everybody will want that'. The young man in question was costing £1900 just to sit there, so an extra £10 to be spent on extra food was seen as 'really a drop in the ocean, these are attitudes which need to be challenged' (Wilson, 2005).

For a short-stay patient on a normal diet, nutrition might not be deemed very important either by the patient or the food chain, but it is. Patients requiring special diets and long-stay patients could be viewed as more important but it is to be hoped that all patients' nutritional needs are met on every level. However, as it has been reported that the total number of untouched/unserved patient meals in 2005/06 was 13 053 065 (Written Answers, 2007b) it cannot be assumed that this will be the case. Indeed this figure could be higher as the data provided had not been collected on a mandatory basis and was therefore incomplete (Written Answers, 2007b).

Everybody should understand the importance of food and therefore nutrition, which requires simple messages to raise awareness and simple questions to ensure the awareness is facilitated at the point of delivery – with the patient.

What cannot be ignored is the fact that although the profile of food has never been higher, fuelled by the media, radio, television and cookery books, one of our most important institutions, the NHS, still has a poor catering record. This could be explained by the diversity amongst the Trusts and what they believe they are capable of and, more to the point, what help is available in the form of funding and personnel, which is lamentable. Perhaps it is time to remove the continual uphill struggle to improve catering that most hospital food chains face by placing proper budgets with experts who can provide personnel to educate the right people giving them the wherewithal to deliver a catering service that will no longer be the butt of jokes.

As has been noted:

'Food provision has a humble profile in the perennial struggle for resources and that is something we have to change ... food is good value for money ... food is the best form of nutritional support. It is the most nutritionally complete, the most physiologically appropriate, the most psychologically supportive and the most socially acceptable and I commend it to you as the best way forward'. (Wilson, 2005)

Notes

1 Workhouses have been included as many were developed into hospitals, taking their catering facilities with them.
2 Parenteral (intravenous) nutrition provides a complete blend of nutrients in liquid form which is fed straight into the vein.
3 2nd edition published in 1980 (DHSS, 1980b).
4 Enteral tube feeding: patient receives a nutritionally complete feed through a feeding tube straight into the stomach or small intestine.
5 New deal involved, amongst others, improving catering for junior doctors (DH, 1998).
6 NHS PASA is an executive agency of the DH, offering expertise on purchasing and the strategic direction of procurement, setting up contracts and framework agreements for goods and services used by the NHS.
7 All information on the BHF programme is available from: http://www.betterhospitalfood. com.
8 This first 'benchmarking' report did not use the 'Essence of Care Benchmarks' as published by the DH in 2001.
9 This was an internal review resulting in a paper to the NPSA board (private email NPSA).

10 These were subsequently updated in 2003 but the benchmarks themselves regarding nutrition remained the same except the term 'client' which was omitted: for brevity the term 'patient' was used.

11 Significance tests have been applied to all response options between surveys with significant differences that exist indicated by the following symbols: a = significant difference between 2002 and 2005, b = significant difference between 2002 and 2006 and c = significant difference between 2005 and 2006. Bonferroni correction was used for multiple comparisons with significance at the 5% level ($p<0.05$) (Boyd & Donovan, 2007).

12 Good Food and the Public Plate details all aspects of sustainable procurement in the UK (Soil Association, 2003).

13 e-auctions are internet-based procurements that are operated as reverse auctions whereby bidders place successively lower prices for the contract.

14 Available from: http://www.sd-commission.org.uk.

15 For more information see www.foodforlife.org.uk.

16 Cornwall has benefited from access to EUOO funding to support the regeneration of its rural economy. EUOO has provided financial support for the feasibility study, including support for the building of the CPFU and has galvanised local farmers and food companies to work in partnership. This commitment has been put in some doubt as reconfiguration of the health service has merged the three PCTs into one new organisation, still at an early stage of development. Ensuring fairness and complicity with European procurement regulations, the CFPU will have to tender for a contract to supply food to other establishments run by the Cornwall PCT on a purely commercial basis.

17 More information about the SDC can be found at http://www.s-dcommission.org.uk.

18 Information on Food in Hospitals (2) can be found at http://www.dietandhealthforum. co.uk.

19 Dysphagia relates to any difficulty, discomfort or pain when swallowing.

20 Providing this information is mandatory for NHS Trusts but not for Foundation Trusts.

21 OFNoSH is now available online: http://www.bapen.org.uk.

22 It was noted that some of the private contractors would not supply cost information for commercial confidentiality and some of the in-house catering providers could not supply suitable cost information.

23 Net costs are the total costs of the catering service including non-patient catering, less income generated from catering.

24 Full details of the requirements, rationale and criteria for each standard together with a simplified version for patients can be found at http://www.nhshealthquality.org/nhsqis.

25 A term often used for the sick where eating to improve their health may require a different intake of nutrients to those recommended for the general population.

26 The DHPSS mission is to improve the health and social well-being of the people of Northern Ireland by ensuring the provision of appropriate health and social care services, both in clinical settings, and in the community through nursing, social work and other professional services. It also leads a major programme of cross-government action to improve the health and well-being of the population and reduce health inequalities.

References

Abel-Smith, B. (1964) *The Hospitals 1800–1948: A Study in Social Administrations in England and Wales.* London: Heinemann Educational Books Limited.

Age Concern (2006) Hungry to be heard. The scandal of malnourished older people in hospital. London: Age Concern.

Allison, S.P. (1999) Hospital food as treatment. *A Report by the Working Party of the British Association of Enteral and Parenteral Nutrition.* Maidenhead: BAPEN.

Association of Community Health Councils for England and Wales (1997) *Hungry in hospital?*

Audit Commission (2001) Acute Hospital Portfolio. Review of National Findings. AC.

Audit Commission (2002) Food for thought on hospital catering in Wales. Available from http://audit-commission.gov.uk/reports. Accessed July 2007.

Audit Scotland (2003) Catering for patients. AS.

Audit Scotland (2006) Catering for patients. A follow up report. AS.

BBC News (2002a) Grossman defends NHS Menus. 18 April. Available from http://www.bbc.co.uk. Accessed February 2007.

BBC News (2002b) Poor response to hospital food drive. 12 February. Available from http://www.bbc.co.uk. Accessed February 2007.

BBC Radio 4 (2006) You and Yours: Better hospital food programme disbanded. 4 May.

Barratt, J. (2001) Diet-related knowledge, beliefs and actions of health professionals compare with the general population: An investigation into a community Trust. Journal of Human Nutrition & Dietetics, 14:25–32.

Baum, T. (2006) Food or facilities? The changing role of catering managers in the healthcare environment. Nutrition & Food Science, 36(3):138–152.

Beck, A.M., Balknas, U.N., Furst, P. et al. (2001) Food and nutritional care in hospitals: How to prevent undernutrition – Report and guidelines from the Council of Europe. Clinical Nutrition, 20(5):455–460.

Bistrian, B.R., Blackburn, G.L., Vitale, J., Cochran, D. & Naylor, J. (1976) Prevalence of malnutrition in general medical patients. Journal of the American Medical Association, 235(15):1567–1570.

Bond, S. (1997) Eating Matters. Newcastle upon Tyne: Centre for Health Services Research, University of Newcastle upon Tyne.

Boyd, J., Graham, C. & Powell, C. (2006) The key findings report for the 2005 inpatients survey. Oxford: Picker Institute Europe. Available from http://www.nhssurveys.org. Accessed June 2006.

Boyd, J. (2007) The 2006 Inpatients Importance Study. Oxford: Picker Institute Europe.

Boyd, J.E. & Donovan, S. (2007) The Key Findings Report of the 2006 Inpatient Survey. Oxford: Picker Institute Europe.

Bristow & Holmes (1864) The Hospitals of the United Kingdom. HMSO. In: Abel-Smith, B. (1964) The Hospitals 1800–1948: A Study in Social Administrations in England and Wales. London: Heinemann Educational Books Limited.

British Association for Parenteral and Enteral Nutrition (BAPEN) (2007a) Available from http://www.bapen.org.uk. Accessed October 2007.

British Association for Parenteral and Enteral Nutrition (BAPEN) (2007b) BAPEN welcomes launch of 10 point 'Mission Statement' for hospitals to improve nutritional care. Available from http://www.bapen.org.uk. Accessed October 2007.

British Association for Parenteral and Enteral Nutrition (BAPEN) (2007c) Organisation of Food and Nutritional Support in Hospitals. Available from http://www.bapen.org.uk. Accessed October 2007.

British Association for Parenteral and Enteral Nutrition (BAPEN) (2007d) Nutrition Screening Week. Available from http://www.bapen.org.uk. Accessed October 2007.

British Association of Parenteral and Enteral Nutrition (BAPEN) (2007e) BAPEN conference 2007 report. InTouch No. 48. BAPEN.

British Dietetic Association (BDA) (1993) Dietetic Standards of Care for the Older Adult in Hospital. Produced in conjunction with the Nutrition Advisory Group for Elderly People (NAGE) in liaison with the Mental Health Group and the Parenteral & Enteral Nutrition group of the British Dietetic Association.

British Dietetic Association (BDA) (2006) Delivering care through food and beverage services. BDA.

British Dietetic Association (BDA) (2007) Available from http://www.bda.uk.com.

Bullen, N. & Reeves, R. (2003) Acute Inpatient Survey. National Overview 2001/02. Oxford: Picker Institute Europe. Available from http://www.dh.gov.uk/en/index.htm. Accessed March 2007.

Butterworth, C.E. (1974) The skeleton in the hospital closet. *Nutrition Today*, 9(2):4–8.

Carlson, E. & Kipps, M. (1990) What do caterers know about nutrition? *Nutrition and Food Science*, 110:10–11.

Chambers, N. & Jolly, A. (2002) Essence of care: Making a difference. *Nursing Standard*, 17(11): 40–44.

Colagiovanni, L. (2006) Interviewed on BBC Radio 4 'You and Yours': Better hospital food programme disbanded. 4 May.

Cole, A. (2008) How many doctors does it take to turn off a lightbulb? *British Medical Journal Career Focus*, 336:27–28.

Commission for Patient and Public Involvement in Health (CPPIH) (2006) PPI forums joining forces to tackle NHS Food. Food Watch August – October 2006. CPPIH.

Coubrough, H.A. (1978) The role of dietitians in hospitals. *Proceedings of the Nutrition Society*, 37:65–70.

Council of Europe (CoE) (2003) Committee of Ministers. Resolution Res AP(2003)3 on food and nutritional care in hospitals.

Davenport, P. (1985) Chicken source of poison that led to 19 deaths, inquiry told. *The Times*, 27 February, p. 4.

Davis, A.M. & Bristow, A. (1999) *Managing Nutrition in Hospital. A Recipe for Quality*. London: The Nuffield Trust.

Dealey, C., Moss, H., Marshal J. *et al.* (2007) Auditing the impact of implementing the Modern Matron role in an acute teaching trust. *Journal of Nursing Management*, 15:22–33.

Deer, B. (1985) Food poison deaths probe may reveal NHS flaws. *The Sunday Times*, 24 February 1985. Available from http://www.briandeer.com. Accessed March 2007.

Department of Health (1981) *Catering for Minority Groups*. Southampton: HMSO.

Department of Health (1984) Nutritional aspects of cardiovascular disease. *Report of the Cardiovascular Review Group Committee on Medical Aspects of Food Policy* (Report on Health and Social Subjects: 46). London: HMSO.

Department of Health (1989) Chilled and Frozen. *Guidelines on Cook-Chill and Cook-Freeze Catering Systems*. London: HMSO.

Department of Health (DH) (1994) Nutrition and health. *A Management Handbook for the NHS*. Great Britain: DH.

Department of Health (DH) (1995) *Nutrition Guidelines for Hospital Catering*. Great Britain: Nutrition Task Force. Hospital Catering Project Team.

Department of Health (DH) (1996a) *Nutrition Guidelines for Hospital Catering a checklist for audit, Guidance Notes*. Nutrition Task Force hospital catering project team. Wetherby: DH.

Department of Health (DH) (1996b) The patients charter for England. Catering services. Patients Charter Unit.

Department of Health (DH) (1996c) Nutrition for medical students. Nutrition in the undergraduate medical curriculum. Report from a workshop, Metropole Hotel, Birmingham, 15–16 November 1995. DH.

Department of Health (DH) (1998) HSC 1998/240: Reducing junior doctors' hours continuing action to meet new deal standards rest periods and working arrangements, improving catering and accommodation for juniors, other action points. DH.

Department of Health (DH) (2000) The NHS Plan: A plan for investment, a plan for reform. DH.

Department of Health (DH) (2001a) Essence of Care: Patient-focused benchmarking for health care practitioners. DH.

Department of Health (DH) (2001b) Implementing the NHS Plan – Modern Matrons. Health Service Circular 2001/010. DH.

Department of Health (DH) (2001c) Caring for older people: A nursing priority. Report by the Nursing and Midwifery Advisory Committee. DH.

Department of Health (DH) (2003) Modern matrons – improving the patient experience. DH.

Department of Health (DH) (2004a) *Standards for Better Health*. Available from http://www. dh.gov.uk/en/publicationsandstatistics.

Department of Health (DH) (2004b) Government hits target of housekeepers in over half of all NHS hospitals. Press Release Ref 2004/0461. DH.

Department of Health (DH) (2004c) *Better Hospital Food Programme*. Speech by Lord Warner, Parliamentary Under-Secretary of State in the Lords, 21 January. DH.

Department of Health (DH) (2004d) *The Changing Face of Hospital Food*. Speech by Lord Warner, Parliamentary Under-Secretary of State in the Lords, 29 April. DH.

Department of Health (DH) (2005a) Choosing a better diet: A food and health action plan. DH.

Department of Health (DH) (2005b) *Creating a Patient-led NHS*. Delivering the NHS Improvement Plan. DH.

Department of Health (DH) (2006) A stronger local voice: A framework for creating a stronger local voice in the development of health and social care services. DH.

Department of Health & Social Security (DHSS) (1968) *Relieving nurses of non-nursing duties in general and maternity hospitals*. A report by the Sub-Committee of the Standing Nursing Advisory Committee. London: HMSO.

Department of Health & Social Security (DHSS) (1975a) *Nutrition Education*. Report of a working party. London: DHSS.

Department of Health & Social Security (DHSS) (1975b) *Health Service Catering. Nutrition and Modified diets*. London: DHSS.

Department of Health & Social Security (DHSS) (1977) *Health Service Catering. Standard Recipes Vol. 3*. London: DHSS.

Department of Health & Social Security (DHSS) (1980a). *Best Buy Hospitals Mark 1*. Evaluation report. London: DHSS.

Department of Health & Social Security (DHSS) (1980b) *Health Service Catering. Nutrition and Modified Diets*, 2nd edn. Great Britain: DHSS.

Department of Health & Social Security (DHSS) (1980c) *Hospital Meal Survey. Ward Issues*. Breakfast-lunch-supper. London: DHSS.

Department of Health & Social Security (DHSS) (1980d) *Strategic Planning for Catering Services*. Management guidelines Part II. London: DHSS.

Department of Health & Social Security (DHSS) (1983) *NHS Scrutiny Programme. The Cost of Catering in the NHS*. London: DHSS.

Department of Health & Social Security (DHSS) (1984) *Diet and Cardiovascular Disease*. Report on health and social subjects, No. 28. London: HMSO.

Department of Health & Social Security (DHSS) (1985) *Catering Services – Competitive Tendering*. Great Britain: Coopers & Lybrand Associates.

Department of Health & Social Security (DHSS) (1988) *Catering for Health. The Recipe File*. London: HMSO.

Department of Health & Social Security and the Welsh Office (1986) *Health* Building Note 10. Catering Department. London: HMSO.

Department of Health & Social Security and the Welsh Office (1976) *The Organisation of the In-Patient's Day*. Report of a committee of the Central Health Services Council. London: HMSO.

Department of Health, Social Services and Public Safety (2003) *Catering Services in Northern Ireland*. Accessed June 2007. Available from http://www.dhsspsni.gov.uk.

Donelan, A. (2000) Dietitians and caterers: An uncertain but critical relationship. *Nutrition & Food Science*, 3:123–127.

Edwards, J.S.A. & Nash, H.M. (1999) The nutritional implications of food wastage in hospital food service management. *Nutrition & Food Science*, 2:89–98.

Elia, M. (Professor) (2005) Speaking at the Westminster Diet & Health Forum Food in Hospitals seminar. 8 December.

Elia, M. (Professor) (2006) *Guidelines and More Guidelines*. In Touch No. 44. BAPEN.

Ellis, E. (2006) All inclusive benchmarking. *Journal of Nursing Management*, 14(5):377–383.

Enloe, F. (1974) "Dietitians' Lib" (editorial). *Nutrition Today*, 9(3):14.

European Nutrition for Health Alliance (2007) Prague Declaration: A call for action to fight malnutrition in Europe. Available from http://www.european-nutrition.org. Accessed December 2007.

European Nutrition for Health Alliance (2008) *Malnutrition – The Silent Killer*. Available from http://www.european-nutrition.org. Accessed January 2008.

Evans, E. (1974) Quality of diet received by the patient. *Proceedings of the Nutrition Society*, 37:71–77.

Food Standards Agency/Department of Health (2001) *Catering for Health. A Guide for Teaching Healthier Catering Practices*.

Food Standards Agency (2003) *Catering for Health Evaluated*. Available from http://www.food. gov.uk/news/newsarchive/2003/jul/cateringforhealthevaluated. Accessed 17/10/2007.

Food Standards Agency (2007a) Consumer attitudes to food standards. Accessed December 2007. Available from: http://www.food.gov.uk.

Food Standards Agency (2007b) *Guidance on Food Served to Adults in Major Institutions*. Available from http://www.food.gov.uk. Accessed December 2007.

Garrow, J. (1994) Starvation in hospitals. *British Medical Journal*, 308:934.

Geary, G. (2004) *The Mind Guide to Food and Mood*. London: Mind.

Gershon, P. (Sir) (2004) Releasing resources to the front line. Independentreview of the public sector efficiency. Available from http://www.hm-treasury.gov.uk. Accessed March 2007.

Gibson, A.G. (1926) *The Radcliffe Infirmary*. Oxford. In: Abel-Smith, B. (1964) *The Hospitals 1800–1948: A Study in Social Administrations in England and Wales*. London: Heinemann Educational Books Limited.

Grossman, L. (2006) Interviewed on BBC Radio 4 'You and Yours': Better hospital food programme disbanded. 4 May.

Hayward, J. (2003) Ward nutrition coordinators to improve patient nutrition in hospital. *British Journal of Nursing*, 12(18):1081–1108.

Health Inspectorate Wales (2007) *How Good is the NHS in Wales?* Available from http://www. hiw.org.uk. Accessed January 2008.

Heath Promotion Wales (1997) *The National Standard for Hospital Caterers*. Cardiff: HPW.

Healthcare Commission (2004) Inspection guide. Core standard C15a & C15b. HC.

Healthcare Commission (2005) Commission begins 120 visits and spot checks on NHS core standards. HC.

Healthcare Commission (2006) How trusts assessed themselves in 2005/2006 HC.

Hill, G.L., Blackett, R.L. Pickford, I. *et al.* (1977) Malnutrition in surgical patients. An unrecognised problem. *Lancet*, 261(8013): 689–692.

Hockridge, E. & Longfield, J. (2005) *Getting More Sustainable Food in London's Hospitals. Can it be Done? And is it worth it*? London: Sustain.

Hospital Caterers Association (2004) Protected Mealtimes Policy.

Hospital Caterers Association (2006) Press releases. The Hospital Caterers Association response to the PPI food watch survey. HCA.

House of Commons, 372 (1866) In: Abel-Smith, B. (1964) *The Hospitals 1800–1948: A Study in Social Administrations in England and Wales*. London: Heinemann Educational Books Limited.

Hwang, L.J.J., Descombe, T., Eves, A. & Kipps, M. (1999) An analysis of catering options within NHS acute hospitals. *International Journal of Health Care Quality Assurance*, 12(7): 293–308.

Hwang, L.J.J. (2003) Gap analysis of patient meal service perceptions. *International Journal of Care Quality Assurance*, 16(3):143–153.

Jochelson, K. (2005) Speaking at the Westminster Diet & Health Forum Food in Hospitals seminar. 8 December.

Jochelson, K. *et al.* (2005) *Sustainable Food and the NHS*. London: King's Fund.

Johnson, V.J. (1985) *Diet in Workhouses and Prisons 1835–1895*. New York: Garland Publishing Inc.

Lennard-Jones, J.E. (1992) A positive approach to nutrition as treatment. King's Fund. Report of a working party on the role of enteral and parenteral feeding in hospital and at home. London: King's Fund Centre.

Kelliher, C. (1996) Competitive tendering in NHS catering: A suitable policy. *Employee Relations*, **18**(3):62–76.

Kelly, I.E., Tessier, S., Cahill, A. *et al.* (2000) Still hungry in hospital: Identifying malnutrition in acute hospital admissions. *Quarterly Journal of Medicine*, **93**(2):93–98.

Kemp, A. (2005) Speaking at the Westminster Diet & Health Forum Food in Hospitals seminar. 8 December.

King Edwards Hospital Fund for London (1931) Patients waking hours in London Voluntary Hospitals. In: Abel-Smith, B. (1964) *The Hospitals 1800–1948: A Study in Social Administrations in England and Wales*. London: Heinemann Educational Books Limited.

King Edwards Hospital Fund for London (1943) Memoranda on hospital diet. In: Platt, B.S., Eddy, T.P. & Pellett, P.L. (1963) *Food in Hospitals. A Study of Feeding Arrangements and the Nutritional Value of Meals in Hospitals*. London: Oxford University Press (for the Nuffield Provincial Hospitals Trust).

King Edwards Hospital Fund for London (1986) *A Review of Hospital Catering*. England: Hollen Street Press.

Kitson, A. (Professor) (2005) Speaking at the Westminster Diet & Health Forum Food in Hospitals seminar. 8 December.

Kipps, M. & Middleton, V. (1990a) Hospital catering. *Nutrition and Food Science*, **123**:2–4.

Kipps, M. & Middleton, V. (1990b) Hospital catering. *Nutrition and Food Science*, **124**:8–9.

Lancet Commission Report (undated). In: Abel-Smith, B. (1964) *The Hospitals 1800–1948: A Study in Social Administrations in England and Wales*. London: Heinemann Educational Books Limited.

Lord Warner (2004) The Changing Face of Hospital Food: Speech by the Parliamentary Under-Secretary of State in the Lords. 29 April. DH.

Lyons, M. (2004) *Well Placed to Deliver? Shaping the Pattern of Government Service. Independent Review of Public Sector Relocation*. London: HMSO.

McCree, A. (2005) Speaking at the Westminster Diet & Health Forum Food in Hospitals seminar. 8 December.

McKie, D. (2000) 'How ministers exercise arbitrary power'. *The Guardian*, 6 December.

McKinley, A. (2006) The Scottish food, fluid and nutritional care standards: progress but a long way to go. in Touch no. 44. BAPEN.

McWhirter, J.P. & Pennington, C.R. (1994) Incidence and recognition of malnutrition in hospital. *British Medical Journal*, **308**:945–948.

Marson, H., McErlain, L. & Ainsworth, P. (2003) The implications of food wastage on a renal ward. *British Food Journal*, **105**(11):791–799.

Matykiewicz, L., Ashton, D. & Cook, J. (2005) Essence of care benchmarking: putting it into practice. *Benchmarking*, **12**(5):467–481.

May, D. & Smith, L. (2003) Evaluation of the new housekeeper role in UK NHS Trusts. *Facilities*, **21**:7/8.

Mitchell, H. (1999) Nutrition audit at a community hospital. *Journal of Human Nutrition and Dietetics*, **12**:425–432.

Morgan, G. (2006) Interviewed on BBC Radio 4 'You and Yours': Better hospital food programme disbanded. 4 May.

National Assembly for Wales (2001) *Improving Health in Wales*.

National Audit Office (2006) *Smarter Food Procurement in the Public Sector*. London: The Stationery Office.

National Health Service (1979) Report on a review of the national trainee scheme for cooks in hospitals. National staff committee for accommodations, catering and other support services staff.

National Health Service Estates (2001a) www.betterhospitalfood.com.

National Health Service Estates (2001b) *Housekeeping. A first guide to new, modern and dependable ward housekeeping services in the NHS*. NHSE.

National Health Service Estates (2002) *Better hospital food partnership sites club interim benchmark report, April*. NHSE.

National Health Service Estates (2003) *Better hospital food partnership sites club 2nd benchmark report, February*. NHSE.

National Health Service Estates (2007) *Better Hospital Food. PEAT 2002 & 2003*. Available from: http://www.nhsestates. Accessed August 2007.

National Health Service Estates Hospitality (2005) *Managing food waste in the NHS*. DH.

National Health Service Executive (1996) *Hospital Catering: Delivering a Quality Service*. London: HMSO.

The National Health Service Plan (2000) *A Plan for Investment. A Plan for Reform*. London: HMSO.

National Health Service Quality Improvement Scotland (2003) *Clinical standards. Food, fluid and nutritional care in hospitals*. NHS QIS.

National Health Service Quality Improvement Scotland (2006) *National overview. Food fluid and nutritional care in hospitals*. NHS QIS.

National Institute for Health and Clinical Excellence (2006) *Nutrition Support in Adults. Oral Nutrition Support, Enteral Tube Feeding and Parenteral Nutrition*. London: National Collaborating Centre for Acute Care.

National Patient Safety Agency (NPSA) (2007) *NPSA announces continued improvement in hospital food and cleanliness*. Available from http://www.npsa. Accessed March 2007.

National Patient Safety Agency (NPSA) (2007) *Key recommendations focus on hospital nutrition as new data highlights safety issues*. 4 Oct. Available from http://www.npsa. Accessed October 2007.

Nicholls, G. (Sir) (1898) *A History of the English Poor Law*. In: Johnson, V.J. (1985) *Diet in Workhouses and Prisons 1835–1895*. New York: Garland Publishing Inc.

Nightingale, F. (1859) *Notes on Nursing: What it is and What it is Not*. London: Harrison.

Paisley, C.M. & Tudor-Smith, C. (2001) Food and catering policies in NHS hospitals in Wales. *Health Education Journal*, **60**:327–338.

Parliamentary Papers 1867–68, xxxiii (4039). Twentieth Report of the Poor Law Board. In: Johnson, V.J. (1985) *Diet in Workhouses and Prisons 1835–1895*. New York: Garland Publishing Inc.

Platt, B.S., Eddy, T.P. & Pellett, P.L., (1963) *Food in Hospitals. A Study of Feeding Arrangements and the Nutritional Value of Meals in Hospitals*. London: Oxford University Press (for the Nuffield Provincial Hospitals Trust).

Rayner, J. (2006) Hospital food – it's enough to make you sick. *Observer Food Monthly*, September 24. Accessed December 2006. Available from: http://www.guardian.co.uk/society.

Read, S. & Ashman, M. (2004) The University of Sheffield and Scott, C. & Savage, J. (2004) Royal College of Nursing Institute and Evaluation of the modern matron role in a sample of NHS Trusts. Final report to the DH.

Reeves, R., Coulter, A., Jenkinson, C. *et al*. (2002) *Development and Pilot Testing of Questionnaires for Use in the Acute NHS Trust Inpatient Survey Programme*. Oxford: Picker Institute Europe.

Reeves, R., Ramm, J., Cornelius, V. *et al*. (2005) Patient Survey Report 2004 – adult inpatients. Oxford: Picker Institute Europe. Available from http://www.healthcarecommission.org.uk. Accessed June 2007.

Richardson, R. & Hurwitz, B. (1989) Joseph Rogers and the reform of workhouse medicine. *British Medical Journal*, **299**:1507–1510.

Richmond, J. (2007) Developing the role of a ward housekeeper within a multidisciplinary team. *British Journal of Nursing*, **16**(1):56–59.

Rivett, G. (1998) *From Cradle to Grave. Fifty Years of the NHS*. London: King's Fund Publishing.

Robbins, R. (1990) Healthy catering is healthy business. *Nutrition and Food Science*, **127**:16–17.

Royal College of Nursing (2007a) *Nutrition now. Principles for nutrition and hydration*. Available from http://www.rcn.org.uk/nutritionnow. Accessed October 2007.

Royal College of Nursing (2007b) *Hospital Hydration Best Practice Toolkit*. Available from http://www.rcn.org.uk/nutritionnow. Accessed October 2007.

Royal Society of Health (1966) *Modern Hospital Catering*. Report of the RSH conference on hospital food. London: Cox & Wyman Limited.

Russell, C. (2007) *A Fresh Approach to Hospital Food*. Bristol: Soil Association.

Salmon, B. (1966) Report of the committee on senior nursing staff structure Ministry of Health, Scottish Home and Health Department.

Savage, J. & Scott, C. (2005) Patients nutritional care in hospital: An ethnographic study of nurses' role and patients' experience. A report to NHS Estates.

Seton, C. (1984a) Hospital food poisoning spread by beef left out on warm day. *The Times*, 11 September, p. 3.

Seton, C. (1984b) Union chief denies beef claim in hospital poisoning. *The Times*, 14 September, p. 3.

Shanley, O. (2004) Measuring the impact of the modern matrons in the ward Setting. *Nursing Times*, **100**(44): 28–29.

Scottish Office (1996) *Eating for health – a diet plan for Scotland*.

Sheen, A. (1875) *The Workhouse and its Medical Officer*. Cardiff. In: Abel-Smith, B. (1964) *The Hospitals 1800–1948: A Study in Social Administrations in England and Wales*. London: Heinemann Educational Books Limited.

Shepherd, R. (1990) The psychology of food choice. *Nutrition and Food Science*, **124**:2–4.

Silk, D.B.A. (1994) *Organisation of Nutritional Support in Hospitals*. Maidenhead: BAPEN.

Soil Association (2003) Peckham, P. & Petts, J. (eds) *Good Food on the Public Plate: A Manual for Sustainability in Public Sector Food and Catering*. Watton: East Anglia Food Link.

South East Thames Regional Health Authority (SETHRA) (1983) *NHS Scrutiny Programme. The Cost of Catering in the NHS*. Great Britain: DHSS.

South East Thames Regional Health Authority (SETHRA) (1993a) *Nutritional Guidelines: Menu Planning*. SETHRA.

South East Thames Regional Health Authority (SETHRA) (1993b) *Service Standards. Nutritional Guidelines. The Food Chain*. Recommendations produced by a Nutritional Service Standards Working Party. SETHRA.

South Manchester Health District Hospitals (1981) *Catering for Health in Hospitals*. The report and recommendations for the working party on Healthy Nutrition in South Manchester Health District Hospitals. Manchester: The Health Education Centre.

Staff Reporters (1984) Hospital kitchen closed by salmonella in drains. *The Times*, 29 September, p. 1.

Stratton, R.J. & Elia, M. (2000) How much undernutrition is there in hospitals? *British Journal of Nutrition*, **84**:257–259.

Stroud, M. (2004) Speaking at Food as treatment: Making the links conference, at the Queen Elizabeth II Conference Centre, London. 21 January.

Sustainable Development Commission (2007) *Progress in Practice. Nottingham*. University Hospitals NHS Trust's City Hospital Campus' Sustainable Catering Project. Available from http://www.s-dcommission.org.uk. Accessed December 2007.

The Hospital (1924) In: Abel-Smith, B. (1964) *The Hospitals 1800–1948: A Study in Social Administrations in England and Wales*. London: Heinemann Educational Books Limited.

The Hospital (1930) In: Abel-Smith, B. (1964) *The Hospitals 1800–1948: A Study in Social Administrations in England and Wales*. London: Heinemann Educational Books Limited.

The Hospital (1931) In: Abel-Smith, B. (1964) *The Hospitals 1800–1948: A Study in Social Administrations in England and Wales*. London: Heinemann Educational Books Limited.

Tiddy, M. (2005) Speaking at the Westminster Diet & Health Forum Food in Hospitals seminar. 8 December.

Waters, A. (2007) *Nutrition now – campaign*. Available from: http://www.nursing- standard. co.uk/professionaldevelpment/nutritionnow.Accessed 1st October 2007.

Wearmouth, P. (2001) Letter to chief executives of NHS trusts and primary care trusts, trust catering managers. NHS Estates.

Weinreb, B. & Hibbert, H. (eds) (1985) *London Encyclopedia*. In: Hibbert, C. (1987) *The English. A Social History 1066–1945*. London: Harper Collins.

Welsh Assembly Government (2005a) Healthcare Standards for Wales. Available from http:// www.wales.nhs.uk. Accessed December 2007.

Welsh Assembly Government (2005b) Beefing up hospital food in Wales. Available from http:// new.wales.gov.uk/news/archivepress. Accessed August 2007.

Which? (2006) *Off the trolley*. November.

Wilson, R. (2005) Speaking at the Westminster Diet & Health Forum Food in Hospitals seminar. 8 December.

Wilson, R. & Lecko, C. (2005) Improving the nutritional care of patients in hospital. *Nursing Times*, **101**(32):28–30.

Written Answers (2001a) Health: Hospital Food. Hazel Blears, 15 October. Available from http:// www.theyworkforyou.com. Accessed April 2007.

Written Answers (2001b) Health: Hospital Meals. Hazel Blears, 8 November. Available from http://www.theyworkforyou.com. Accessed April 2007.

Written Ministerial Answers (2007a) Northern Ireland: Health and Social Services Estates Agency. Lord Rooker, 26 April. Available from http://www.theyworkforyou.com. Accessed April 2007.

Written Answers (2007b) Health: Hospitals Food. Ann Keen 8 October Available from http:// www.theyworkforyou.com. Accessed December 2007.

Young, R. (1985) Hospitals 'harmed' by prosecution immunity. *The Times*, 9 May, p. 5.

3 Care homes for the elderly

Barbara MacDonald

3.1 Introduction

> '*What do you see nurses, what do you see?*
> *What are you thinking when you are looking at me*
> *A crabbit old woman not very wise,*
> *Uncertain of habit with far-away eyes,*
> *Who dribbles her food and makes no reply,*
> *When you say in a loud voice*
> '*I do wish you'd try*'.
> *Who seems not to notice the things that you do,*
> *And forever is losing a stocking or shoe,*
> *Who unresisting or not lets you do as you will*
> *With bathing and feeding the long day to fill,*
> *Is this what you're thinking, for is this what you see?*
> *Then open your eyes nurse,*
> *You're not looking at me ...*' (Bonart, 2005)[1]

This poem is a sad indictment of what many elderly people might experience in care homes (or any other institution) not just in the UK but across Europe. For these vulnerable individuals, moving into a care home wouldn't have been an easy decision: consider the fact that amongst the general, younger, population, moving house is known to be one of the most stressful activities. Therefore, the impact of moving into a care home on every facet of an elderly person's life can only be imagined. In fact, moving into a care home has been described as a kind of bereavement for the elderly, who are often vulnerable, with staff having to rely on unreliable evidence from relatives who may describe them as more independent than they actually are (Herne, 1994).

And, let us not forget just how vulnerable these elderly people are: In a study of 2573 individuals, the main reasons for social workers admitting them into care homes were (Bebbington *et al.*, 2001):

- Physical health problems
- Mental health problems
- Functional disablement
- Stress on carers
- Lack of motivation
- Present home physically unsuitable
- Family breakdown (including loss of carer)
- Need for rehabilitation
- Fear of being the victim of crime
- Abuse
- Loneliness or isolation
- Homelessness

The care of elderly individuals who can no longer cope alone, has its origins in the work houses, with care homes themselves evolving in a haphazard way, with the badly needed reforms for this forgotten elderly generation, seemingly to be almost inconsequential, often superseded by the needs of younger groups of people (Townsend, 1962).

Reform for the elderly institutionalised was notable in the 1940s in as much as some of the work houses were closed but many were just renamed with many of their inherent problems unchanged, compounded by a lack of funding (Townsend, 1962). New care homes were built but the building programme did not keep up with demand, with the plight of the increasing elderly population viewed later as a 'growing burden upon the community' (DHSS, 1972).

As for nutrition, the nutritional requirements of the elderly were largely unknown until the 1960s when it was realised that there was a connection between ageing, ill health and poor nutrition (Exton-Smith & Stanton, 1965). Further studies confirmed these findings and it was also recognised that malnutrition existed amongst the elderly. In addition inequalities were exposed, with differences not only in the diets but the weight of free living elderly individuals compared to those who were institutionalised (Finch *et al.*, 1998). Many homes offered both inadequate catering and dining facilities (Townsend, 1962) with the notion of 'institutional starvation' reported (DH, 1992a).

The care of the elderly in these homes still remained largely unregulated until 1984 when there was a requirement for homes to be both registered and inspected and a code of practice was issued to assist homes in achieving certain standards, including those concerned with 'diet and food preparation' (Registered Homes Act).

There were many publications aimed at improving the nutrition of the elderly but it wasn't until 2002 that Minimum Standards for care homes were introduced in England, with each standard having a specific requirement. Care homes were now inspected and expected to reach certain standards with the standard on Meals and Mealtimes itself containing nine requirements. Again, there has been criticism of the way in which the homes are inspected but the sheer magnitude of the inspection process is evidenced by the fact that as on 31 March 2007, there were 18 577 registered care homes for adults, providing 441 958 places, including residential homes, nursing homes and non-medical nursing homes (CSCI, 2008).

The actual problems of feeding the elderly cannot be ignored, but it has to be remembered that they are individuals with their own attitudes, influencing what they will and will not eat. Also, let us not forget those elderly with dementia, who present particularly difficult 'feeding' challenges. These challenges can be compounded by problems with staff, many of whom are untrained and therefore unsuitable for dealing with the elderly.

Currently, the ownership of care homes falls into the independent sector or the Local Authority, with the latter being publicly funded and managed and largely in the residential care sector. In the independent sector, care homes can be privately owned by anyone from large-for profit companies down to small one person businesses or owned by charities or other voluntary organisations (Bajekal, 2000).

The number of elderly individuals in care homes will keep increasing and, like the rest of the population, they have a right to decent food and therefore decent nutrition. Old age is always beckoning and it is to be hoped for those who have reached this celebrated age and for those yet to experience it that their carers do not forget who they are: the elderly have both identities and nutritional needs and are at this stage in their life when they often have no choices and are, in reality, often completely dependent upon their carers, in whom they can only trust.

3.2 Workhouses

The care of the elderly has its origins in the workhouses: during the 1830s and 1840s hundreds of workhouses were built, housing many elderly people who were supposed to be 'deserving and of blameless character' even though there were many aged workhouse residents who were viewed as 'undeserving' and deemed fortunate to be looked after by these austere institutions. Indeed, the 'deterrent discipline' of the workhouse was felt to be necessary even for the aged with a presumption that they must have led an 'improvident or dissolute life'. Despite their obvious presence in the workhouse, little reference was made to this elderly population until the end of the nineteenth century. Such classification as there was, led to some of the elderly being separated from other workhouse inhabitants, but in 1909, the Royal Commission complained that out of 140 000 elderly residents in Poor Law institutions in England and Scotland, only a thousand or two were in separate establishments with none at all in Ireland with many crowded into dormitories and day rooms and deprived of work, simple comforts and civilised amenities.[2] The fact that individuals aged 60 and over accounted for around 45% of the workhouse population, showed the enormity of the problem with the rise in the numbers of the elderly in the general population increasing more than any other age group. Although it was envisaged that this increase would continue, little was done to extend separate provision for the elderly as recommended by the Royal Commission: in schemes for social reform, problems of the sick, the unemployed and children gained priority (Townsend, 1962).

3.3 Reform and the development of care homes

Any reform aimed at the elderly was not necessarily the result of policy aimed at those living in institutions but seen as a by-product of independent policies, with the needs of the infirm aged in the workhouses being grossly neglected. Indeed there was less information on these individuals made available to the public between 1910 and 1946 than between 1834 and 1909:

'For almost four decades there was what amounted to a conspiracy of silence on the subject yet during this period the population aged 65 and over more than doubled and by 1946 the number of old people who were by then living in workhouses or former workhouses, run as general or chronic sick hospitals, was greater than what it was at the turn of the century'. (Townsend, 1962)

Many of these former workhouses, renamed public assistance institutions, had harshly administered rules such as forbidding aged male and female residents to be in the garden together: 'the residents tend to sit round the walls, unoccupied and merely waiting for the next meal or for bedtime', all this representative of over a century of 'reform'.

During the 1940s, the Nuffield Survey Committee had advocated reform for 'normal' old people with a suggestion that they should be accommodated in small homes with 30–35 beds, rather than large institutions, with an estimated several thousand of these smaller homes required. In the interim, some of the highly classified institutions might have been suitable for housing up to 200 aged residents but not many of the old workhouses were deemed suitable for this purpose. The idea of small homes was not new but they were more likely to have been found in the voluntary sector with few administered by local authorities. However, in its report of 1948–1949, the Ministry of Health reported that local authorities were planning and opening small comfortable homes for a maximum of 25–30 persons, providing accommodation likened to hotels that had previously been enjoyed by 'well to do people', where old people could live with dignity.

More reform was evidenced with health care being defined within the National Health Service Act of 1946 and social care determined under the 1948 National Assistance Act. The distinction between health and social care was based on an explicit assumption that it was possible to make a distinction between 'the sick or infirm' (people with health needs who should receive care from the NHS) and the 'frail and old' (people with social needs). These differences meant that the former received care free of charge and the latter would be called upon to pay (Dudman, 2007).

The 1948 National Assistance Act set out in broad terms the responsibilities of local authorities which were largely concerned with residential provision. Section 21 of the Act stated that the duty of every local authority was:

'... to provide residential accommodation for persons who by reason of age, infirmity or any other circumstances are in need of care and attention which is not otherwise available to them'.   (Sutherland, 1999)

It was also stipulated that local authorities were required to register and inspect homes run by charitable organisations and private individuals.

By 1949 there were nearly 400 public assistance institutions (former workhouses) housing 130 000 people in England and Wales with less than 100 of them being transferred for use entirely as hospitals. Approximately 200 of them became 'joint user establishments' housing 'sick and other persons'. The remaining institutions were owned by local authorities and used for residential accommodation. This redefining of the use of these institutions was seen as an attempt to 'distinguish between the aged who were sick and those who were in need of care and attention'.

Although, the provision of residential accommodation during the 1950s suffered from a lack of both funding and drive, substantial improvements did take place in residential services as many homes were built, with many others converted from large houses where the amenities and standards of comfort were 'often satisfactory'. Good use was also made of the homes run by voluntary organisations such as the Red Cross, the Salvation Army and the Women's Voluntary Service. Despite this, the government's earlier aims had not been realised: most local authorities were reconciled to keeping the old workhouses for 'the foreseeable future'. It was argued that the workhouses could 'be modernised out of all recognition and that, for the very frail, these large premises serve a useful function' (Townsend, 1961). Few were closed: in 1949, of the 42 000 residents in local authority accommodation there were approximately 39 000–40 000 in public assistance institutions and by 1960 the figure had only been reduced to 35 000. The actual number of homes that were opened for the 'old and handicapped' can be seen in Table 3.1, which shows that more homes opened in the years after the 1948 Act, than latterly.

3.3.1   1960s

By 1960, in England and Wales, there were 95 500 residents of pensionable age with two thirds living in former public assistance institutions and the remainder split between local authority, voluntary and private premises.

Following a study to investigate and assess residential institutions and homes for old people in England and Wales it was shown that the food and dining facilities across the whole spectrum varied considerably (Townsend, 1962).

Table 3.1 Number of homes opened for old and handicapped persons in England & Wales 1948–1960.

Year	Number of homes opened	Of which newly built
1948	97	0
1949	103	0
1950	138	1
1951	112	5
1952	130	5
1953	119	17
1954	99	15
1955	57	13
1956	73	22
1957	72	29
1958	53	26
1959	55	27
1960	76	47
Total	1184	207

Source: Townsend (1962).

Box 3.1 An example of meals in a public assistance institution.

Breakfast:	Porridge, boiled egg, sausage or bacon, bread and butter and tea.
Dinner:	Lancashire hot pot or roast lamb, stewed steak or cottage pie, cabbage and potatoes. This was followed by rice, tapioca or bread and butter pudding, prunes and custard or jam tart.
Tea:	Fried haddock or cold luncheon meat and beetroot, bread and butter, Swiss roll or fruit cake and tea.
Supper:	Bread and butter or biscuits and meat paste, cheese spread or jam and tea, cocoa or Bovril.

Source: Townsend (1964).

3.3.1.1 *Public assistance institutions*

In these former workhouses, conditions were often far from ideal: dining rooms were comparatively few in number with some accommodating up to 300 people for each meal with those institutions accommodating less than 40, being in the minority. In some of these institutions, residents ate and slept in the same room.

Breakfast was usually served at 7.30 or 8 a.m., dinner between 11.45 and 12.20 p.m., tea between 4 and 5 p.m. and supper between 6.30 and 7 p.m. An example of what each meal might consist of is shown in Box 3.1.

There were reported examples of meat that was too tough for residents to eat, tapioca pudding made without milk and little sugar, with fish and vegetables uneaten. One attendant commented: 'It's surprising how many of them don't like fish. You can always tell on a Friday. The pail of scrapings is always full'.

The diets were reportedly sufficient in quantity for frail persons but there were complaints from those who were more active who sometimes said they were hungry, especially in the evenings, reflected by the early timing of tea and the 'small' supper. Seven per cent of residents were on special diets (e.g. salt free, fat free, high protein or vegetarian) but in the main there was, no choice of menu and little attempt to cater for individual needs or taste. Many of the residents drew on their private stores of biscuits, jam, chocolate and sugar which they bought with their pocket money or was supplied by relatives. Some articles of food could also be bought from trolleys taken around by voluntary organisations such as the WVS or the Red Cross.

Staff shortages also played a part in how much food the residents received: some of the residents were put to bed before supper: '*We have to start getting a lot of them to bed early because the staff wouldn't get through*'. In other instances early morning tea was sometimes served in bed by the night attendants or with the help of one of the residents and many infirm elderly could be found an hour or two before breakfast in day rooms where fires had been unlit, with another example of an uncaring attitude shown below:

'*They get angry if someone sits in their chair. They like routine and don't like change. Yesterday one old man refused to eat his meals because I had moved him to another table. He'll get hungry though and I expect he'll eat tomorrow*'.

3.3.1.2 Purpose-built homes

Although many post-war homes were more comfortable than the workhouses their standards were still lower than the desired levels and it was the purpose-built homes which showed the optimum standards being aimed at by the government and local authorities. One was described as having a dining room with small tables for three or four residents with bright checked cloths, table napkins, blue crockery and glasses of water for the midday meal. However many were built without much forethought or consultation with matrons and staff resulting in poorly designed buildings and equipment not conducive to the comfort of the elderly population they were, supposedly, catering to.

Some of the residents received an early morning cup of tea in bed and in about a third of the homes some were allowed to stay in bed for breakfast either through illness or choice. Their diets tended to be more varied and more attractively presented than in the old workhouses but again there was little choice except for those on special diets. The supper was described as 'extremely light' often consisting of no more than biscuits and cheese with a cup of milk or cocoa. There were complaints about insufficient amounts of food and the long period between the last meal at 5 p.m. until 8–8.30 a.m. the following day. Cooks were not available in the evenings and residents could not cook their own meals which largely explained why they kept packets of biscuits in their rooms and went to bed so early. A menu for a typical Local Authority home is shown in Table 3.2.

Table 3.2 Menu for a typical Local Authority home.

	Breakfast	Dinner	Tea	Supper
Sunday	Cereal or porridge, boiled eggs, bread & butter	Roast lamb, potatoes, runner beans. Fruit jelly, Ideal milk	Bananas, bread & butter, jam	
Monday	Cereal or porridge, tomatoes, bread & butter	Cold ham & chips, mashed potatoes, baked jam roll, custard	Welsh rarebit bread & butter, jam	
Tuesday	Cereal or porridge, toast & marmalade	Stewed steak, potatoes, cabbage, tapioca	Sardines, bread & butter, jam	
Wednesday	Cereal or porridge, sausage, fried bread, bread & butter	Liver & bacon, potatoes, onions, baked jam sponge, custard	Hot buttered scones, bread & butter, jam	Coffee, cocoa, milk, sandwiches or cheese & biscuits
Thursday	Cereal or porridge, bacon, bread & butter	Steak & kidney pudding, green beans, potatoes, baked egg custard & stewed fruit	Cheese and pickles, bread & butter, jam	
Friday	Cereal or porridge, scrambled eggs, bread & butter	Salt silverside, pease pudding, greens & potatoes, semolina & jam	Finnan haddock, bread & butter, jam	
Saturday	Cereal or porridge, bacon, bread & butter, marmalade	Cold beef salad, pickles, potatoes, steamed date pudding, custard	Boiled eggs, bread & butter, jam	

Source: Townsend (1964).

3.3.1.3 Voluntary homes

Some of the voluntary homes did not have dining rooms with residents taking their meals in their rooms or on trays in a lounge whilst others had communal rooms for both dining and sitting. (This was all the reporting there was on these homes with no reports on the actual food itself.)

3.3.1.4 Private homes

There were said to be striking differences in private homes with one kitchen described as a *'Harrods showpiece with everything down to an extractor fan and a "Dishmaster"* with another described as *unclean with residents eating their meals in a tiny conservatory whilst the kitchen in another was described as being "dishevelled and strewn with dirty utensils"'.*   (Townsend, 1962)

The more expensive homes supplied food which was 'more varied and plentiful' with supper, for example, tending to be more substantial than in local authority premises: one home provided soup or eggs, a light sweet, cheese and biscuits and a hot drink. As the homes were often smaller, meals could also be adapted more easily to individual tastes and in some instances meals times could be varied to suit individual requirements, with cakes being prepared for birthdays.

This study, aptly named *The Last Refuge*, concluded that homes existing in England and Wales did not '*adequately meet the physical, psychological and social needs*' of the elderly and that '*alternative services and living arrangements should quickly take their place*'.

Worrying words, compounded by the DHSS who later said that although there might not be any change in the willingness of relatives to care and feed the elderly who could not manage for themselves, '*a growing burden would be placed upon the community*', warranting more up-to-date information to '*devise ways and means of caring for those in need efficiently and economically*' (DHSS, 1972).

The report *The Aged in the Welfare State* (Townsend & Wedderburn, 1965) shed more light on why this 'burden' was growing, reasoning that an understanding of family structure was important in comprehending the reasons for the elderly being institutionalised: far more of the old people in institutions were unmarried, lacked children or brothers and sisters: of those who had children, some only had one child and sons rather than daughters. People who had relatives but found themselves in institutions, had more often than not led their lives in seclusion from these relatives. Therefore, '*in family structure and propinquity the elderly institutional population differs sharply from the rest of the population*'. This information was the result of a survey undertaken throughout Britain of over 6000 people aged 65 and over in 1962/1963.

Institutionalised or not what were elderly people eating? In 1962 the nutritional needs of old people were not known. This prompted a study undertaken by the King Edwards Hospital Fund (Exton-Smith & Stanton, 1965), which attempted to discover the levels of nutritional intake, compatible with health, in the elderly. Sixty women, living alone, were involved, with an average age of 75.9, living alone in North London.

The results, published in 1965, showed that the findings for the whole group did not support the popular idea that old people existed entirely on bread, butter, jam and sweetened cups of tea. In the main they ate a varied diet, cooked at least one meal a day and frequently ate fruit and vegetables. A clinical assessment showed that three quarters of the women enjoyed normal or excellent health with the subjects' own evaluation of their health often slightly better than that of the medical observer. However, marked differences occurred with advancing age: by the end of the eighth decade the mean skin fold thickness of the 'normal' subjects was approximately half that in the early 70s, the mean body weight of the subjects in the highest age group was 14% less than that of the subjects in their early 70s, with 'this remarkable reduction in intakes of calories and nutrition' seen as 'unexpected'. The correlation between diet and health was said to be 'striking' with, in general, a better than average diet resulting in better than average health.

Owing to the nature of this cross-sectional study, it was not possible to assess the relative importance of some of the factors discussed above so the results were followed up by a longitudinal study on the remaining group of women, nearly seven years later (Stanton & Exton-Smith, 1970). So that diet and health could be analysed, the groups were split into two. Group I comprised those who had showed a minimal change in their dietary intake during the intervening period between the two studies and Group II who had shown a marked decrease in both protein and calorie intake. The constancy of the dietary intake in Group I was associated with a similar state of both health and weight, whilst in Group II the association between a lower intake of food and a deterioration in health was in evidence. The report concluded:

> '*It must be emphasised that old people are not just random survivors of a general population, nor are those who attain extreme old age merely random survivors of the population of seventy-year-olds. They are, in fact, people whose special characteristics have enabled them to outlive their contempories*'. (Stanton & Exton-Smith, 1970)

Up until the mid-1960s, no clear-cut indication of malnutrition among the elderly had been established, although a Panel on Nutrition of the Elderly set up by the Committee on Medical Aspects of Food Policy (COMA) in 1967, had reported that although overt malnutrition rarely occurred there might be a wider incidence of sub-clinical nutrition. However, the Panel acknowledged that 'evidence is too patchy and unrepresentative to enable a comprehensive picture to be obtained'.

Thus, a nutrition survey of the elderly performed during 1967–1968 was designed to fill in some of the gaps of knowledge regarding these unknown areas of malnutrition. It was undertaken in six towns in England and Scotland on 764, elderly, non-institutionalised people, revealing geographical and sex differences in energy and nutrient intakes, with 'only' 3% of those surveyed diagnosed as having malnutrition and in three quarters of these cases it was in association with clinical disease. The survey also reasoned:

> '*The sort of food that old people want; is the same as other people have. Further provided it is properly prepared and suitably varied, it is also what they need to prevent the development of malnutrition. What is less simple, once an old person has been identified as being at risk, is to ensure that he or she does receive such food*'. (DHSS, 1972)

It was also shown that inefficient dentures, although not seemingly to result in 'any obvious evidence of disability' did mean that patients who experienced difficulty in chewing had to avoid certain types of food. Adapted diets, requiring less mastication were available but were usually unappetising:

> *'And since elderly subjects frequently have few pleasures left in life their ability to enjoy to the full a wide variety of foodstuffs is important to them'.* (DHSS, 1972)

Although these surveys were about the elderly who did not live in care homes, they provided an insight into what the elderly were actually eating, perhaps influencing what food was provided once institutionalised: would they be provided with the same food?

3.3.2   1970s

There was a further study *Nutrition and Health in Old Age*[3] (DHSS, 1979a) in 1972/3 of 365 surviving people who had participated in the former survey and who could be traced. This showed that 7% were considered to be malnourished and this condition was more prevalent in those over 80 years of age. The diets of the malnourished were generally poor with several medical and social risk factors being identified of which the most important was being housebound. A major conclusion of the survey was that provided individual elderly people were in good health, their dietary patterns and the foods eaten were no different from what was known about those of younger people.

In 1972 there was also a survey to assess the nutritional status of the housebound and to compare their dietary intake with those of more active old people. The results added further evidence to the facts that low intakes of nutrients were associated with a deterioration in physical and mental health in old age but there was no decline in intake with age *per se*. With regards to incidences of malnutrition, the authors recommended that subgroups should be defined for groups in which risk was particularly high, as prevention in these groups was more manageable than in the whole elderly population (Exton-Smith *et al.*, 1972).

In 1979 the Department of Health & Social Security (DHSS) published a report from COMA[4] on the Recommended Daily Amounts (RDAs) of food energy and nutrients for different groups of healthy people in the United Kingdom (DHSS, 1979b). It replaced an earlier report from 1969 whose figures were confusing and although intended to apply to groups of people, had been used mistakenly as recommendations for individuals. This new report provided updated recommendations, where possible, but it was acknowledged that over the past decade there had been relatively little new information which could alter the figures. RDAs were seen as being valuable for planning food supplies and diets, as a yardstick in the assessment of information about food supplies by means of which differences between groups of individuals and trends in time could be described and for directing attention to sub-groups who may be at risk of under-nutrition. At this time there were 150 000 people over the age of 65 living in residential homes.

3.3.3   1980s

In the 1980s there were changes in funding by the DHSS which opened doors to new providers with the bulk of older peoples' long-term provision moving into the independent sector: 'private, i.e. for profit and voluntary, i.e. not for profit' (Dudman, 2007). This brought with it the start of more regulation for care homes through the Registered Homes Act 1984 (RHA) covering independent residential care homes, nursing homes, mental nursing homes and private hospitals. Residential care homes, which provided residential accommodation with both board and personal care by reason of old age, disablement, past or present dependence on alcohol or drugs or past or present mental disorder were to register under Part I. Nursing homes used for nursing persons suffering from any sickness, injury or infirmity were to register under Part II. Some homes chose to be dual registered[5] both as a residential care home and as a nursing home to enable residents to remain in one home if their condition changed after admission (DHSS, 1984).

Regulation 18 of the Act empowered inspection of a registered home at least once every twelve months. This was regarded as a minimum and authorities were advised to inspect more frequently where warranted. The registration and inspection process was 'more than a negative policing procedure': authorities could 'actively endeavour to maintain and improve standards of care as well as facilities'. Local Authority homes were inspected by social services and nursing homes by health authorities, although 'elsewhere, health and local authorities have less formal arrangements but do liaise closely' (DHSS, 1984).

The publication *Home Life*[6] (Centre for Policy & Ageing, 1994) was a code of practice seen as an integral part of the Government's measures to regulate the establishment and conduct of private and voluntary residential care homes registered under the 1984 Act.

The Working Party which developed the Code faced two principal challenges, firstly the wide range of establishments and secondly the need to address one audience in one document. The legislation encompassed large homes, the voluntary, charitable and commercial sector, homes providing specialist care and nursing homes. The Working Party's concern was to 'ensure that the care provided in a home accurately reflects the stated aims and objectives of that home and that it satisfactorily responds to the needs of the residents'. They argued that the quality of care was shaped to a large extent by the attitudes of owners, managers and staff at all levels and therefore the Code of Practice attached considerable weight to the underlying philosophy of care and:

'to the tenets which gave substance to the philosophy. Concepts such as privacy, autonomy, individuality, esteem, choice and responsible risk taking provide the foundations and reference points for good practice and observance of these concepts in all possible circumstances is in itself good practice'. (Centre for Policy & Ageing, 1994)

Within the Code 'Diet and Food Preparation' were under the remit of Physical Features which advised that the attitudes of those responsible for the running of the home were reflected in the style of catering and the variety and presentation of food. Seen as integral to the 'philosophy of the home' was the consideration of residents' dietary needs and wishes, allowing choice and flexibility:

- Meals must be varied, properly served and nutritious and should provide choice
- Ready-plated meals should be avoided
- The timing of meals should be flexible and provision made for residents to prepare snacks and drinks for themselves
- Attention to residents with eating difficulties should be given discreetly
- Homes should be prepared to cater for special diets, whether these are medically advised, of cultural, religious or philosophical significance or the result of strong preference
- Residents should never be deceived into eating foods they would not otherwise take
- Staff training should include the cultural and social importance of meals, their content and preparation
- Proprietors should ascertain residents' dietary needs on admission, seeking advice from the community dietitian or religious advisers where necessary in order to meet these needs

Some local authorities did provide nutritional standards (Hertfordshire Health Authority, 1996) in accordance with Regulation 10(1) of the Registered Homes Act, which required the registered person to 'supply, suitable, varied and properly prepared wholesome and nutritious food in adequate quantities for the residents' (Read & Worsfold, 1998) but research on the system of regulating standards of care and food in residential care had shown considerable weaknesses in both the inspection and registration of homes by social services and environmental health teams. Particularly pertinent was the fact that although food was simultaneously acknowledged to be a highly important facet of the homes' operation in official literature such as *Home Life*, it was, in practice, regulated to a lowly position (Herne, 1994).

There were also several studies carried out to monitor the implementation of the Registered Homes Act and one in particular, in 1986, involved a question-naire being sent to all social service departments in England and Wales requesting information on their policies regarding private and voluntary residential homes. This was to establish what sort of policies and standards individual local authorities had developed to 'implement a piece of legislation which was silent in many issues important to both suppliers and consumers of residential care'. It was reported that homes for elderly people greatly outnumbered homes for 'mentally disordered' or 'younger physically handicapped client groups' (Laing & Bouisson, 1987). In addition, allowing for the possible ambiguities of questionnaire responses, the status of standards adopted by different local authorities were varied: some saw the minimum standards as a minima below which homes may not fall, other than in exceptional circumstances, without putting their registration at risk. Others saw standards more as indicators of good practice, applied with a correspondingly larger measure of *'flexibility and exhortation'* (Laing & Bouisson, 1987).

As for the impact of the 1984 Act, one of the points raised by the British Association of Social Workers (BASW) was:

> *'Like it or not, private residential care is a fact of life and an integral part of what some might call the new welfare "pluralism". It is not only with us but growing and in some areas at least, has virtually replaced local authority residential care. In short then it will not go away'.*   (BASW, 1986)

In 1987, more information on nutrition and dietetics was provided for those involved in catering for any group of elderly people via *Eating a Way into the 90's*[7] (NAGE, 1987), which was published by the Nutrition Advisory Group for Elderly People of the British Dietetic Association.

NAGE considered the timing of meals as very important as 'they are often high spots in the daily routine of many residents', with a recommendation that tea should not be any earlier than 5.00 p.m., as even with supper it was a long time to wait until breakfast. The suggested meal times were as shown in Box 3.2.

The importance of food for physical and social well being was emphasised, with information given on the nutritional requirements and food requirements of the older adult, general guidelines on food for health, factors affecting nutrition and the aims of menu planning. It stated *'remember – a little of what you fancy does you good'* suggesting that staff should *'be prepared to encourage and support people who are easily discouraged … nutritional problems are easier to prevent than cure'* (NAGE, 1997).

At this time, 13% of the male population and 19% of the female population of England and Wales were aged 65 or over, with 210 000 people (over 65) living in residential homes (DH, 1992a). Private residential home places increased rapidly in the 1980s from 39 253 in 1981 to 159 000 in 1990 (Read & Worsfold, 1998) and more than ever before, the 1990s saw more elderly people in the UK being cared for in institutions run as businesses, responsible for the nutritional well being of many elderly and physically handicapped people (Herne, 1994). By 1992 there were just

---

Box 3.2   Suggested meal times.

Early morning drink	7.00 a.m.–7.30 a.m.
Breakfast	8.00 a.m.–9.00 a.m.
Mid-morning drink/snack	10.00 a.m.–10.30 a.m.
Lunch	12 noon–1.00 p.m.
Mid-afternoon drink/snack	2.45 p.m.–3.15 p.m.
Evening meal	5.00 p.m.–6.00 p.m.
Bedtime snack	8.30 p.m.–9.30 p.m.

Source: NAGE (1997).

over a quarter of 85 year olds living in residential care homes, most of them run by private or voluntary organisations (Read & Worsfold, 1998).

This increase in the elderly population was discussed by the National Dairy Council (NDC) (National Dairy Council, 1992), who reported that life expectancy had been extended in most populations of the world due to changes in the main causes of death and improvements in infant mortality. This had resulted in an increase of old people in the population with the current average life expectation being approximately 72 years for men and 78 for women. They also anticipated that over the next ten years there would be an even greater expansion of elderly people especially those classified as 'very elderly' (over 75 years age) 'encompassing an extremely heterogeneous group'. At this time the accepted definition of an elderly person was one aged above the chronological age for retirement, 60 for women and 65 for men but it could extend to over 100 years of age. This age range included people who were chronologically old but biologically healthy, the chronologically sick and those who were frail because of advanced chronological age.

The NDC also expressed concern that there was a lack of information about the specific nutritional requirements of elderly people, with dietary recommendations frequently derived from the extrapolation of data from younger age groups. They recognised that there was a need for better biochemical and nutritional reference data for elderly people and there was 'good evidence' that institutionalised old people were particularly at risk of poor nutrition. They provided a suggested eating plan and a sample menu for the elderly (see Table 3.3 and Box 3.3).

3.3.4   1990s

There were more changes in funding arrangements for residential care through the NHS and Community Care Act 1990, resulting in the transfer of state funding to cash-limited local authority budgets. The act also required local authorities to inspect their own in-house residential care provision and to make their inspection reports openly available, ensuring that any recommendations and

Table 3.3 Suggested eating plan for an elderly person.

Food group	Daily servings
Lean meat, poultry, fish, eggs, pulses, nuts	2–3
Milk, cheese, yogurt	3 or more (extra portions for those advised to increase calcium intake may be necessary)
Bread, rice, pasta, breakfast cereals (choose a greater proportion of wholegrain) potatoes	4 or more to satisfy appetite
Vegetables (fresh or frozen), salad, fruit and fruit juices	4 or more
Spreading and cooking fats	In small amounts
Sugar and confectionery	In addition to basic foods to add variety, not as substitutes. Caution if subject is overweight

Source: National Dairy Council (1992).

Box 3.3   Sample menu for an elderly person.

Breakfast	Bowl of porridge or wholegrain cereal with milk. Glass of orange. Wholemeal toast thinly spread with butter or margarine and marmalade. Tea or coffee.
Mid-morning	Tea or coffee with milk. A banana
Midday meal	Shepherds pie, frozen peas, carrots. Stewed fruit and custard
Mid-afternoon snack	Cup of tea. Wholemeal scone or bread, lightly spread with butter margarine and/or jam
Evening meal	Sandwiches made with wholemeal bread filled with chopped hard boiled egg, sliced tomato and a little grated cheese. A yogurt or some fruit
Bedtime snack	Milky drink and digestive biscuit

Quantities of food and the number of between meal snacks will depend on the levels of activity and therefore energy needs of each individual

Source: National Dairy Council (1992).

requirements resulting from the reports were carried out (OFT, 1998). At this point, the majority of old people living in care homes lost specialist support from multidisciplinary teams within NHS units as they were not costed into the care provided (Dudman, 2007).

On the nutritional front, progress about the populations' nutrient requirements were evidenced through revised Dietary Reference Values (DRVs), as determined by COMA in 1991 (DH, 1991). The DRVs replaced RDAs and differed from the previous recommendations in the range of nutrients covered: previously COMA had only considered 10, now it was around forty. In addition, fat and carbohydrates were considered for the first time in the context of their relation to energy requirements and DRVs for those aged over 50 years of age were also presented.

COMA also produced *The Nutrition of Elderly People* (DH, 1992a), which replaced their 1970 study in which they had concluded that the quality of the diet did not change with age but that quantity tended to decrease. COMA acknowledged that it had been 20 years since they had last examined this subject, commenting that 'the base of scientific knowledge had enlarged'.

This new report defined elderly people as being over 65 years and over, young elderly as those aged 65–74 and older elderly aged 75 and over. COMA recommended that the majority of people aged 65 or over, should adopt, where possible, similar patterns of eating and lifestyle to those advised for maintaining health in younger adults: physical activity improved muscle tone and power, leading to higher energy expenditure. Therefore, a diet which provided an adequate intake of all nutrients could be more easily obtained if the energy intake remained at a level close to that recommended for younger adults.

An area of particular concern was the impact of illness and disability on the nutritional status of this aged group with an acknowledgement that there was little data on their energy and nutrient requirements. In addition there were cases of inadequate intakes, evidenced by low body weight, particularly among very disabled old people being cared for in institutions. In addressing the possibility of 'institutional starvation', research was recommended in this area. Moreover, the anthropometric measurements used in nutritional surveys were of 'questionable value' when used in elderly populations, an issue that also needed to be addressed.

Other recommendations included:

- Further studies to quantify energy requirements for elderly people which took individual health status into account with particular emphasis on those who were thin
- Dietary intakes of elderly people should tend to be generous except for those who were obese
- Elderly people deriving their dietary intakes from a diet containing a variety of nutrient dense foods
- Steps being taken to increase the awareness by health professionals of the importance of being both underweight and overweight in elderly people
- The micronutrient requirements of the elderly population to be determined more accurately
- Increased intakes of vitamin C & fibre
- Encouraging exposure to sunlight to produce vitamin D

It was also reported that the Working Group were disappointed that all too often, their work was constrained by a lack of data. Disappointment about this limited evidence was also expressed in an article from a British Nutrition Foundation bulletin:

'Perhaps those bulletin readers who have any influence over nutrition research policy and can identify themselves as the one person in four who hopes to be over 65 in the year 2030 can persuade scientists to make an effort to study the nutritional status of people other than students and young colleagues. Only in this way will future COMA panels make any greater progress'.   (Groom, 1993)

But even knowing the nutritional requirements of the elderly, institutionalised or not, just how problematic care home catering could be was shown in 1994 by the Food Policy Research Unit who published the findings of a study resulting from interviews with care home managers.

Although it was acknowledged that elderly people were often afraid to complain for fear of retribution it was believed that even if the quality of meals was a target for complaint this was often an attempt to draw attention to a general dissatisfaction with their lifestyle: the only way they could express this dissatisfaction was to complain about the food. 'Battles of will' could occur after admission with residents feeling lonely and frustrated:

'She was determined that she wouldn't settle here. She has not accepted that she needed care. For weeks all she would have was stewed apple every day.

We couldn't get her to eat anything else. Even now the only vegetables she'll eat are carrots and cabbage'. (Herne, 1994)

Residents could also be highly intolerant of each other with mealtimes, the main communal occasion, seen as the most obvious time for intolerances to manifest themselves with eating habits a common bone of contention:

'Sometimes her table manners are disgusting because of her dementia. She takes her teeth out in the middle of lunch to look at them'. (Herne, 1994)

These difficulties surrounding the social aspects of eating were probably underestimated with homes that refused dementia patients mentioning this type of disruptive behaviour as the basis for separating mentally and physically ill people:

'When his dementia became apparent we couldn't cope. He wandered into other residents' rooms, helped himself to their food and frequently went naked. Our old ladies in particular found it very distressing'. (Herne, 1994)

With regard to choices at mealtimes, purported to be the most important aspect of catering to the elderly, choice was offered at breakfast, tea and supper but only 38% of homes were able to offer a choice at the main lunchtime meal. This was due to costs, lack of staff to make and serve several dishes and the inability of some residents to make choices, particularly those in various stages of dementia. It was the smaller homes that were most likely to have a restricted choice, with 'emergency supplies' in the freezer such as burgers, frozen fish, chops and pies, for those who did not like what was being offered: these items could be easily prepared alongside the main menu (Herne, 1994).

The use of laxatives was widespread, akin to a 'wide scale addiction'. To reduce the amount of laxatives taken, placebos such as vitamin tablets or, in one case, soda water were administered. It was pointed out that dietary therapy could have been used but even if staff agreed with healthy eating, actually persuading residents to change their eating habits was 'no mean feat':

'We try brown (sic) bread, prunes and bran but you have to get them used to the idea. Most of them have never eaten brown bread in their lives. It's a slow process'. (Herne, 1994)

This issue of healthy eating prompted criticism for the authors of *The Nutrition of Elderly* People (DH, 1992a) and the *Health of the Nation* (DH, 1992b) for failing to acknowledge that older people come from a generation 'good at ignoring health education'. As a result some of the healthy eating policies brought out by suppliers such as NHS Regional Supplies, had failed to impress their target audience:

'They wouldn't supply grapefruit in syrup because it's healthier to have it in its own juice. Our old ladies refused to eat it or else they put piles of sugar on it'.

'They like plain, basic food – you can't try new things. We gave them plaice rolled and stuffed with prawns. Because it didn't look fish-shaped they just pushed it around their plates'.   (Herne, 1994)

Forcing the issue was not considered to be a viable option as it was seen as breach of rights: 'if they've got to 80 on fish and chips, all power to them' with managers contenting themselves with the successes they had achieved: only a small proportion of residents still insisted on a cooked breakfast – most had taken readily to the idea of eating prunes or grapefruit, toast and cereals including high fibre versions such as Weetabix and muesli. It was men requiring low cholesterol diets who had presented the greatest problems because they were more fiercely attached to their fried breakfasts: *'As for the rest of the meals, for the moment at least, it seemed that the COMA recommendations will have to take a back seat to food as enjoyment'* (Herne, 1994).

The 'real problem' was getting residents to stick to special diets, especially if they were a recent introduction. Although diabetics and 'slimmers' knew why they were on diets, food was their main source of enjoyment and so they felt they were being denied some of the pleasure of eating. Under these circumstances and on the understanding that it was only 'occasional' residents were allowed treats:

'E hates her diet – she loves her puddings. We have to let her have treats or life would be so boring for her'.   (Diabetic)

'We have to keep telling him how well he's doing and let him have the odd treat to keep him going'.   (Slimming diet)

However, the elderly could not be underestimated:

'Residents proved to be extremely resourceful when they wished to abandon their special diets. Tactics included late night raids on food cupboards, swapping plates of diabetic cakes for normal ones and persuading relatives to bring in "extras". Most old ladies are very attached to their handbags but we did wonder why these two took them absolutely everywhere until we found they were full of sweets'.   (Herne, 1994)

Success rates varied: diabetics tended to stabilise because they were given regular meals and drug treatment, while the slimmers were less successful because homes had a real problem deciding how strict they should be:

'If it was a case of lose weight or die then of course we would insist he stuck to it but he does love food and it seems such a shame'.   (Herne, 1994)

Introducing more fibre into the diet was easier than any other regime. Apart from the success of breakfast cereals the use of white bread with added bran was a successful halfway house. Discretion was the key: *'if they did not realise they were eating it they did not object. We try to make sure they have enough bran in the diet. Often we will mix a bit in things like mashed potato'.* (Herne, 1994).

Sixty-two per cent of homes had at least one patient who needed help with feeding. Policies on how to conduct feeding varied: homes that were of a sufficient size had two sittings for the main meal, feeding the dependent residents separately from the others. Others chose to feed dependent residents in a different room or put people of mixed abilities on a table, more able residents then helped their frailer counterparts, which relied on the goodwill and tolerance of the residents. The input ranged from cutting food to full spoon feeding. The actual act of feeding an individual was a potential minefield as it exposed the disabilities of the residents:

'Now we take the food to her in its original state. We then ask her if she'd like a little help. It would be so easy to take it over to her already cut up but she found it very offensive that we didn't even give her the chance to try'.   (Herne, 1994)

The mechanics of feeding an individual were also complicated: what position should the care assistant take? How much should they put in each fork/spoonful? How long should they allow between mouthfuls?

'Helping someone to drink is incredibly difficult. Get it wrong and you spill it all over the resident or cause them to choke'.   (Herne, 1994)

It was explained that the requirement for soft or pureed diets was often the result of conditions which had destroyed the swallowing reflex. Initially the staff who prepared pureed food were 'revolted': they had experimented with the presentation of purees but using tactics such as the use of food colourings had only made the food look synthetic. They were more successful when they used soft food such as making potato with plenty of milk and butter. Other items considered to be 'revolting' were special bread and cakes used for a low protein diet (Herne, 1994).

On a positive note, contrary to what might have been expected, it was also reported that for some of the residents not having to plan, budget, shop or prepare foods was one of the more pleasurable aspects of care. Around a quarter of the residents said they like the food: 'I like the food it's beautiful. It's like Christmas every day'. Being 'pleased' with meals and enjoying the socialising around the table that accompanied them has been reported elsewhere (Connor, 1999): in this study the constant complaint was against the unresolved problem of large portion sizes. In addition many of the respondents had heard of healthy eating and although happy with the menu, would have liked more wheaten bread, wholemeal bread and fresh fruit.

Taking all these issues into account, it is remarkable that as late as 1995, reference was again being made to the fact that there were:

'no guidelines on appropriate nutritional standards for older people available in a readily accessible form for the many thousands who have responsibility for producing food for older people in residential nursing homes and for community meals'.

This observation came from the Caroline Walker Trust (CWT) who subsequently published *Eating Well for Older People* (CWT, 1995) providing guidelines for food in residential and nursing homes and for community meals.

As *Eating Well for Older people* was being compiled, the members of the expert working group were acutely aware that they had not looked at the specific requirements for older people with dementia who merited special consideration because of the link between weight loss and dementia and their poor nutritional status.

Thus a further expert working group was established with the support of the CWT and the Department of Health under the aegis of Voluntary Organisations Involved in Caring in the Elderly Sector. The resulting publication *Eating Well for Older People With Dementia* (VOICES, 1998) gave facts on dementia itself, nutrition and dementia, how a good diet could help, practical guidelines for achieving a good diet, strategies to encourage older people with dementia to eat well and the eating environment. Characteristics associated with dementia which may affect eating habits are shown in Box 3.4, with examples of why these strategies, based on reported comments, are so important to all concerned with those involved in their nutritional care, shown in Box 3.5.

In 1998, a nutritional analysis of the weekly menus from 24 residential homes revealed that the menus complied with the recommendations from *Eating Well for Older People* (1995), providing different main course items, familiar traditional home-cooked dishes, a variety of vegetables and a selection of puddings: if the meals were eaten they would provide sufficient energy and nutrients to meet most of the dietary needs of the elderly residents. However, the menus did not provide an adequate amount of starch, fibre and vitamin D, plus they contained a higher than recommended level of sugar and salt (Read & Worsfold, 1998). In addition, adequate drinks and snacks were provided between meals, but for many residents

---

Box 3.4 Characteristics associated with dementia which may affect eating habits.

Practical physical changes – whereby the person may be unable to use cutlery, have problems with tremor or lack of coordination in getting food to their mouth, be unable to unwrap or unpeel items, be unable to sit for meals, be extremely slow in eating

Physiological changes – the person may lose their sense of smell and taste, lose their appetite, have difficulty swallowing, be unable to chew, have mouth or tooth pain, show a preference for sweet foods

Emotional/cognitive changes – the person may be distracted from eating, forget to eat or forgotten having eaten, have difficulty making choices, eat food with their hands, be unable to communicate hunger or thirst

Changes associated with depression/paranoia – the person may lose interest in eating or eat constantly, be suspicious about food, refuse to eat.

Source: VOICES (1998).

Box 3.5   Why strategies to encourage older people with dementia to eat well are important.

One **carer** gave the example of a home that always served a woman who required puréed food last at mealtimes, explaining: (Alzheimer)

> *'They had to blend her food for her but she was always served last and she cried every day. And they just said "she's crying again, she knows every day she's going to get her food." Now anyone would put it on her table first to stop her getting distressed everyday'.*   (Alzheimer)

Whilst a **relative** said: *'Mum's non-verbal are quite good if they would just spend a bit more time with her, especially at meal times'*. (Alzheimer)

Source: Alzheimer's Society (2007).

---

a choice of meals was not provided, meals were pre-plated and there was a lack of variety with weekly repeated meals (Read & Worsfold, 1998).

With regard to the high levels of sugar, one of the main sources came from sweetened beverages. Other sources included sweetened breakfast cereals, puddings, cakes and biscuits, with sweet biscuits being the most popular sweet items. However, it was pointed out that sugar could provide a significant source of calories for residents with poor appetites and could make the food more palatable to those with diminished taste perception. COMA had previously stated that if large amounts of foods rich in simple sugars were consumed, appetite for a more varied and nutrient-rich diet might be blunted (DH, 1992a), but in terms of overall nutritional intake, other advice has suggested that attempts to over restrict the amount of sugar and salt in an elderly persons' diet might be counter-productive, leading to a reduction in the palatability of food with the notion that limiting extrinsic sugar intake to avoid dental caries was unwarranted in old age (National Dairy Council, 1992).

It was also indicated that the residents enjoyed their food but there were difficulties experienced in persuading some residents to eat an adequate quantity of food, thought to be the result of apathy, confusion, the effects of medication and problems with chewing and swallowing. Residents were generally reluctant to try unfamiliar foods such as pasta and rice, making it difficult to introduce new dishes. There was also a difficulty in presenting pureed foods attractively but it was noted that commercial thickening agents and food-shaped moulds were now available to improve the texture and appearance (Read & Worsfold, 1998).

The study concluded that staff in residential homes should ensure that their 'clients' should have enough to eat through the provision of varied, appetising, well-presented meals, served at the right temperature, in pleasant surroundings with appropriate utensils and adequate feeding assistance.

Therein might have lain one of the problems for the 'clients': in 1997, the Office of Fair Trading (OFT) announced that it intended to undertake an inquiry on care homes 'focusing solely on the experience of residents as consumers in care homes within the public, private and voluntary sectors'. The resulting report, *Older People as Consumers in Care Homes* (OFT, 1998) confirmed fears that vital information was not reaching those who not only needed it but when they needed it most:

> *'We have an interest therefore, in ensuring that older consumers are offered the best possible deal. Part of that deal means clear and comprehensive information of what can be expected in a care-home environment'.* (OFT, 1998)

It has been intimated that the reports 'unusual source' is what made it so 'refreshing' but although it was made available free of charge it has been suggested that few care homes managers or owners have seen it with the reality of 'grey power' having only been recognised fleetingly in the UK (Burton-Jones, 2000).

Yet more information on the elderly was soon to be gathered when the largest and most detailed survey undertaken of the diet and nutritional status of older people living in Britain, in both the community and institutions, was undertaken: the *National Diet and Nutrition survey of people aged 65 and over* was published in 1998, split into two volumes which covered the diet and nutrition survey and the oral health survey respectively (Finch *et al.*, 1998; Steele *et al.*, 1998). From the diet and nutrition survey, for those living in institutions, some of the findings showed:

- 35% had facilities to make a hot drink
- 22% had facilities for preparing a light snack
- 72% were sometimes able to order a different meal from that offered
- 51% of men and 69% of women received food or drink from their visitors

The institutionalised also tended to have a more traditional eating pattern with energy intakes, on average close to the estimated average requirements (EARs), with the energy sources, compared to the free living group, higher from cereal-based milk puddings and lower from meat and meat products. Average intakes of protein were well above the recommended nutrient intake (RNI) with 18.4% of food energy derived from non-milk extrinsic factors (NMES) which was above the COMA recommendations of 11%, with table sugar alone providing 38% of the total intake. The average daily intake for non-starch polysaccharide (NSP – dietary fibre) was below the COMA recommendations and saturated fat intake exceeded the recommendations.

Other findings showed that in the institutionalised group:

- Intakes were below the lower recommended nutrient intake (LRNI) for zinc and iron
- Average intakes of magnesium and potassium were below both the RNIs and the LRNIs
- 7% had low intakes of riboflavin and folate

- 40% had low vitamin C, folate and riboflavin biochemical status, 10% for thiamine and 37% for vitamin D
- 52% of men and 39% of women had haemoglobin levels below the WHO defined level for anaemia
- Up to 11% had low serum ferritin concentrations, indicating low iron stores

Moreover, free living men and women were, on average, significantly heavier than those living in institutions, two thirds of free living individuals were classified as overweight or obese compared to just under half of those institutionalised with few free living classified as underweight compared to one in six of those in institutions.

Similar findings about these low intakes of dietary fibre, vitamins A and D, and folic acid were also found to be very low in another survey with the surprising finding of the over consumption of vitamin C derived from large tumblers of orange and grapefruit juice. There were also excessive intakes of calcium derived from the use of milk in puddings, sauces and in the cups of tea for which there was an average consumption for each resident of eight cups of tea per day (Connor, 1999).

These findings could suggest a lack of actual dietary understanding itself as in this latter study, all the catering staff themselves had a good knowledge of cooking. However, only one home had sent the catering staff on a course specialising in catering for the elderly: *'this home was also the most progressive and efficient of those surveyed'* (Connor, 1999).

Towards the end of the 1990s, the funding of care for the elderly in general was on the agenda with the appointment of a Royal Commission with the following terms of reference:

'To examine the short and long term options for a sustainable system of funding of Long Term Care for elderly people, both in their own homes and in other settings, and, within 12 months, to recommend how, and in what circumstances, the cost of such care should be apportioned between public funds and individuals'. (Sutherland, 1999)

The resulting document *With Respect to Old Age* (Sutherland, 1999), published in 1999 said that the Commission had begun from the point of view that old age should not be seen as a problem, but a time of life with fulfillments of its own. To provide security in old age and proper care for those who needed it, the main recommendations were:

- The costs of long-term care should be split between living costs, housing costs and personal care. Personal care should be available after assessment, according to need and paid for from general taxation: the rest should be subject to a co-payment according to means.
- The Government should establish a National Care Commission to monitor trends, including demography and spending, ensure transparency and accountability in the system, represent the interests of consumers, and set national benchmarks, now and in the future.

The British Dietetic Association was involved in submitting evidence for *With Respect to Old Age*, evidence which was prepared through the Nutrition Advisory Group for Elderly People (NAGE) (Eaton, 1999). Their resulting document, *How Nutrition Relates to Cost of Long-term Care* contained seven sub-sections: nutrition requirements, the impact of malnutrition, food as treatment, food as care, provision of food service, ethical matters and training. The following suggestions were offered:

- Adequate staff training of an agreed standard to include such topics as the importance of food, helping people to eat and drink, the importance of good nutrition to recovery, food hygiene.
- Registration and monitoring of services. A national minimum standard for food provision to meet nutritional requirements should be agreed for community meals and nursing and residential homes and hospitals.
- Sufficient staff must be available to facilitate eating and drinking (Eaton, 1999).

However, the Royal Commission worked around a specific definition of care, excluding most food from personal care costs suggesting that the work of the Commission was about funding personal care and not about practicalities of subsistence, including food: the nutrition implications of age and disability were not seen to be within the remit of the funding enquiry. This meant that physical rehabilitation, that is the work of physiotherapy and occupational therapy was considered while diet therapy fell outside their remit, reflected too in the composition of the Commission's Reference Group. It was also predicted that the report had less immediate use for practising dietitians with a suggestion that '*once again the lack of core nutritional input to social services at the highest level of public food policy is highlighted by its absence.*' (Eaton, 1999)

As the Commissioners assured:

'*When Royal Commissions are created, the cynical view is that either a difficult issue is being kicked into the long grass so that someone other than Government can take the blame for problems which are impossible to solve or unpalatable in their solution, or that a seemingly independent body will be told by Government to deliver an unpalatable response it does not want to take responsibility for itself. In the first case we can expect a Royal Commission to take years to reach its conclusions, and in the second the Government of the day will tell it when to report. Neither of these views apply in our case*'.

This lack of 'core nutritional input' could have added to the nutritional inequalities for residents in care homes, highlighted in the *Health Survey for England* (Bajekal, 2000) report which showed that the proportion of men and women eating fruit (fresh, tinned or frozen) and red meat six or more times a week in care homes was about half that in private households. Additionally, for individuals with a valid body mass index (BMI) measurement, those in care homes had a lower BMI than older people in private households, reflected in higher proportions of underweight individuals in the care homes population with the prevalence of anaemia being on average two and a half times higher in care homes than in private households: 43% of men in care homes compared to 16% in private households and for women 28% and 11% respectively. All this at a time when more pressure was being put on care homes with the announcement of plans to move elderly patients to private nursing homes to ease the congestion of 'bed blocking' in NHS hospitals. There was concern that homes would not have the staff to support these plans with Age Concern calling for private homes to be more tightly regulated and monitored (News, 2000).

Yet another document, *Fit for the Future?* (DH, 1999) reiterated the governments' commitment to improving protection for vulnerable people through new inspection systems and stronger safeguards, stating that the present regulatory arrangements were 'incomplete and patchy and have developed in a piece-meal fashion'.

At the time, responsibilities for regulating various services for adults and children were divided between health authorities, local authorities and the DH centrally. Other services, such as LA care homes and small children's homes were not subject to any regulation meaning that people in local authority care homes did not benefit from independent regulation. This meant that there was not enough scrutiny of nursing care in residential homes and social care in nursing homes and due to a lack of consistency there was uncertainty for both providers and service users. In terms of the standards that care homes must meet, the still current, *Registered Homes Act 1984* and its regulations did not set out much detail in terms of the standards.

Thus, the Centre for Policy on Ageing (CPA) was commissioned to advise on the proposed standards for residential and nursing homes for older people, seen as the largest category of care homes.

The resulting draft standards were organised around a number of main topics which contained sub-topics, any relevant legislation/regulations, national required standards, evidence of the standard having been met and outcomes. Under the main topic of Policies, Procedures, Records and Protocols was sub-topic Nutrition (4.9), which stated that the home must have a written food policy including:

- Standards of nutrition
- Standards of catering
- Dining arrangements
- How cultural, religious and personal preferences were catered for
- How special dietary needs were catered for
- The home's contract with residents which stated whether the provision of, and charges for all meals, and food and drink, were wholly or partly included

In addition, under the main topic of Food Preparation, Meals and Mealtimes, there were 27 National Required Standards split into the sub-topics Food Policy, Resident's Food, Menus, Mealtimes and Food Purchase, Storage and Preparation.

Age Concern (2000), welcomed this consultation document and in a detailed response to the DH they considered the effects of the proposed standards, whether they were at the right level, their timescale for implementation and whether the government should wait for the Regional Care Commissions to be established before implementing the standards. Amongst these issues, they argued that *Fit for the Future?* was inconsistent in its objectives and outcomes indicators and although most of the outcomes were measurable, they were not, in the main, pass or fail indicators. There was also concern that there was 'little emphasis on actively encouraging residents to participate in day to day activities'. For example, with regard to Standard 7.2 which referred to the availability of hot and cold drinks and snacks at all times, it was suggested that the standard should place an onus on homes to enable residents to make their own drinks or snack if this was preferred.

Concerns had also been voiced about the fact that the new standards would require sufficient numbers of both catering and health care staff to ensure that the requirements for meal provision and nutrition were fully met. In addition, staff would require training to enable them to perform the required nutritional assessments and provide feeding assistance for residents with complex eating problems (Stanner, 2002).

It was also pointed out that few care home providers would be able to meet the new standards without professional catering and support staff with more independent care homes having to turn to specialised contractors to provide catering services. It was also suggested that the problems associated with the current skills shortage amongst the hospitality industry could be overcome by 'growing one's own' from within, along with the notion of encouraging those who thought that catering in the health sector had little to offer, to actually join it: this sector did not have a glamorous image but managers of homes could ask themselves if catering qualifications really mattered, particularly as there was no legal or registration requirement for catering staff to be qualified in anything other than food safety, with hands on experience often worth far more than somebody having just coming out of college. In addition, managers of homes could be confused by the various qualifications of catering staff which were often in the form of NVQ's which focused on hotel and restaurant catering, with basic nutrition not being part of the syllabus. Although other courses were available, there was still a gap in the provision of bespoke courses for health care catering: in 2000 there was only one association supporting the care home caterers, which was the Advisory Body of Social Services Caterers (ABSSC) (Innes–Farqhar, 2000).

With these concerns in mind, the extent of the actual numbers of people needing a certain nutritional standard is evidenced by the fact that in 2001, there were a reported 341 200 older people living in residential care accommodation with a further 186 000 in nursing care. In addition, about a quarter of people over the age of 85 lived in long-stay care, which was forecast to rise because of the particularly rapid increase in the number of over-85s (CWT, 2004a).

3.4   Current decade

3.4.1   National Minimum Standards

Concerns aside, the DHs *National Minimum Standards and Care Homes Regulations for Care Homes for Older People*[8] (DH, 2006) were published in 2002, in accordance with section 23 of the Care Standards Act[9] (CSA) 2000 (for England & Wales), forming the basis on which the new National Care Standards Commission (NCSC) 'will determine whether such care homes meet the needs and secure the welfare and social inclusion of the people who live there'. The NCSC was an independent non-governmental public body, regulating social and health care services previously regulated by local councils and health authorities:

> 'In assessing whether a care home conforms to the Care Homes Regulations 2001 which **are** mandatory, the National Care Standards Commission take standards into account. However, the Commission **may** also take into account any other factors it considers reasonable or relevant to do so. Compliance with national minimum standards is not in itself enforceable, but compliance with regulations is enforceable subject to national standards being taken into account. The Commission may conclude that a care home has been in breach of the regulations, even though the home largely meets the standards. The Commission also has discretion to conclude that the regulations have been complied with by means other than those set out in the national minimum standards'. (DH, 2006)

There are 38 core National Minimum Standards (NMS), which apply to all care homes providing accommodation and nursing or personal care for older people under the general headings of Choice of Home, Health and Personal Care, Daily Life and Social Activities, Complaints and Protection, Environment, Staffing and Management and Administration. The standards are not themselves legally binding but operate in tandem with the *Care Home Regulations 2001*, which are legally enforceable.

With regard to the NMS relating to nutrition, Standard 8 (8.9), Health Care, states that:

> 'Nutritional screening is undertaken on admission and subsequently on a periodic basis, a record maintained of nutrition, including weight gain and loss and appropriate action taken'

Under the heading Daily Life and Social Activities (Standards 12–15) are Standard 12, (12.2) Social Contact and Activities and Standard 15, Meals & Mealtimes:

Standard 12.2 states that:

> 'Service users have the opportunity to exercise their choice in relation to ... food, meals and mealtimes'

The requirements of Standard 15 are:

15.1   The registered person ensures that service users receive a varied, appealing, wholesome and nutritious diet, which is suited to individual assessed and recorded requirements and that meals are taken in a congenial setting and at flexible times.

15.2   Each service user is offered three full meals each day (at least one of which must be cooked at intervals of not more than five hours)

15.3   Hot and cold drinks and snacks are available at all times and offered regularly. A snack meal should be offered in the evening and the interval between this and breakfast the following morning should be no more than 12 hours.

15.4   Food, including liquefied meals, is presented in a manner which is attractive and appealing in terms of texture, flavour and appearance, in order to maintain appetite and nutrition.

15.5   Special therapeutic diets/feeds are provided when advised by health care and dietetic staff, including adequate provision of calcium and vitamin D.

15.6   Religious or cultural dietary needs are catered for as agreed at admission and recorded in the care plan and food for special occasions is available

15.7   The registered person ensures that there is a menu (changed regularly), offering a choice of meals in written or other formats to suit the capacities of all service users, which is given, read or explained to service users.

15.8   The registered person ensures that mealtimes are unhurried with service users being given sufficient time to eat

15.9   Staff are ready to offer assistance in eating where necessary, discreetly, sensitively and individually, while independent eating is encouraged for as long as possible.

The outcome for this standard is: 'Service users receive a wholesome appealing balanced diet in pleasing surroundings at times convenient to them'.

In addition, Standard 27 (27.7), Staff Complement, states:

'Domestic staff are employed in sufficient numbers to ensure that standards in relation to food, meals and nutrition are fully met'

with 'Records to be kept by a care home', including Regulation 17(2):13 stating:

'Records of the food provided for service users in sufficient detail to enable any person inspecting the record to determine whether the diet is satisfactory, in relation to nutrition and otherwise, and of any special diets prepared for individual service users'.

It has been suggested that the new NMS clearly recognised that food and nutrition were essential to the quality of life of older people in long-term care.

This was important because psychological and social discomfort could be experienced by individuals offered meals that were inappropriate for their social, cultural or religious needs, thereby causing distress, even to those who were otherwise healthy (Stanner, 2002).

In terms of reform, the Independent Healthcare Authority (IHA) welcomed improved regulation for the independent health and social care sector as it had been calling for amendment to the 1984 Registered Home Act for over ten years. In addition it would be seen as a relief for many care providers as it would hopefully remove the idiosyncrasies which organisations working in more than one local authority had experienced when dealing with registration and inspection units (Fermoy, 2000).

However, because the NMS also had rules on issues such as room sizes[10] (Standard 23) there were concerns that this would impact financially on smaller care homes who were already struggling to keep their heads above water:

'I am sick of having my business interfered with by people who do not understand the difficulties in trying to make a livelihood for a group of people who the state seems to have simply been willing to wash its hands of'. (Readers Letters, 2000)

Another Standard with a potential to create problems was Standard 27 (27.7) regarding staff: it has been reported that although care homes standards had improved since 2002/03 there were still many concerns, amongst others, about the lack of trained staff (Robinson & Banks, 2005), making it difficult to ensure that all staff understood the importance of good nutrition and hydration (OFT, 2005).

As has been suggested, many care home staff are committed to their work but many who are employed by small care organisations in the independent sector experience particular difficulties in accessing training leading to National Vocational Qualifications (NVQs). This situation is the same for care home staff who have English as a second language and those who have poor literacy and numeracy skills (Robinson & Banks, 2005).

Problems with staff are also affected by differing geographical areas: in London, the continuity of care for older people is adversely affected by the high staff turnover and the well above average vacancy rates for care staff in residential care. London is also affected by the large amount of ethnic minority care workers, who make up around 60% of the work force. Many of these carers are well qualified in their own countries but speak English as a second language. There are clear benefits to having a multi-ethnic workforce but problems such as racism can be experienced by staff with poor communications between staff and service users (Robinson & Banks, 2005).

These issues aside, how did care homes perform? In their 2004 report, *How do we care?* (Dalley, 2005/06) on care homes and their performance against the NMS for 2002–03, the National Care Standards Commission (NCSC) reported that 50% of the Standards were met by 68% of care homes for older people and that in many cases the scores were representative of relatively minor problems which could be overcome readily. With regard to Meals and Mealtimes, 78% of care homes met the Standard.

Homes meeting or attempting to meet the NMS could refer to more updated information though the Caroline Walker Trust (CWT), who published a second edition of *Eating Well for Older People* (CWT, 2004) in 2004. This provided a practical tool for those planning menus for older people, used extensively across the UK.

The CWT recommended that:

- The nutritional guidelines should become minimum standards for food prepared for older people in residential care accommodations and for community meals. Cost considerations should not override the need for adequate nutritional content in the planning and preparation of food for older people.
- Local authorities should adopt these nutritional guidelines and insist on them being maintained in residential and nursing homes with which they contract for long-term care, and in the provision of community meals.

The CWT also reported that many older people in residential care accommodation were undernourished either through previous poverty, social isolation, personal or psychological problems or due to the effects of medication. Furthermore, since its original publication in 1995, there had been a number of recommendations made relating to the food service for older people in residential and nursing care, but there was still a need to provide practical information on how managers of residential or nursing homes could achieve appropriate nutritional content in the food they served (CWT, 2004).

The CWT also produced a computer menu programme called the *CORA*[11] – *Menu Planner* (CWT 2004b). Table 3.4 shows sample menus provided by the CWT and the *CORA Menu Planner* for older people living in residential or nursing homes.

By now there were an estimated 410 000 people living in residential and nursing homes across the UK, with approximately 15 700 in private, voluntary and Local Authority care homes, providing care at an estimated value of more than £8 billion per annum (OFT, 2005).

3.4.2 Inspection

Meanwhile, the comments of one author on the fact that the National Care Standards Commission (NCSC) had not been provided with many of the powers which were then common place among other regulators and the likelihood that they would 'soon cast an envious eye toward the powers of those other regulators and return to government for future reform' (Kerrison & Pollock, 2001) turned out to be prophetic: in 2004, the NCSC was replaced by the Commission for Healthcare Audit and Inspection (CHAI) and the Commission for Social Care Inspection (CSCI). During 2004/2005 the CSCI spent 70% of its budget on inspection with 80% of its time allocated to care homes (Furness, 2008).

Table 3.4 Sample menus provided by the CWT and CORA.

	CWT	CORA
Breakfast	Prunes, porridge or high fibre cereal with milk. Toast (white or wholemeal) with butter/ polyunsaturated margarine and marmalade or jam, tea or coffee with milk [a]	Choice of high fibre cereals. Fresh citrus or cranberry juice. Scrambled eggs, or baked beans, or grilled bacon, or grilled kipper, or grilled tomatoes with toast. Tea or coffee
Mid-morning	Tea or coffee with milk and digestive biscuit	Choice of fresh fruit slices (apple, pear, banana, orange, melon etc.) as in season. Tea or coffee
Lunch	Fruit juice. Roast pork and apple sauce, cabbage, sweetcorn, roast potatoes. Rhubarb crumble and custard. Water	Kidney turbigo, braised rice, celery, green beans. Queen of puddings and custard. Water or fruit juice
Mid-afternoon	Tea or coffee with milk. Jam sponge	Tea or coffee. Choice of apple and cinnamon cake, banana tea bread, date and raisin tea bread, farmhouse sultana cake, fruit scones with butter, sticky prune cake or lemon cake
Evening meal	Fish cakes and tomato. Cherry pie. Fresh orange. Water or fruit juice	Lentil soup, smoked mackerel pate and toast. Fruit yogurt. Water or fruit juice
Bedtime	Milky drink: Horlicks, Ovaltine, hot chocolate, milky tea or milk shake	Milky drink: Horlicks, Ovaltine, hot chocolate, milky tea or milk shake.

[a] Residents should be offered additional drinks after meals: 8 cups of fluid a day are recommended.
Source: CWT (2004).

As part of their inspection process, the CSCI monitor care home processes for assessing and reviewing older people's nutrition, weight and dietary requirements, although they have stated:

> '*inspectors are not tasked with, nor qualified to, assess for malnutrition. This is a task for trained healthcare professionals who are best placed to provide advice and nutrition support and assess for malnutrition*'. (CSCI, 2006)

In 2005, the Nutrition Advisory Group for the Elderly (NAGE) identified inconsistencies in the way nutrition standards were being interpreted between different geographical areas of England by different inspectors. NAGE suggested that it should be obligatory for all inspectors to receive appropriate training, or at the least, guidance notes on interpretation of the standards. However, the CSCI were reportedly unable to make this a priority which meant that NAGE could not take this issue further forward, despite working in partnership with BAPEN and the National Association of Care Caterers (NACC) (Smith, 2007).

Priority or not, it has been reported that CSCI inspectors normally have a background in either nursing or social care, hold relevant qualifications, are trained

Table 3.5 Percentage of homes by owner type meeting the meals and mealtimes NMS in 2002/03 and 2004/05.

	Independent (%)	Local authority (%)	Voluntary (%)	All services (%)
31 March 2003	77.3	81.6	83.4	78.2
31 March 2005	82.6	85.2	88.7	83.4
Difference in % points	5.3	3.6	5.3	5.2

Source: CSCI (2006).

Table 3.6 Percentage of homes by type meeting the meals and mealtimes NMS in 2002/03 and 2004/05.

	Personal care only (%)	Care homes (with nursing) (%)	All homes (%)
31 March 2003	79.9	74.5	78.2
31 March 2005	85.5	78.9	83.4
Difference in % points	5.6	4.4	5.2

Source: CSCI (2006).

in the NMS and are expected to attend professional development training (Furness, 2008). However, they currently, do not receive specific training regarding nutrition or how to interpret the standards relevant to nutrition, making their figures on care homes meeting or exceeding requirements questionable (Smith, 2007).

Findings from the CSCI 2006 report, *Highlight of the day?* (CSCI, 2006) stated that as at March 2005, 83% of care homes met or exceeded the requirements of the meals and mealtimes standard, meaning that one in six care homes in England were known to be failing to meet the standard. This translated into 1916 care homes which provided approximately 70000 places. In addition there had only been a slight improvement since 2003 when 78% of all care homes met the standard (see Table 3.5).

In 2005 the greatest difficulty in meeting the meals and mealtimes Standard seemed to be experienced by care homes with nursing: 79%, compared with 86% of care homes providing personal care (see Table 3.6). This could be explained by the amount of residents with conditions such as dementia or problems with staff: with adequate staffing levels, 89% of care homes for older people met the Meals and Mealtimes Standard, with insufficient staffing levels, only 65% of the homes met the Standard.

There was also an issue of complaints: within the Care Standards Act, the CSCI does not have expressed powers to take action in response to interpersonal disputes between the care home provider and the complaint. However, it must make enquiries to establish whether the allegation/complaint is an indication that the registered manager and the provider are not adhering to their legal requirements and/ or national minimum standards. The type of complaint determines what approach the CSCI takes with the care home providers to resolve the problem.

From April 2004 to October 2005 there were 453 complaints about food across *all* regulated care services that were found not to adhere to the legal requirements and the standards. The number of complaints from older people in care homes *per se* could not be determined 'due to the limitations in the way the data was categorised'. Nevertheless examples were provided which illustrated ways in which care homes could fail to meet the standard on meals and mealtimes:

'The chef/staff do not seem to be aware of (person's name) likes and dislikes. There is no cook at weekends and not all staff who prepare meals have the basic food hygiene certificate'. (Anonymous)

'When my dad was in a home he wasn't getting any food – he was terminally ill – so I went to get a sandwich for him, but there was only cheese and it was three days old'. (Family member)

'When visiting my Mum at a mealtime I found her with some sandwiches in front of her covered in a paper napkin. When I asked her why she had not eaten them she said they were not fit to eat. I checked them and the bread was stale, very hard and only fit to put out for the birds. I think that my Mum has lost weight since being in the home because she is not getting proper food'. (Son of resident)

'Most evenings, the dinner consists of sandwiches. There is no alternative, no choice. Some users would like something cooked or warm. The preferences of Caribbean service users are not taken into consideration. Very rarely there is a choice of suitable cold drinks for diabetics. They are, at times, given sugary drinks, in the absence of anything else but water. The cook is not qualified and does not understand about special diets, for example for diabetics'. (Anonymous)

'I have raised concerns with the staff about my mother not receiving a proper vegetarian diet with protein. I have observed on six to eight occasions just peas, carrots, potatoes and Bisto gravy served as her main meal. This has led to my mother losing weight'. (Daughter of resident)

'I have provided menu sheets but these are not used. There is no choice regarding the menu. There used to be a choice of vegetables, but not now. There's only a basic choice of sandwiches for tea'. (Daughter of resident)

However, as *Highlight of the Day* was designed to assist care home managers and their staff to improve the delivery of meals to older people and, particularly, to improve their experiences of mealtimes in care homes, it also provided good practice examples, along with recommendations on guidance on how to achieve these aims:

• *Empower people to choose*: When care home staff understood the reason for choice being important they were willing to improve their consultation time with older people and themselves:

'There was an issue of contention between a number of residents regarding the addition of salt in the cooked food. Some residents were complaining that the

food was too salty and others were saying that they felt salt should be added at the table and not during cooking. The manager promptly organised a residents' meeting to seek the views of the residents on this issue and included the cook in the meeting'.   (Inspector)

'Everyone has their own booklet about themselves. It tells people what someone likes and dislikes, as well as what hopes and dreams people have for the future. The residents have support to write these booklets on themselves'.   (Resident of a care home)

- *Involve people in developing meals*: Good performing care homes use creative ways to include older people in meal planning and preparation, consider the risks of this involvement and then manage them well:

'A care home for older people made meals with vegetables and ingredients that some residents did not like. The residents worked together to produce a recipe booklet for the cook to follow'.   (Inspector)

'An Asian woman moved into a home where all other residents were white. The home assumed the Asian woman enjoyed the British food provided; however, this was not the case. She was unable to cook but was able to observe and offer advice on how to best prepare the food of her choice. The woman then watched the cook prepare food that was culturally appropriate for her. This event took place twice a week and the home arranged to make extra meals and bases for sauces which could be frozen, to be used in the preparation of her food in the coming week. This became a valued activity for the Asian woman'.   (Inspector)

- *Cater for diversity*: Cultural awareness is important but there is no substitute for simply asking an older person what they want:

'One tribunal case included concerns about the poor variety and quality of food, with potato and gravy regularly served to a vegetarian resident'.   (Inspector)

'An Asian man moved into a care home for Asian lifestyles. His partner was white and it was stated that he had enjoyed a diet of Asian and British food throughout his life. Whilst in the home it was assumed that the man would only want and enjoy Asian food. His partner argued that the home was "knocking the Englishness out of him". When the care home asked the man what food he would like to eat, he responded stating both British and Asian food'.   (Inspector)

'A home accommodating one Afro-Caribbean resident did not recognise that people from this cultural background may require culturally appropriate food other than British food. When the home decided to put jerk chicken and other Caribbean food on the menu for all residents, there was a high uptake including from white residents. The home then recognised that all their residents enjoyed food from around the world and satisfied the cultural preferences of the Afro-Caribbean resident'.   (Inspector)

- *Keep people healthy*: Joining up activities between catering and general care improve the ability of a care home to meet older peoples needs, challenging for larger homes who use contract caterers: although this provides greater choice and variety, the service can become budget driven or lose touch with the needs of the residents. The staff in smaller homes face the challenge of having to undertake a wider range of tasks:

'There can be a failure to recognise the benefits of "little and often" approaches. Staff frequently feel that this is greedy or too much trouble, yet it is often the best way to ensure people at risk take in enough nutrients'. (Inspector)

'Older people who are constantly on the move often lose weight much more quickly and therefore need higher calorie foods to compensate'. (Inspector)

'Menus sometimes fail to include a balanced diet across a day, or sometimes staff deviate from the menu with insufficient thought. Heavy reliance on convenience foods can mean that meals are deficient in vitamins, particularly C and D, and this can affect their health'. (Inspector)

'Some homes use highly technical calculations to carry out nutritional assessments, but all staff need to know is how these can be translated and work in practice. Even the most complicated nutritional assessments are only as good as the staff are at interpreting them'. (Inspector)

'One care home brought in a specialist to assist them train staff and review meals, so they were tailored for people with dementia. The training included the provision of nutritious finger foods, additional meals rather than biscuits, regular fluid intake and meals delivered in a timely fashion'. (Inspector)

- *Respond to changing needs*: Staff should be actively involved in care planning and this should be conveyed to the catering staff:

'There have been times when I have seen a brown splodge on a plate and that has been all the food liquidised together. There are other good providers who liquidise each item separately and present this as an appetising meal, with three or four different portions or colours of food on the plate'. (Inspector)

'In some care homes, the type of crockery isn't suitable – for example, cups have small finger holes, heavy cups that spill or plastic mugs used for hot drinks. Just providing a dessert fork helped people in one home, who were afraid to risk spilling food but couldn't grapple with cutting up pie or larger pieces of fruit'. (Inspector)

'We encourage homes to recognise signs which suggest likes and dislikes, for example tasting different foods and the reactions of the resident, asking the resident to blink or squeeze the carer's hand if they like the food and showing residents pictures of meals to select what they would like to eat'. (Inspector)

'Visual aids are very good at stimulating recognition for a person with communication difficulties'.   (Inspector)

- *Put good management systems in place*: Although some knowledge of catering is useful, clear management systems and sufficient staffing levels seem to be critical for improving the quality of meals:

'An unannounced inspection of a care home (with nursing) with over 50 older people found that many hadn't been served breakfast by 11am, others had been left with the remains of the meal in front of them and had fallen asleep. The service hadn't thought through the manner of service (trolleys on each floor, the number of staff needed) and the individual needs of residents'.   (Inspector)

'Some providers rush mealtimes because the cook wants to get the kitchen tidied and ready for the next meal. There are some care staff that condone the rush to finish the meal. When assisting the feeding of residents, some staff seem to be shovelling food into residents to get the mealtime over and done with'.   (Inspector)

'It is not uncommon for meals to be provided either in their rooms on trays, in isolation, or in lounges using cantilever tables. This makes it difficult for some people to actually feed themselves as positioning can be difficult'.   (Inspector)

'I was concerned to find that cleaning substances were placed on service users' tables, next to their drinks, without staff having any apparent realisation of the possible consequences'.   (Inspector)

'Some homes adhere rigidly to fixed shopping days, with stocks dwindling to a dangerous level, leaving no choice at the end of the week. Often fruit and vegetables have gone off by then!'   (Inspector)

With these points to hand, it could be argued that there seems to be a two-tier system whereby some of the residents have a voice and are duly acknowledged and others who do not have the wherewithal to do anything about untenable conditions. On this latter level, perhaps, this would appear to be indicative of staff who are not behaving responsibly to people in their care.

3.4.2.1   Changes to inspection

Like some of the Standards themselves, there have already been changes to the inspection process itself: inspections originally took place at least once or twice a year, but from April 2006 there has been a reduction in inspections, of which there are currently three types:

- *Key inspections* are major assessments of the quality of a service and any risk that it might present
- *Random inspections* are shorter, usually unannounced and take place if there is a specific issue that needs to be followed up. They happen in addition to the key inspection.

Table 3.7   Care home star rating and inspection rate.

Quality rating	Key inspection frequency
3 Star Excellent	One **at least** every 3 years
2 Star Good	One **at least** every 2 years
1 Star Adequate	One **at least** once a year
0 Star Poor	Two a year

Source: CSCI (2008).

- *Thematic* inspections will focus on a theme, for example nutrition, the findings of which will go towards an individual report on a service. There have been two since 2006, with the first looking at the information given to people to choose the right care home and whether they knew what to expect when they moved in with the findings contributing to the report on *Fair Contracts for Older People*. Findings from a thematic inspection on the care that people with dementia receive will be published in 2008 with a third sample of thematic inspections in the spring.

In addition every new service gets a key inspection in its first six months. Table 3.7 shows the key inspection frequency rate which is linked to the star rating of a care home.

But if these themed inspections do specifically look at nutrition, it has been perceived 'unlikely' that there will be a rise in standards due to a lack of understanding among the inspectors about the nutritional needs of the elderly, together with less frequent inspections (Smith, 2007).

With regard to the reduced inspection times the Relatives & Residents Association (R&RA) have expressed concern, asking how inspectors would know what a 'good' home was in order to reduce the number of times they inspected. They argued that the quality of care homes could go downhill very rapidly and questioned how this deterioration would be picked up, the reliability of the care homes' self-assessment and whether residents and their relatives really wanted fewer standards to be laid down. In addition the R&RA felt that the changes were being proposed for financial reasons – the need to reduce the cost of regulation rather than to improve the regulatory process (Dalley, 2005/06). Furthermore, the R&RA did not accept that the alleged burden of regulation needed to be reduced:

> '*Older people in receipt of residential care are far older, more confused and more isolated from mainstream services ... health and social care providers must be subject to external regulations in a market where they are providing care for people who are in the later stages of their lives, who cannot manage for themselves, who may lack capacity, who are very old and often very frail*'.   (Dalley, 2005/06)

Action on Elder Abuse (AEA) and the Directors of Adult Social Services (DASS) have also expressed concern that these inspections can leave vulnerable people dependent on a new, untried and untested inspection system which is based on risk assessment (Furness, 2008).

In addition, the United Kingdom Home Care Associates (UKHCA) have described the proposed publication of star ratings as 'premature' and 'inconsistent'. They argue that the national picture of star ratings is encouraging but a deeper analysis of the figures show a 'wildly variable picture' across the country and between CSCI offices in the same region. Moreover, they argued that 2 star providers will have no chance to increase their star rating for up to two years and the CSCI are also preventing any new care service from receiving a 3 star rating at is first key inspection because it doesn't have a long-term track record. UKHCA also questioned the use of 3 stars when the public are more familiar with the 5 star system operated by hotels (Angel, 2007).

An add-on to the inspection process was put in place in 2007, when the CSCI required homes to provide Annual Quality Assurance Assessments (AQAAs) consisting of two parts:

- A self-assessment that asks you to tell us how well you think you are meeting the needs of the people who use your service. (We will be using the current outcome groups contained in the national minimum standards for your type of service.)
- A data set that asks you to give us some basic facts and figures about your services.

Once the CSCI have received an AQAA they will carry out an annual service review which assures the CSCI and the public that the quality of service has not changed since the last key inspection. If the service is still performing as well since the last key inspection then inspection plans will remain unchanged. However, if the quality of service has worsened 'we will probably visit you to do an inspection and write a report on what we find'.

The completed assessment is seen as the main way in which care homes will let the CSCI know how well their service is delivering good outcomes for the people using their service, provide a comparison of what the home says about their service with what the inspectors already know and help the inspectors choose which people using the service to send a survey to, enabling more information about how well a service is performing. The data set will inform the national view of social care (CSCI, 2008).

It has been suggested that the CSCI should think carefully about the type of data asked and how best to share this information with the public to avoid 'putting in place cumbersome monitoring mechanisms that mask the realities of life in care homes and do little to address any shortfalls' (Furness, 2008).

So, have things improved? In 2006, 79% of all care homes met the NMS with 80% in 2007. The Meals and Mealtimes standard was met or exceeded by 88% and 87% respectively (CSCI, 2008), indicating little change.

Reports for individual care homes can be accessed from the home themselves and online at http://www.csci.org.uk.

3.5   Other initiatives

As with many other public health issues, there are often other initiatives contributing to overall outcomes, which although not contained within legislation are still subject to debate and perhaps, implementation. Two examples of these initiatives are explored below.

3.5.1   Water

The Caroline Walker Trust recommended that older people should drink 1.5 litres of fluid a day (just over 2½ pints or about 8 teacups) (CWT, 2004), with research showing that most elderly residents in UK care homes only consume 2–4 glasses (Water UK, 2007).

The CWT recommendation was, in the main, commended by Water UK, who in 2005, created a toolkit, *Water for Healthy* Ageing (Water UK, 2007). This contained fact sheets, checklists and advice to enable improved water consumption for older people. Carers were seen to have a vital role in supporting older individuals to maintain healthy hydration levels by ensuring fluids were freely available and accessible with a suggestion that if difficulty was experienced in increasing fluid intake, it might be possible to maintain adequate hydration levels by increasing the amount of moisture-containing foods such as fruit and vegetables.

At the time the Care Standards only recommended that hot and cold drinks and snacks be available throughout the day and offered regularly. It was deemed likely that this would change to include water provision when the Standard (15) was reviewed in 2006 (Water UK, 2007). In light of this, the following recommendations were made:

- Wholesome fresh water should be included as a central part of the diet
- As a primary and essential nutrient, fresh drinking water should be made available as part of a varied appealing wholesome and nutritious diet and its consumption encouraged throughout the day
- As care standards now begin to consider the clear benefits of drinking water, it is likely that in the future care homes will be asked to ensure that fresh drinking water is available to residents throughout the day, free of charge.
- Staff should also consider extending guidance on assistance and independent eating to ensure that residents are encouraged and reminded to drink appropriately

The importance of good hydration for older people is that it can assist in preventing or treating ailments such as:

- Pressure ulcers
- Urinary infections and incontinence
- Heart disease
- Diabetes (management of)
- Dizziness and confusion leading to falls
- Skin conditions

- Constipation
- Kidney stones
- Low blood pressure
- Cognitive impairment
- Poor oral health

The importance of all this advice on adequate fluid intake cannot be disputed but, as shown in the comments below, the practicalities could prove to be more difficult:

> 'Gosh I find it really odd to think of our Dad drinking that much water. He never used to drink that much at home. Mind you, he never liked fruit or chocolate either, and he seems to like it now. I don't like the idea of them forcing him to drink, even if it is healthy, but he kind of does what he's told now, so maybe it'll be OK. I hope they take him to the toilet enough though'.   (Private interview with relative of care home resident, December 2007)

> 'Dad hated drinking water anyway. Whether or not the care-workers tried to give him water is not known. What I do know that he was always terribly thirsty at any time I visited with quite obvious dry lips and I always either got him tea or fruit juice. Tea he would drink readily but not the fruit juice. Even when the dementia was very advanced he still had the ability to decide whether to drink or not. So I suppose that if the staff **did** try and he refused, then that's why he was always thirsty'.   (Private interview with relative of former care home resident, January 2008)

> 'I am not sure what all that water would have done to his dignity ... he had managed to stay dry during the daytime with regular timed toilet trips when a member of staff would escort him to the loo and help him do what he had to do. He would never indicate that he wanted to go. How many more trips would he need to the toilet if the water was markedly increased or how many accidents would occur? ... no think I'd rather him have some dignity'.   (Private interview with daughter of former care home resident, January 2008)

To date, the standards in relation to meals and mealtimes have not changed but there are changes due to the NMS inspectorate when the Care Quality Commission (CQC) will replace the CSCI in spring 2009. As the CQC is set up, the care home regulations and the National Minimum Standards will be extensively reviewed and updated. The CQC will provide new criteria for care home evaluation which will operate as an equivalent 'checklist' to the current standards. The Department of Health and the CQC will consult extensively with providers and stakeholders as the regulations and assessment criteria are prepared (private email DH).

3.5.2 National Association of Care Catering and Sustain

Again in 2005, the National Association of Care Catering (NACC) and Sustain, the alliance for better food and farming wrote a briefing paper in which the opportunities for sustainable food procurement in care catering were explored. The NACC were aware of Sustain's *Good Food on the Public Plate* project which aims to increase the amount of sustainable, local, seasonal, fresh food used in the public sector and the resulting pilot project focused on residential care homes for older people as a 'manageable starting point'.

Currently, Sustain continue to work with the NACC sustainability working group but plans to enrol the services of a project officer, specifically working with care homes, have been put on ice until they can find funding. Meanwhile they are still working closely to bring together 'easy to replicate' case studies (relating not just to food but schemes such as energy reducing and recycling) that can be forwarded to all NACC members (private email Rosie Blackburn, Sustain).

During the course of the *Good Food on the Public Plate* project, officers have started to work with a couple of care home providers in London and the South East, who although keen, have faced difficulties in persuading their procurement teams/management that using sustainable, local food is not going to be more expensive or generally onerous and that the benefits far outweigh the initial start up issues. This is enormously frustrating for the keen, enthusiastic people within the organisations who contacted the project to begin with – individuals who are very passionate about food and who care about the quality and sustainability of the food they serve. Sadly, that motivation doesn't seem to be widespread across public sector catering: people are recruited into catering without catering experience or training; there is generally very little investment in catering training or equipment; agency staff are relied upon but because they don't stay in one place very long they, generally, have no 'connection' with the place or the patients, which would explain why motivation and standards are typically low (private email, Rosie Blackburn, Sustain).

Sustain also coordinate courses for public sector catering and procurement staff in London to teach them about the use of sustainable food. This is funded by the London Development Agency and the Greenwich Cooperative Development Agency. More information on Sustain and sustainability is available from http://www.sustainweb.org.

3.6   Developments in 2007

In 2007, there were many developments focused on the nutrition of the elderly, some of which are detailed below.

3.6.1   British Association for Parenteral and Enteral Nutrition

BAPEN's Nutrition Screening Week (NSW) was held in September 2007. The NSW was a joint venture between BAPEN, the Royal College of Nursing and the British Dietetic Association, supported and endorsed by the National Patient Safety Agency, the DH, the Welsh Assembly Government, the Scottish Government and the Chief Nursing Officer in Northern Ireland.

The purpose of NSW was to complement the data collected during the European Nutrition Day audits and inform the DH, other government departments, other organisations and the media of the current magnitude of the problem of malnutrition on admission to care homes (and hospitals). In addition, data from participating centres would be returned to reporters to enable local data to be compared with national figures with the survey results forming the basis of launching or promoting other initiatives such as the education and training of health professionals, including nurses, who usually perform nutritional screening.

A total of 1610 care homes took part and the results showed that there was:

- A 28% overall risk of malnutrition
- In the age betwee <70 years and >90 years malnutrition risk ranged from 26% to 36% (a significant increase with age)

3.6.2 Food Standards Agency

The Food Standards Agency (FSA) published *Guidance on Food Served to Older People in Residential* Care (FSA) aimed specifically at 'care homes for older people (aged 75 and over) who do not have nutritional requirements due to illness or disease'. It was assumed by the FSA that breakfast would contribute 20% of daily intake, lunch and evening meals contributing 30% each, and foods consumed between meals (snacks) contributing 20%. The FSA also said that carers should ensure that water and other forms of liquid were freely available throughout the whole day and residents who had difficulty in drinking should be supported in getting a good fluid intake. There was advice on procurement in relation to whether food had high, medium or low amounts of fat, sugars and salt in 100 g of the food, which corresponded to the Agency's signpost traffic light labelling system.

Food-based guidelines gave guidance on how often a particular food should be served, why, what the food was included in, tips on choosing foods, cooking and serving foods, food-related customs, allergies, food safety and general tips on feeding older people. This advice was based on:

- Bread, rice, potatoes, pasta and other starchy foods
- Fruit and vegetables
- Milk and dairy products
- Meat, fish, eggs, beans and other non-dairy sources of protein
- Foods and/or drinks high in fat and/or sugar

Examples of two 7-day menus and a nutritional analysis were also provided (see Table 3.8 for sample menus).

The National Association of Care Caterers (NACC) has said that the FSA standards are not suitable for older people in care because they are written for healthy 75-year-olds who are rarely found in care. The NACC have published their own advice on how the nutritional needs of adults in care can be met through a new manual *Menu Planning and Special Diets for Care Homes* (see page 367).

Table 3.8 Sample menus for care homes.

	Tuesday Week 1	Tuesday Week 2
Early morning	Tea or coffee, water	Tea or coffee, water
Breakfast	Grapefruit segments, cereals/ porridge, toast with butter/ spread, preserves, tea or coffee, water	Grapefruit segments, cereals/ porridge, toast with butter/spread, preserves, tea or coffee, water
Mid-morning snack	Tea or coffee + water, biscuits	Tea or coffee + water, biscuits
Lunch	Spaghetti bolognaise, tuna pasta bake, vegetarian lasagne (v) side salad, rhubarb crumble & custard, fresh pear, tea or coffee	Roast pork & apple sauce, spaghetti bolognaise, vegetarian lasagne, roast/new potatoes, spinach/carrots, side salad, rhubarb crumble & custard, fresh pear, tea or coffee
Afternoon tea	Tea or coffee + water, malt loaf, biscuits, fresh pear	Tea or coffee + water, malt loaf, biscuits, fresh pear
Evening meal	Tomato rice soup & bread roll, jacket potato & baked beans, sandwiches – turkey/egg, side salad, stewed apple, yogurt, tea or coffee, water	Tomato rice soup & bread roll, jacket potato & cheese & coleslaw, sandwiches – beef/egg, side salad, peaches & yoghurt, peaches & rice pudding, tea or coffee, water
Night-time snack	Hot drink, jam sandwich/ biscuits water	Hot drink, jam sandwich/biscuits water

Note: Hot drink for night-time snack is a choice of tea, coffee, hot chocolate, malted milk drink or Ovaltine (V) – Vegetarian option.

Source: Food Standards Agency (2007).

Its aim is to '*exceed the national minimum standards by providing nutritional and wholesome solutions to common menu-planning problems and special dietary requirements*' (Harmer, 2007).

3.6.3   Nutrition Action Summit & Action Plan

The DH, with 28 named key stakeholders, held a summit on Nutrition in the Care of Older People in Health and Social Care Health. It was organised in response to a need to address the current issues around peoples' experiences of food and drink in care settings. In the resulting report *Improving Nutritional Care* (DH, 2007), an Action Plan[12] was delivered detailing, the importance of nutrition, progress in improving nutritional care, key priority areas for tackling nutrition, covernance arrangements and suggestion for how 'you' would tackle issues around nutrition and hydration. The action plan section itself, provides a valuable resource for anybody wanting to access the commitments of the stakeholders to address the five key priorities:

(1) To further raise awareness of the link between nutrition and good health and that malnutrition can be prevented

(2) To further ensure that accessible guidance is available across all sectors and that the most relevant guidance is appropriated and user-friendly

(3)   To further encourage nutritional screening for all people using health and social care services

(4)   To further encourage provision and access to relevant training for front-line staff and managers on the importance of nutrition for food health and nutritional care

(5)   To further clarify standards and strengthen inspection and regulation

A progress report from the Nutrition Action Plan Board is expected in summer 2008.

3.7 Scotland

3.7.1 Care standards

In Scotland it was recommended that nationally recommended guidelines and quality of care standards should be produced by the Scottish Office through a National Consultative Committee. Scottish Ministers set up the National Care Standards Committee (NCSC) and following a consultation process with working groups the National Care Standards (NCS) were developed. The Regulation of Care (Scotland) Act 2001 set up the Scottish Commission for the Regulation of Care (also known as the Care Commission) who register and inspect all the services regulated against the NCS. The act also resulted in there being no legal differences between residential and nursing homes.

There are 20 revised Standards (Scottish Government),[13] grouped under four headings with 'Eating Well' under the umbrella of day-to-day life (standards 12–19). An introduction to the standard stated:

'Good, nutritious food and drink are important in keeping and improving your health. Individual choices of food and drink vary, as do dietary needs. Enjoying your food and having your own needs and choices met is an important part of the quality of day-to-day life'.

Eating well (Standard 13) states: 'Your meals are varied and nutritious. They reflect your food preference and any special dietary needs. They are well prepared and cooked and attractively presented':

(1)   Catering and care staff get to know your food choices and preferences, including ethnic, cultural and faith ones. Any special diet (for example, vegetarian, low fat or high protein) is recorded in your personal plan.

(2)   You are offered a daily menu that reflects your preferences. The menu varies regularly according to your comments and will always contain fresh fruit and vegetables.

(3)   You have a choice of cooked breakfast and choices in courses in your midday and evening meals.

(4)   Meals are nutritionally balanced for your dietary needs, for example, if you are diabetic or have poor kidney function.

(5) You can have snacks and hot and cold drinks whenever you like.

(6) If you are unable to say if you are getting enough to eat or drink, staff will keep an eye on this for you. If there are concerns, staff will explain them to you or your representative. With your agreement, staff will take any action needed, such as seeking advice from a dietician or your GP.

(7) Your meals are well prepared and presented. All food handling follows good food hygiene practices.

(8) You are free to eat your meals wherever you like, for example in your own room or in the dining room. You can eat them in your own time.

(9) You must be able to eat and enjoy your food. If you need any help to do so (e.g., a liquidised diet, adapted cutlery or crockery, or help from a staff member), staff will arrange this for you.

(10) Staff will regularly review anything that may affect your ability to eat or drink, such as your dental health. They will arrange for you to get advice.

Compared to England, the Scottish standards appear to be more personalised, addressing the person who is (hopefully) reading them. Their content is largely the same but it might be more appropriate if they were standardised, even in their numbering: surely the nutritional requirements or the elderly and how these are achieved are the same, regardless of where they might happen to live?

The results of inspection reports for each individual care home are available from the care home themselves and are also published on the website of the Scottish Commission for the Regulation of Care. Available from http://www.care-commission.com.

3.8 Wales

3.8.1 National Minimum Standards

The National Minimum Standards (NMS) for Care Homes for Older People were issued by the Welsh Assembly Government (WAG) under Section 23 of the Care Standards Act (2000) in 2002 (revised 2004). Also in 2002 the Care Standards Inspectorate for Wales took over the inspection of all care homes. There are 32 Standards with Meals and Mealtimes (Standard 16) under the heading of Section 4, Quality of Care and Treatment whose outcome is that:

'service users receive a wholesome, appealing, balanced diet in pleasing surroundings at times convenient to them'.

16.1 The registered person ensures that service users receive a varied, appealing, wholesome and nutritious diet which is suited to individual assessed and recorded requirements, in a congenial setting and at flexible times.

16.2 Each service user is offered three full meals each day (at least two of which must be cooked) at intervals of not more than five hours during the day time.

16.3   The interval between the evening meal and breakfast should not normally be more than 14 hours. Hot and cold drinks and snacks should be available at all times.

16.4   Food, including liquified meals, is presented in a manner that is attractive and appealing in terms of texture, flavour, and appearance, in order to maintain appetite and nutrition.

16.5   Special therapeutic diets/feeds are provided when advised by health care and dietetic staff, including adequate provision of calcium and vitamin D.

16.6   Religious or cultural dietary needs are catered for as agreed at admission and recorded in the care plan; food for special occasions is available.

16.7   The registered person ensures that there is a changing menu offering a choice of meals in written or other formats to suit the capacities of all service users. This is given, read or explained to service users. This requirement will not apply to homes with three residents or fewer.

16.8   The registered person ensures that mealtimes are unhurried with service users being given sufficient time to eat.

16.9   Staff are ready to offer assistance in eating where necessary, discreetly, sensitively and individually; independent eating is encouraged for as long as possible.

Most of the Welsh standards are exactly the same as those in England, with the same impersonalised style. One of the main differences is the time between the evening meal and breakfast which in Wales 'should not be more than 14 hours' and in England 'not more than 12 hours'. How these timings are deemed to be adequate is unknown but it is to be hoped that the 'freely available snacks' in Wales are available and the 'snack after the evening meal' in England is eaten. If an elderly resident has the wherewithal to ask for a snack in the evening, the gap between the evening meal and breakfast might be perfectly reasonable: if they can't ask, perhaps it isn't.

The standards are currently inspected by the Care and Social Services Inspectorate Wales (CSSIW[14]) and inspection reports for individual care homes are available from the care homes themselves and online: http://www.wales.gov.uk/cssiwsubsite. The *Care Standards Inspectorate for Wales Report 2006–7* is also available online at http://www.assemblywales.org.

3.9   Northern Ireland

3.9.1   Minimum standards

Following the issue of the consultation paper *Best practice – Best care* by the Department of Health Social Services and Public Safety (DHSSPS) in 2001, the Health and Personal Social Services (Quality, Improvement and Regulation) (Northern Ireland) Order 2003 ('the Order') was issued. The Order allowed for the establishment of the Northern Ireland Health and Personal Social Services Regulation and Quality Improvement Authority (now known as the Regulations and Quality Improvement Authority (RQIA) who regulate establishments and agencies in both the Health and Social Care (HSC) and the independent sector.

The Order conferred powers on the DHSSPS to prepare, publish and review statements of mandatory Minimum Standards (MS) of which, for residential homes, there are 35, with Standard 12, Meals and Mealtimes, coming under the heading of Quality Care (standards 1–18) (DHSSPS, 2008a).

Standard 12: Residents receive a nutritious and varied diet in appropriate surroundings at times convenient to them.

Criteria:

12.1   Residents are provided with a nutritious and varied diet, which meets their individual and recorded dietary needs and preferences. Full account is taken of relevant guidance documents or guidance provided by dietitians and other professionals and disciplines.

12.2   Residents are involved in planning the menus.

12.3   The menu either offers residents a choice of meal at each mealtime or when the menu offers only one option and the resident does not want this, an alternative meal is provided. A choice is also offered to those on therapeutic or specific diets.

12.4   The daily menu is displayed in a suitable format and in an appropriate location so that residents and their representatives know what is available at each mealtime.

12.5   Meals are provided at conventional times, hot and cold drinks and snacks are available at customary intervals, and fresh drinking water is available at all times.

12.6   Residents can have a snack or drink on request or have access to a domestic style kitchen.

12.7   Menus provide for special occasions.

12.8   Residents are consulted and their views taken into account regarding the home's policy on 'take away' foods.

12.9   Meals are served in suitable portion sizes, and presented in a way and in a consistency that meet each resident's needs.

12.10   Staff are aware of any matters concerning residents' eating and drinking as detailed in each resident's individual care plan, and there are adequate numbers of staff present when meals are served to ensure:

- Risks when residents are eating and drinking are managed
- Required assistance is provided
- Necessary aids and equipment are available for use.

12.11   A record is kept of the meals provided in sufficient detail to enable any person inspecting it to judge whether the diet for each resident is satisfactory.

12.12   Where a resident's care plan requires, or when a resident chooses not to eat a meal or is unable to eat a meal, a record is kept of all food and drinks consumed. Where a resident is eating excessively a similar record is kept.

Such occurrences are discussed with the resident, and reported to the registered manager or senior staff in charge of the home. Where necessary, a referral is made to the relevant professionals and a record kept of the action taken.

12.13   Menus are rotated over a three-week cycle and revised at least six-monthly, taking into account seasonal availability of foods and residents' views.

12.14   Variations to the menu are recorded.

There are also 40 MS for nursing homes (HSSPS, 2008b) with Meals and Mealtimes (Standard 12) being the same as residential homes but with the term 'patient' instead of 'resident'. What is additional is Standard 8, Nutrition.

Standard 8: Nutritional needs of patients are met

8.1   Nutritional screening is carried out with patients on admission, using a validated tool such as the MUST (see Box 2.9, page 151) tool or equivalent.

8.2   Nutritional screening is repeated monthly or more frequently depending on individual assessed need, and nutritional support is implemented according to the screening protocol.

8.3   There are referral arrangements for the dietitian to assess individual patient's nutritional requirements and draw up a nutritional treatment plan. The nutritional treatment plan is developed taking account of recommendations from relevant health professionals, and these plans adhered to.

8.4   There are up-to-date nutritional guidelines that are used by staff on a daily basis.

8.5   There is nutritional information in an accessible format for patients, and their representative.

8.6   Nurses have up-to-date knowledge and skills in managing feeding techniques for patients who have swallowing difficulties, and in ensuring that instructions drawn up by the speech and language therapist are adhered to.

8.7   Nurses have up-to-date knowledge and skills in the provision of enteral tube feeding, and ensuring that feeding regimens drawn up by the dietitian are adhered to.

There are more standards in Northern Ireland than elsewhere which appear to include the involvement of the elderly in this particular aspect of their care, for example, by involving them in menu planning. The two types of standards seem to be aimed at those elderly who are 'able bodied' and those with eating difficulties. In addition the availability of 'fresh water' is mentioned. This different approach to the standards might be indicative of the fact that the standards were only published early in January 2008 and therefore, perhaps, reflect a more modern approach to these elderly individuals.

The MS are used by the RQIA as part of their programme of registration and inspection of care homes with their reports available direct from the care homes themselves or the RQIA. They will be available online, sometime in 2008: http://www.rqia.org.uk.

3.10   Europe

3.10.1   European Nutrition Day

The project European Nutrition Day (END) was designed 'to improve nutritional care based on knowledge, information exchange and awareness of all relevant stakeholders. The central element is a harmonised multi-lingual data acquisition tool in Europe to be used by patients and caregiver. END took place in January 2007, all across Europe.

The preliminary results of (END)[15] 2006–7 showed that only Austria and Germany took part in the Nursing Home Pilot. The principle findings showed that a key risk factor for undernutrition was cognitive impairment, particularly apparent in patients in tube feeding regimens. Of concern was the fact that although 25% of patients were nutritionally screened if it was thought to be necessary, staff did not classify 60% of patients with a BMI <20 kg/m^2 as being malnourished. The study also showed the significant amount of time involved in supporting patients who needed help with eating, there were no additional staffing resources available to meet this need. Although no UK units took part in the pilot, the results showed that 'these problems are universal' (Howard, 2007).

The problems in care homes in other European countries seem to indicate that it is not the problem of food *per se*, but staffing levels for those elderly who require assistance with eating. As these problems 'are universal', perhaps it is time for them to be addressed Europe-wide to reverse the whole situation of malnutrition in care homes for the elderly.

3.10.2   Forum on undernutrition in care homes and home care

An event which might have helped to address this issue was held in Europe, in November 2007 when an international two day workshop *Forum on Undernutrition in Care Homes and Home Care*, was held in Brussels (European Nutrition for Health Alliance, 2006). A report from the workshop is pending.

3.11   Useful resources

The Alzheimer's Society *Food for Thought* project, aims to ensure that people with dementia are healthier by examining issues related to eating and drinking and providing advice and information on these topics. There are a range of downloadable leaflets available in which carers share their experiences and offer tips and suggestions to help overcome some of the difficulties related to feeding people with dementia. Their publication, *Eating and Nutrition, Top Tips for Carers and Finger Food Ideas*, is available from http://www.alzheimers.org.uk.

Malnutrition Among Older People in the Community, by the European Nutrition for Health Alliance addresses issues around the fact that many elderly people are malnourished before they enter institutions.

Menu Planning and Special Diets in Care Homes by The National Association of Care Catering (NACC) Available from http://www.thenacc.co.uk.

The National Minimum Standard for Care Catering – Care Homes for Older People and – Care Homes for Adults 18–65 by the NACC. Available from http://www.thenacc.co.uk.

Eating for Health in Care Homes – A Practical Nutrition Handbook by the Royal Institute of Public Health (RIPH). Available from http://ww.riph.org.uk.

In *Home from Home, Alzheimers* the Alzheimer's Society discuss the difficulties for carers in dealing with dementia. Available from http://www.alzheimers.org.uk.

Help the Aged have launched a new website, allowing care home professionals across the UK to share best practice in key topics within care homes, including staff training. See: *My Home Life. Quality of Life in Care Homes. A review of the literature.* Available from www.myhomelife.org.uk.

3.12 Conclusion

As has been shown, for many elderly people, moving into a care home is their only option. The challenges that face both these elderly individuals and their carers can be daunting to say the least.

Having moved into a home, the elderly are more than likely to face limitations of care brought about by inadequate staffing levels. This is not a new phenomenon as there were reported staffing problems back in the original care homes – the workhouses – and this was still in evidence by the 1960s when it was reported that there were high turnovers of staff mainly due to the poor salary levels with institutions in the cities suffering more than those in towns. In addition, there were often misgivings about the 'quality of the staff with many recruited from immigrant groups who had little or no training (Townsend, 1962). It would seem that little has changed as many of these issues still remain (Robinson & Banks, 2005) and if this is the case then it would appear that there is a fundamental problem, in many cases, of not just having enough staff but recruiting those who are actually trained. But is training all that is required to enable a carer to care? True it can raise levels of awareness of issues such as nutrition but surely many of the issues around the care of the elderly are common sense and require a level of sensitivity and respect from the carer of an elderly person who, in turn, is often entirely dependent on them. The points below, from an online survey to hear directly from the public about their experiences of being treated with dignity in care or about care they had seen given to others in 2006 (DH, 2006), show that is often not the case:

- Vulnerable patients were being left alone at mealtimes
- People were too weak to cut up their food or lift cutlery to their mouth
- Carers did not seem to have time to spend with individuals at meal times or were unobservant
- Mealtimes seemed to be a process to get over with as quickly as possible rather the potentially a social opportunity

- Service users may be embarrassed to ask for help so care staff should be more aware
- If a vulnerable adult was seen not to eat their own meals there was a worry that it was a sign of neglect in some institutions

This kind of reporting is not an isolated event: in the same year, in a residential care home, it was reported that despite adequate food provision, under nutrition was not only prevalent but in the majority of cases, unidentified and untreated: given the low-energy consumption in this particular setting, the results were unsurprising. There was also a lack of awareness on the part of the staff with regard to the nutrient requirements of residents (Leslie *et al.*, 2006). Arguably, some of these points could be the result of understaffing and a lack of training but it could be just a lack of general humanity towards others.

For those care homes with staff who do care, things can be so different:

'My husband and all the patients were weighed weekly, I saw this happen. He put on weight for a while and then it became stable'.   (Private interview with wife of former care home resident 2008)

'Meals were taken at a set time and appeared varied. I did not see anyone pushing food away in distaste. The feeding of patients was done very patiently and independent eating was encouraged for as long as possible'.   (Private interview with wife of former care home resident 2008)

Although the food was perfectly acceptable to the relative, there was still a slight concern about the timing of the last 'meal':

'I think they had porridge for breakfast which my husband (when he was capable of telling us) said he liked. Lunch at 12 noon smelled very appetising and consisted of 2 courses, quite a substantial pudding. 4–4.30 sandwiches and cake. I hoped they had something about 7pm but I was never there to see'.   (Private interview with wife of former care home resident 2007)

If a relative in this situation is left wondering but not actually questioning, how would a lone elderly resident fare?

The nutritional care of the elderly who are particularly vulnerable, for example, those with dementia, has been shown to be difficult but again, there are ways of addressing the issue, but they involve both an awareness of the problem and appropriate actions from people who care enough to sanction it: in 1998, VOICES was advocating the good practice example of 'quiet and calm in the dining room' and more recently an example of this was demonstrated in a home in Liverpool which was trying to ensure dementia residents could focus their attention on enjoying their meals by providing a calm atmosphere, free from distractions (VOICES, 1998). This introduction of 'protected mealtimes' was reported to have made an 'unbelievable difference' with the comment below summing up the situation:

'This simple measure illustrates how meeting the nutritional needs of care home residents is more than a matter of providing wholesome food'. (Caring Times, 2006)

Staffing requirements are included in the NMS under Standard 28, with an explanation of the numbers and types of staff qualified to NVQ level 2, or equivalent, which should have been put in place by 2005. In addition, Standard 27 of the NMS refers to the fact that there should be sufficient numbers of staff to *'ensure that standards relating to food, meals and nutrition are fully met and that the home is maintained in a clean and hygienic state, free from dirt and unpleasant odours'* (DH, 2003). Therein might be one of the reasons, why, for the 'untrained', nutrition is not that high in the pecking order: it is mentioned in the same breath as 'unpleasant odours'. Anybody who has ever been inside a care home understands that this latter point is often a priority, for obvious, but incomparable reasons.

There are publications available which are aimed at helping care homes meet the nutritional requirements of the elderly, backed by many organisations, but as discussed earlier, the problems of actually getting the elderly to eat nutritious food is not always easy even if they are fully able to do so and aware of the reasons why they should (Herne, 1994). Another angle to consider is the suggestion that 'health education and more specifically nutrition education has neglected the elderly consumer' with the message being that the damage 'was already done'. Therefore, 'it is not surprising that older people have felt that health education is not relevant to them with their health problems a natural consequence source of getting older' (Herne, 1994).

In addition, because this *'homogenous group'* are as *'individually different as the rest of the population'* (Herne, 1994), it could be that it is not appropriate to take a *'prescriptive approach'* for their dietary advice and, *'perhaps the most important advice about food for elderly people is that it should be enjoyed'* (National Dairy Council, 1992).

There is no disputing that conditions in many care homes have improved and continue to improve. However, the continuity of the inspection process has been interrupted by changes in the inspectorate with the CSCI themselves stating that rather than engaging and listening to service users, they concentrate on the details of the NMS and the regulations, which they view as a main weakness of the inspection process (Furness, 2008).

In addition, the CSCI has been criticised for taking Standard 15, Meals and Mealtimes, as a starting point because it is only a minimum standard and therefore *'not very ambitious in its demands'*. Furthermore, it has been suggested that the CSCI should be looking towards an ideal standard of care and not just *'rock bottom levels of service'* below which nobody should fall (Smith, 2006).

As discussed, more changes are due in 2009, when the care home regulations and the NMS will be extensively reviewed and updated. Hopefully these changes will bring more improvements both in the inspection process and the NMS themselves but, as has been noted, the NMS might be more achievable if the government *'stopped moving the goal posts'* (Furness, 2008).

Another issue to consider is the general publics' awareness of these inspection reports in deciding which home to choose for an elderly person. As some relatives have recently noted:

*'We took it home to read before Dad was admitted. It was more an open-policy document about rules and regulations governing the running of the home, and the actual care of the patients – as opposed to a report **after** inspection. The document was clear and transparent, stressing the policies of total frankness between all staff and families. It also stressed that everything was being worked within the government guidelines – there may have been references but I can't remember'.* (Private interview with daughter of former care home resident 2007)

'I was unaware of inspection reports but I'm not sure it would not have made any difference as at the time we were relieved that the home didn't smell as much as others we had seen. I have read an inspection report since and the home came out well, thankfully, and I agreed with the comments on the good food'. (Private interview with relative of former care home resident 2007)

And the future for nutrition in care homes? It has been suggested that the labelling of the elderly can 'mask the wider value of residents as people with the same needs and rights as those who do not happen to be living in residential care homes' (Centre for Policy on Ageing, 1994). These values include the nutritional needs and rights of the elderly which need to be continually addressed, monitored and regulated to protect this vulnerable population, with the words, quoted below, encompassing some of the current laissez faire attitudes:

'A home which reaches the NMS for food and drink ... should not be congratulating itself and taking a day off but urging its staff ever onwards and upwards. We don't give an employer a rosette for paying the national minimum wage or a railway company an accolade for reaching minimum safety standards, so lets set our sights a bit higher when considering what vulnerable old people deserve from providers and regulators of services'.   (Smith, 2006)

Finally, on a lighter note, this title of a newspaper article might be used as 'food for thought' when remembering just whose nutritional needs are actually being addressed in these, often forgotten, institutions:

'Granny grub: menu ideas for the mature – Tickling the old taste buds' (Clarke, 2006).

Notes

1 'Crabbit Old Woman', 'Kate' or 'Open your eyes'. This is part of a poem whose title prompted 2980 hits an internet search in 2007. There is much speculation and urban myth concerning its creation and the reference used provides a comprehensive insight into its origins.
2 Food in workhouses is discussed in the chapter on Hospitals.

3   A further survey of a representative sample of 1000 elderly people was carried out for the COMA panel on the Elderly in 1973/4 but a report of the study was unpublished. The results of the 1972/3 survey were used in the 1992 COMA report on The Nutrition of Elderly People (DH, 1992a) as they were the most recently published national nutritional data about elderly people.

4   COMA has been superseded by the Scientific Committee on Nutrition (SACN). It is likely that SCAN will review UK nutritional requirements in the near future as they are over 10 years old (British Nutrition Foundation).

5   Since the mid-1990s there was a rise in the number of care homes which were dual registered, tending to be in the independent sector (Bajekal, 2000).

6   Republished in 1994.

7   This was renamed in 1990 to *Eating through the 90s* (NAGE, 1997).

8   The Standards had a second edition in 2003 and a third impression in 2006.

9   Under the Care Standards Act (2000) the terms 'nursing homes' and 'residential homes' were replaced by 'care homes' for institutions which provide accommodation together with nursing or personal care. Care homes (personal) provide only 'broad personal care' whereas care homes (nursing) are intended for those who need regular or constant nursing care (Bajekal, 2000).

10 This Standard was later amended.

11 The *CORA Menu Planner* has been superseded by the Nutmeg UK programme available from http://www.nutmeg-uk.com.

12 The Action Plan details plans for both care homes and hospitals.

13 The NCS were revised in November 2007 but to date do not appear on the website (private email Scottish Government).

14 CSSIW was known as the CSIW until April 2007.

15 The next END was held on 31 January 2008.

References

Age Concern (2000) *Age Concern's Response to the Consultation Document, Fit for the Future? National Required Standards for Residential and Nursing Homes for Older People*. London: Age Concern.

Alzheimer's Society (2007) Home from Home. A report highlighting opportunities for improving standards of dementia care in care homes. Available from: http://www.alzheimers.org.uk. downloads/home_from_home_full_report_2_.pdf

Angel, C. (2007) *CSCI must halt star ratings*. Homecarer, November. United Kingdom Home Care Association Limited (UKHCA).

Bajekal, M. (2000) *Health Survey for England. Care Homes and their Residents*. London: The Stationery Office.

Bebbington, A., Darton, R. & Netten, A. (2001) *Care Homes for Older People. Vol. 2. Admissions, Needs and Outcomes. The 1995/96 National Longitudinal Survey of Publicly Funded Admissions*. Canterbury: Personal Social Services Research Unit (PSSRU).

Bonart, J. (2005) *Empathy and stereotype: the work of a popular poem*. Perspectives on Dementia Care, 5th Annual Conference on Mental Health and Older People, University of East Anglia, Norwich, UK, 3 November. Available from http:///www.uea.ac.uk./swk/pd_care/presentations/ Kate.pdf. Accessed December 2007.

British Association for Parenteral and Enteral Nutrition (2007) *Nutrition Screening Week*. Available from www.bapen.org.uk. Accessed December 2007.

British Association of Social Workers (1986) *The Impact of the 1984 Registered Homes Act*. Birmingham: BASW.

British Nutrition Foundation (2007) *Nutrient requirements and recommendations*. Available from http://www.britishnutrition.org. Accessed November 2007.

Burton-Jones, J. (2000) Are residents' relatives customers, too? *Nursing & Residential Care*, 2(12):598–599.

Caring Times (2006) *Dementia – less noise means better nutrition.* March.

Caroline Walker Trust (1995) *Eating well for older people. Practical and nutritional guidelines for food in residential and nursing homes and for community meals.* Report of an expert working group.

Caroline Walker Trust (2004a) *Eating well for older people. Practical and nutritional guidelines for food in residential and nursing homes and for community meals* (2nd edition). Report of an expert working group.

Caroline Walker Trust (2004b) *CORA Menu Planner.* London: DGAA.

Centre for Policy on Ageing (CPA) (1994) *Home Life: A code of practice for residential care.* Report of a Working Party sponsored by the Department of Health and Social Security and convened by the Centre for Policy on Ageing under the Chairmanship of Kina, Lady Avebury. London: CPA.

Clarke, J. (2006) Granny grub: Menu ideas for the mature – tickling the old taste buds. *The Times*, 3 June.

Commission for Social Care Inspection (2006) *Highlight of the day? Improving meals for older people in care homes.* Issue 1, March. Available from http://www.csci.org.uk. Accessed November 2007.

Commission for Social Care Inspection (2008) *State of Social Care in England* 2006–07. Available from http://www.csci.org.uk. Accessed January 2008.

Connor, R.J.G. (1999) Is healthy eating only for the young? *Nutrition and Food Science*, 99(1):12–18.

Dalley, G. (2005/06) *The Relatives & Residents Association Newsletter*, Winter:1–8.

Dalley, G., Unsworth, L., Keightley, D., Waller, M., Davies, T. & Morton, R. (2004) *How do we care? The availability of registered care homes and children's homes in England and their performance against National Minimum Standards 2002–03.* National Care Standards Commission.

Department of Health (DH) (1991) *Dietary Reference Values for Food Energy and Nutrients for the United Kingdom.* A report of the Working Group on the Nutrition of Elderly People of the Committee on Medical Aspects of Food Policy. Report on Health and Social Subjects No 41. London: HMSO.

Department of Health (DH) (1992a) *The Nutrition of Elderly People.* A Report of the Working Group on the Nutrition of Elderly People of the Committee on Medical Aspects of Food Policy. Report on Health and Social Subjects 43. London: HMSO.

Department of Health (DH) (1992b) *The Health of the Nation. A Strategy for Health in England.* London: HMSO.

Department of Health (DH) (1999) *Fit for the Future? National Required Standards for Residential and Nursing Homes for Older People.* Consultation Document. DH.

Department of Health (DH) (2003) *National Minimum Standards and The Care Homes Regulations 2001* (3rd edition, 3rd impression 2006). London: TSO. Available from http://www.dh.gov.uk. Accessed December 2007.

Department of Health, Older People and Disability Division (2006) *'Dignity in Care' Public Survey.* Report of the Survey. DH.

Department of Health & the Nutrition Summit stakeholder group (2007) *Improving Nutritional Care. A Joint Action Plan from the Department of Health and Nutrition Summit Stakeholders.*

Department of Health & Social Security (1972) *A Nutrition Survey of the Elderly.* Reports on Health and Social Subjects No. 3. London: HMSO.

Department of Health & Social Security (1979a) *Nutrition and Health in Old Age. The Cross Sectional Analysis of the Findings of a Survey Made in 1978/3 of Elderly People who had been Studied in 1967/8.* Reports on Health & Social Subjects 16. London: HMSO.

Department of Health & Social Security (DHSS) (1979b) *Recommended Daily Amounts of Food Energy and Nutrients for Groups of People in the United Kingdom.* Report by the Committee on Medical Aspects of Food Policy. Report on Health and Social Subjects 15. London: HMSO.

Department of Health & Social Security (DHSS) (1984) *Registered Homes Act 1984: Guidance Notes on Registration System for Residential Care Homes and on Registered Homes Tribunals.* London: HMSO.
Department of Health Social Services and Public Safety (2008a) *Residential Care Homes Minimum Standards.* Available from http://www.northernireland.gov.uk. Accessed February 2008.
Department of Health Social Services and Public Safety (2008b) *Nursing Homes Minimum Standards.* Available from http://www.northernireland.gov.uk. Accessed February 2008.
Dudman, J. (2007) *Context.* In: *Help the Aged. My Home Life. Quality of Life in Care Homes. A review of the literature.* Prepared by the National Care Homes Research and Development Forum.
Eaton, P. (1999) With respect to old age. A report by the Royal Commission in long-term care. *Journal of Human Nutrition and Dietetics*, 12:481–482.
European Nutrition for Health Alliance (2006) *Malnutrition among Older People in the Community: Policy Recommendations for Change.* In association with BAPEN, International Longevity Centre & The Associate Parliamentary Food & Health Forum.
Innes-Farqhar (2000) Catering in nursing and residential homes. *Nursing and Residential Care*, 2(12):587–590.
Fermoy, P. (2000) Care Standards Act: The health-care perspective. *Nursing & Residential Care*, 2(8):361.
Finch, S., Doyle, W., Lowe, C., Bates, C.J., Prentice, A., Smithers, G. & Clarke, P.C. (1998) *National Diet and Nutrition Survey: People Aged 65 Years and Over, Vol. 1: Report of the Diet and Nutrition Survey.* London: HMSO.
Food Standards Agency (2007) *Guidance on food served to older people in residential care.* Available from www.food.gov.uk. Accessed December 2007.
Furness, S. (2008) A hindrance or help? The contribution of inspection to the quality of care in homes for older people. *British Journal of Social Work*, 1–18.
Groom, H. (1993) COMA report on the nutrition of elderly people. *British Nutrition Foundation Bulletin*, 18:99–101.
Harmer, J. (2007) *Contract catering: Addressing the problem of malnutrition in care homes.* Available from http://caterersearch.com. Accessed January 2008.
Herne, S. (1994) Catering for institutionalized elderly people: The care home's dilemma. *British Food Journal,* 96(9):3–9.
Herne, S. (1995) Research on food choice and nutritional status in elderly people: A review. *British Food Journal*, 97(9):12–29.
Hertfordshire Health Authority (1996) *Guidelines and Procedures for Registration and Conduct of Nursing Homes.* HHA.
Howard, P. (2007) *European Nutrition Day 2006–7. In Touch 48.* BAPEN (British Association for Parenteral and Enteral Nutrition).
Kerrison, S.H. & Pollock, A.M. (2001) Absent voice compromise the effectiveness of nursing home regulation: A critique of regulator reform in the UK nursing home industry. *Health and Social Care in the Community*, 9(6):490–494.
Laing & Buisson (1987) *Implementing the Registered Homes Act 1984. A Survey of Local Authority Policies and Criteria for Registration.* London: Laing & Buisson in association with The National Confederation of Registered Residential Care Home Associates.
Leslie, W.S., Lean, M.E.J., Woodward, M., Wallace, F.A. & Hankey, C.R. (2006) Unidentified under-nutrition: Dietary intake and anthropometric indices in a residential care home. *The British Dietetic Association,* 19:343–347.
National Dairy Council (1992) *Nutrition and Elderly People. Fact File 9.* NDC.
'News' (2000) 'Bed blockers' to be moved into care homes. *Nursing & Residential Care*, 2(6):262.
Nutrition Advisory Group for the Elderly People of the British Dietetic Association (1987) *Eating a Way into the 90s.* NAGE.

Nutrition Advisory Group for Elderly People of the British Dietetic Association (1997) *Eating Through the 90's. A Handbook for those Concerned with Providing Meals for Older People*, 3rd edition. South Yorkshire: NAGE, The British Dietetic Association.

Office of Fair Trading (1998) *Older People as Consumers in Care Homes*. London: OFT.

Office of Fair Trading (2005) *Care Homes for Older People in the UK. A Market Study*. London: OFT.

Read, S. & Worsfold, D. (1998) Catering for older people in residential care homes. *Nutrition & Food Science*, **1**:30–37.

Readers Letters (2000) *Nursing & Residential Care*, **2**(8):398.

Registered Homes Act (1984). London: HMSO. Available from httpl//:www.opsi.gov.uk/acts. Accessed November 2007.

Robinson, J. & Banks, P. (2005) *The Business of Caring. Kings Fund Enquiry into Care Services for Older People in London*. London: Kings Fund.

Exton-Smith, A.N. & Stanton, B.R. (1965) *Report of an Investigation into the Dietary of Elderly Women Living Alone*. London: King Edwards Hospital Fund.

Exton-Smith, A.N., Stanton, B.R. & Windsor, A.C.M. (1972) *Nutrition of Housebound Old People*. London: King Edwards Hospital Fund.

Smith, J. (2006) Making meals more meaningful. *Caring Times,* May. Available from http://www.careinfo. Accessed December 2007.

Smith, A. (2007) What's new in nursing home nutrition? *Complete Nutrition*, **1**(4):5–7.

Scottish Government (2005) (revised) *National Care Standards Care Homes for Older People*. Available from httpl//:www. Scotland.gov.uk. Accessed November 2007.

Stanner, S. (2002) Improving the nutritional status of older residents in care – new National Minimum Standards. *British Nutrition Foundation Bulletin*, **27**:181–184.

Stanton, B.R. & Exton-Smith, A.N. (1970) *A Longitudinal Study of Dietary of Older Women*. London: King Edward's Hospital Fund.

Steele, G. et al. (1998) *National Diet and Nutrition Survey: People Aged 65 Years and Over, Vol. 2: Report of the Oral Health Survey*. London: HMSO.

Sutherland, S. (1999) *With Respect to Old Age: Long Term Care – Rights and Responsibilities. A Report by The Royal Commission on Long Term Care*. London: HMSO.

Townsend, P. (1961) *The Development of Home and Welfare Services for Old People, 1946–1960*. An address given on Friday, 12th May 1961, at the Annual General Meeting of the Association of Directors of Welfare Services in the City of Bath. Leicester: W. Thornley & Son.

Townsend, P. (1962) *The Last Refuge. A Survey of Residential Institutions and Homes for the Aged in England and Wales*. London: Routledge & Kegan Paul.

Townsend, P. & Wedderburn, D. (1965) *The Aged in the Welfare State. The Interim Report of a Survey of Persons aged 65 and over in Britain, 1962 and 1963*. London: G. Bell & Sons.

VOICES (1998) *Eating well for older people with dementia. A good practice guide for residential and nursing homes and others involved in caring for older people with dementia*. Report of an expert working group. Available from httpl//:www.cwt.org.uk.

Water UK (2007) *Water for Healthy Ageing. Hydration Best Practice Toolkit for Care Homes*. Available from www.waterforhealth.org.uk. Accessed January 2008.

Welsh Assembly Government (2004) (revised) *National Minimum Standards for Older People*. Available from: http://www.csiw.wales.gov.uk. Accessed October 2007.

4 Prisons

Maria Cross

4.1 Introduction

'Food is one of the four things you must get right if you like having a roof on your prison'. (Prison governor, NAO, 2006a)

Over 82 million meals are served annually in prisons in England and Wales. Uptake of meals is consistently and predictably high: a prison is a total institution, so those in its custody (with the exception of inmates of open prisons) are totally dependent on the food provided by that institution and cannot choose to take their custom elsewhere.

Food matters a great deal to prisoners. Mealtimes punctuate the day, breaking up the monotony of imposed routine with the possibility of pleasure. When that possibility fails to deliver, disappointment is assuaged by focussing on the next opportunity. It is not difficult to imagine to what extent a prisoner must look forward to his or her next meal. Food matters not just to the individual but to the whole establishment. Along with visits, letters and health services, the provision of satisfactory food is known to be key to the general wellbeing of a prison population (Crow, 1995). Eating is not just about satisfying hunger and meeting health requirements. The value of food extends into issues of control, power, currency, comfort and hope. Those in authority can use food as an instrument of control and power, whilst those being held can exchange food for favours and 'luxury' items. Refusal to eat may be used as a form of protest, when all that a person has left as a means of dissent is his own body.

Many ex-inmates have documented their experiences in prison, and so fundamental to their experiences is prison food that descriptions of it rarely go unmentioned. Even Oscar Wilde's most famous poem, *The Ballad of Reading Gaol,* published in 1898, describes

> *The brackish water that we drink*
> *Creeps with a loathsome slime,*

And the bitter bread they weigh in scales
Is full of chalk and lime. (1978)

Prisons are unique in that, unlike other institutions (as a general rule), mealtimes can be a trigger for aggressive behaviour and riots. The dining area can become a scene of violent outbursts which are not just about the food itself but also about feelings of power and powerlessness (Smith, 2002). Indeed, it is because of so many incidents in dining halls that communal dining halls in men's prisons (but not women's), have been progressively fazed out (Smith, 2002). The importance of food in prisons, as far as keeping the peace is considered, cannot be overstated. Prison riots down the centuries have almost always had food as a central grievance. In the spring of 1817 all the inmates of Millbank prison were involved in 'open mutiny' – the alleged injustice being the issue of a new type of bread which they considered inferior, though it was in fact brown bread (Griffiths, 1884).

When a riot took place in January 1932 at Dartmoor prison, the prisoners temporarily took control of the prison. Later, during the trial, defendants cited staff brutality and inadequate food as their main grievances (Brown, 2007). The only prisoner to defend himself in court declared: '*We were not sentenced to be deliberately badgered into insanity and killed with bad food; and when I say bad food I do not mean distasteful food, I mean food unfit for human consumption, in many cases*' (Brown, 2007).

4.2   The prison population

Caterers not only have the onerous task of ensuring that what they serve up is non-riot forming, but also of producing good, satisfying meals in ever greater quantities. There are 139 prisons in England and Wales and Her Majesty's Prison Service has responsibility for all of them with the exception of eleven which are privately run. England and Wales have the highest imprisonment rate in western Europe – 147 per 100 000 of the population (Prison Reform Trust, 2008). On 16 May 2008 the prison population stood at over 82 600. In Scotland, where there are 16 prisons in the charge of the Scottish Prison Service, that figure was nearly 8000 on 1 August 2008. In Northern Ireland, the Northern Ireland Prison Service oversees three prisons with a total population of over 1500 on 4 August 2008. There are no signs of those figures decreasing and every indication that they will continue to increase.

Adult inmates are placed in one of four security categories, graded from A to D, and the level of security in each individual prison is similarly graded. Category A prisons are maximum security and category D are semi-open or open prisons. Young offender institutions hold prisoners aged 18–21 and juvenile prisons hold prisoners under the age of 18. At the age of 21 prisoners are transferred to an adult institution. In Northern Ireland there is one high security prison housing adult male long term and remand prisoners, a medium security prison and a young offenders centre accommodating young male offenders and all female prisoners.

The vast majority of prisoners in England and Wales are male and relatively young. The average age of those receiving a prison sentence in 2006 was 27, with a quarter aged 22 or under (Prison Reform Trust, 2008). The demography of the population is however changing quickly. The last decade or so has seen a rapid increase in the number of young women and older people given custodial sentences. The number of women has more than doubled over the last decade – on 16 May 2008, the women's prison population stood at 4458 (Prison Reform Trust, 2008). There has also been a rapid rise in prisoners from minority ethnic groups. By 2006, one in five was from such a group. Of those groups, 37% were foreign nationals. Of the British national prison population, 11% are black and 5% are Asian. Around 11% of the total population is Muslim (Prison Reform Trust, 2008). Around 7000 prisoners are Muslim (House of Commons Select Committee on Public Accounts, 2006).

4.3   History of prison food

Until the twentieth century, the history of the provision of food in prisons was one of condemnatory miserliness intended to punish, debilitate and degrade. Severe food deprivation was a punitive measure in itself, and starvation not unusual. The prevailing sentiment was, historically, that prisoners did not deserve to eat, let alone eat half-decently.

The first prisons were built in the twelfth century, on the orders of Henry II. By the thirteenth century prison construction increased rapidly, to accommodate the number of people ordered to be detained. Living conditions were exceptionally grim. In the fourteenth century, prisoners slept on bare earth and were given only bread and water, and then only every other day. If prisoners wanted anything at all, including food, bedding and fuel, they had to pay for it. This was an arrangement which was to endure for centuries. Better-off prisoners who could afford to pay their jailers had a greater chance of survival. Conditions did improve marginally during the sixteenth century when the introduction of the Poor Law of Elizabeth I meant that counties could use public funds to provide for the poorest prisoners.

Prison overcrowding is not a modern phenomenon: by the seventeenth century prison numbers were soaring, thanks largely to the custom of incarcerating debtors, until they were able to pay for their release. But this was nothing compared to the effect that the birth of the Industrial Revolution was to have on the prison population.

4.3.1   The eighteenth century

The Industrial Revolution which began in the late eighteenth century brought with it a rise in petty crime which exacerbated the existing overcrowding in prisons. Even so, few people were actually imprisoned as punishment for their crimes and detention was usually short: most were awaiting trial or the implementation of a non-custodial sentence, such as flogging (McGowen, 1995).

There were basically two types of prison: the jail and the house of correction. The jail and the house of correction had different functions, although distinctions between the two were often ignored and prisoners of different categories would find themselves incarcerated together. Jail was a detention centre rather than a penitentiary and housed debtors and those awaiting trial. Debtors were held until their dues were paid. Jail was also used to hold those awaiting transportation to the Americas or Australia.

The house of correction held those convicted of short term, petty offences, such as itinerants and prostitutes. Any more serious offences were punished by death, transportation, stocks, the pillory, flogging or fining. As a penitentiary, the house of correction was designed to reform as well as punish criminals, idlers and vagrants through hard labour. The first house of correction was located in the former palace at Bridewell in the City of London and opened in 1556. For that reason, these houses were often referred to as bridewells.

Prisons in the eighteenth century continued to be forbidding, squalid places where conditions were almost invariably appalling. Lack of sanitation, air and light coupled with a starvation diet meant that disease was rife, especially scurvy and typhus, then known as gaol-fever. The only food prisoners received from the authorities was an allowance of bread (Drummond & Wilbraham, 1957). If bread prices increased, the daily allowance shrank. Water was rationed, and although that ration varied, it was generally not enough for both washing and drinking purposes (Hinde, 1951). The sale of alcohol, however, flourished and was a lucrative business for the jailer and continued to be so even after it was outlawed in 1784 (Hinde, 1951).

It was generally believed by both the public and the authorities that a restricted diet should form part of the discipline of punishment. Even so, the dietary restriction imposed on a prisoner depended on his or her ability to fund extras. Not surprisingly, starvation was often the fate of the poor (Drummond & Wilbraham, 1957). On entering prison everyone was expected to pay the jailer a 'garnish' to ensure milder treatment. If given enough garnish the jailer would supply the prisoner with extra food. It wasn't just the jailer who expected pay-offs; established prisoners would demand payment from newcomers, and if the newcomer had no money, he would have to relinquish part of his clothing (Howard, 1929). Prisons held many people who had been acquitted of their crimes, but who could not afford to pay the jailer's fee so were forced to remain confined.

Money, friends and family were the life-line of the eighteenth century prisoner. Family and servants could move freely in and out of prison, bringing provisions, so the lucky ones could in fact find themselves well catered for. Others scavenged what they could: if the prison had gratings on the street side, prisoners were able to beg food from passing members of the public (Drummond & Wilbraham, 1957) Prisoners' criminal associates would often keep their colleagues supplied with food and drink, presumably because they knew they might need to have the favour returned in the future. However, most prisoners were not so lucky and were forced to make do with their pitiful allowance of bread and water (Drummond & Wilbraham, 1957).

Prisons were not state-run, but administered by local justices. The result was that conditions and allowances varied from one establishment to another. Conditions, including food rations, were a matter of good or bad luck. There were rare exceptions to the grim norm: for example, prisoners at the Sussex county jail, rebuilt in 1775, enjoyed airy, separate cells, with each room equipped with bed, blankets and clothes. Debtors were allowed a quart of strong beer or a pint of wine a day, but felons fared worse, being allowed only water to drink (McGowen, 1995).

The eighteenth century may have epitomised the very worst of prison conditions, but it did set in motion the impetus for reform, thanks largely to the eighteenth century prison reformer and High Sheriff of Bedfordshire, John Howard (1726–1790). He wrote his famous 'The State of the Prisons', published in 1777, after visiting every prison in England and Wales. He also travelled throughout Europe to see how prisoners abroad fared and push for reform. Today, the Howard League for Penal Reform is named after John Howard, the founder of the penal reform movement.

What Howard saw during his visits shocked and appalled him. He summarised conditions as 'Filthy, corrupt-ridden and unhealthy'. He was particularly concerned by the diseases typhus and smallpox which were rife among the debtors and criminals in prisons, some of whom he described as 'almost totally destitute of the necessaries of life'. Prisoners were found to be 'covered (hardly covered) with rags; almost famished; and sick of diseases, which the discharged spread where they go; and with which those who are sent to the county gaols infect these prisons'. Howard reported that debtors were denied bread (presumably because they had no money to pay for it) which was given instead to criminal inmates. The amount of bread granted to 'felons' varied and in some cases was only given every two days. Being virtually starved meant that prisoners were too ill to work. Many prisons did not provide water so inmates were dependent on whatever their jailers saw fit to give them. These deprivations, when combined with being held in underground dungeons, often in irons and without circulating air would have been unimaginably wretched. Damp floors and walls and little in the way of bedding added to the suffering, as did the absence of sewers in some jails. The lack of air was due to the absence of windows – windows meant window tax. The sum result of these conditions was disease and death.

Howard believed that prisons should be healthy, disease-free institutions and jailers should not charge prisoners for food and other basic commodities. He called for wide-ranging reforms to improve prison conditions. Amongst his proposals was the provision of a proper diet in the form of a daily allowance. 'I plead only for necessaries, in such moderate quantity as may support health and strength for labour' (Hinde, 1951). As well as a daily bread allowance, Howard argued that prisoners should have boiled beef and broth on a Sunday and be given a penny a day to buy cheese, butter, potatoes, peas or turnips or be given a penny's worth of these foods on a daily basis.

The dietary recommendations Howard made for prisoners held in a bridewell were slightly different. 'I have before said, that I am no advocate for luxury in prisons; for I would have no meat diet for criminals in houses of correction, or at *most, only on Sundays. Yet I would plead, that they should have a pound and half of good household bread a day, and a quart of good beer: besides twice a day a quart of warm soup made from peas, rice, milk or barley. For a change they might sometimes have turnips, carrots, or potatoes'* (Howard, 1929).

Transportation of convicts to the Americas and Australia was coming to an end, and from 1776 until 1857 those condemned to hard labour were kept either in convict prisons or on old sailing ships known as hulks. By day they were employed in hard labour and at night kept in appalling conditions, in chains. Little attention was paid to legislation for better conditions in jails, and the hulks gained notoriety as the most brutal and squalid penal institutions of all (Hinde, 1951). Despite that, prisoners held in hulks were considered to be, in theory, slightly better off than their land-based counterparts when it came to food, in that their ration contained a small amount of meat and broth. It wasn't always palatable though. As one commentator observed, *'Their flesh-meat, as they inform me, is not at all times sweet, but even green with rottenness. The biscuit, which is the only bread they have, is made of the third of coarsest part of the flour and is very unwholesome'* (Smith, 1776).

Howard sowed the seeds of reform but they did not bear fruit until much later, despite the passing in 1779 of the Penitentiary Act. Solitary confinement, religious instruction, hard work and a basic diet were to be introduced. However, political inaction meant that the Act was ineffectual. Various other acts were passed, but it was not until the beginning of the nineteenth century, following a national campaign led by the Quakers and others, that reform really got off the ground.

4.3.2   The nineteenth century and the Victorian era (1837–1901)

'The low animal natures of too many of the criminal class, and the admitted efficiency of reductions in food in cases of prison offences, render plain the value of diet as one form of penal correction'.   Earl of Carnarvon (quoted in Priestly, 1999)

So it was that conditions in the early part of the nineteenth century were much the same as they were at the end of the eighteenth. Garnish was still demanded by jailers and other inmates, alcohol was still sold and food was still scant and of egregious quality. The ration allowance continued to be at the whim of county justices of the peace and borough or corporation magistrates, with no centralised control.

A number of select committees were appointed to investigate the conditions of prisons in London and elsewhere. In London jails it was found that the food allowance consisted mainly of bread, which was often a charitable donation, and meat, which was a weekly 'gift' from the sheriffs (Hinde, 1951). Food allowances varied considerably from prison to prison: in Borough Compter each prisoner received 14 oz of bread a day and 2 lb of meat a week; in Bury the allowance was 1½ lb of bread a day, 1 lb of cheese and ¾ lb of meat a week. Millbank Prison, which was built as an experiment to reflect the new 'age of enlightenment', opened in 1816 and combined solitary confinement, hard labour and religious instruction, as recommended by John Howard. Prisoners there were relatively lucky: each received 1½ lb of bread, 1 lb of potatoes and 2 pints of hot gruel a day with either 6 oz of boiled meat or a quart of strong broth mixed with vegetables (Hinde, 1951).

In 1822 there were complaints that the inmates of Millbank were too well fed; as a result, the meat ration was virtually eliminated, along with the daily potato ration. Instead they got soup made of ox heads at a ratio of one head per hundred prisoners. This soup was thickened with vegetables or peas and was rationed to a quart a day, half at midday and half in the evening. Bread was rationed to a pound and a half and breakfast consisted of a pint of gruel (Griffiths, 1884). A year later, there was an outbreak of sickness and debilitation among the prisoners. An investigation revealed that they were suffering from infectious dysentery and scurvy (with the exception of those prisoners who worked in the kitchen). Consequently, the meat ration was restored and each prisoner was given three oranges a day. The scurvy – but not the dysentery – rapidly vanished (Griffiths, 1884).

Reform in the nineteenth century was fragmented and came in waves, but it did eventually result in better ordered and cleaner prisons (McGowen, 1995). The provision of food however saw no real improvement. In most prisons the diet consisted chiefly of bread and thin gruel or broths. Inmates were lucky if once or twice a week they received a small piece of meat or cheese. Disease continued to be rife (Drummond & Wilbraham, 1957).

The Gaols Act of 1823 was passed under the home secretary Sir Robert Peel as part of an effort to impose standards and uniformity in local prisons throughout the country (McGowen, 1995). Alcohol was forbidden, regular visits by prison chaplains were introduced and jailers were salaried, making them no longer dependent on 'fees' from prisoners. Unconvicted prisoners in local prisons could, generally, buy extra food or receive food gifts from visitors. Convict prison diets were similar to those served in local prisons but were on the whole more monotonous than those of the local prison (Johnston, 1985).

In 1835 prison inspections were introduced. Prison diet had become something of a national scandal and continued to vary from prison to prison. In Morpeth, prisoners received 56 ounces of bread a week, whereas the more fortunate inmates of Cambridge County and Borough enjoyed 280 ounces (Tomlinson, 1978). The home secretary, Sir James Graham, requested that prison inspectors report to him on the whole of prison administration, with a special reference to diet. To eradicate the disparities in provisions, the prison inspectors William Crawford and William Whitworth Russell set about devising their own dietary code in 1842 (Tomlinson, 1978). Crawford and Russell were quite radical reformers in that they were probably the first to direct that prison diet should not be made 'an instrument of punishment' – they believed that people should not leave prison suffering, either mentally or physically, through lack of proper food (Tomlinson, 1978). At the same time, they were still guided by the pervading principle of less-eligibility which prescribed that the prisoner should not be better fed than the poorest, honest labourer. They recommended that there should be three meals a day, at least two of which should be hot, and that there should be a variety of foods, much of which should be in solid form, as opposed to slops. They also urged that meat should form part of the diet of prisoners doing hard labour (Tomlinson, 1978).

On the basis of these recommendations, a ration scale (often referred to as the Graham dietaries) was devised for the first time, which consisted of bread, potatoes, meat, soup, gruel and cocoa, with quantities depending upon whether or not the prisoner was subjected to hard labour (Table 4.1) (Hinde, 1951). The rations were drawn up on the principle that they should be '... *sufficient and not more than sufficient, to maintain health and strength, at the least possible cost; and that, whilst due care should be exercised to prevent extravagance or luxury in a prison, the diet ought not to be made an instrument of punishment*' (Home Secretary's Circular, 1843). Solid foods were an important feature as it was thought that excessive 'slops' in the form of gruel and broths were responsible for the sickness so prevalent among prisoners.

Despite the comparatively good intentions which prompted the ration scale, knowledge of nutritional requirements was at the time scant, and the prevailing view was that any generosity in terms of food provision would inevitably lead to an outbreak of crime. According to one visiting justice of the model prison at Reading, '*If they wished imprisonment to deter from crime, they must cease to supply an excessive diet as to afford temptation to a poor man to commit crime in order to get into prison*' (Drummond & Wilbraham, 1957).

It wasn't just that an 'excessive' diet was believed to be responsible for recidivism; public opinion still upheld the principle of 'less-eligibility'. This principle was hard to put into practice, considering that the poorest, honest labourer endured an indigent standard of living, worse than which would have been hard to achieve. It was probably a combination of prejudice and preconceptions that led to the new ration scale being, in the main, ignored – only 63 out of 140 local prisons adhered to it (Du Cane, 1885). Meat and potatoes were often dispensed with and as a result, there were still regular occurrences of scurvy, potatoes being a rich source of vitamin C which would have prevented the disease from occurring.

It is probably safe to assume that those prisoners who did receive their allowance did not rate it very highly. The bread was frequently described as resembling sawdust and the gruel was so repellent that it was often rejected (Priestly, 1999). Potatoes were frequently found to be black inside. The cocoa element of the diet – later deemed too extravagant to merit a place in the prison ration – contained a great deal of oil which tended to float to the surface and form an unsavoury slick (Priestly, 1999).

That prisoners should not be treated too kindly, or fed too well, was very important to the Victorians. They believed that extremely harsh prison conditions, including hard labour, would act as a deterrent against criminal activity. There was a great deal of prison building during this period. Despite the efforts of penal reformers and much legislative activity, conditions were still appalling and far from uniform. Men, women and children were all mixed together and treated similarly; all were at the mercy of the jailer who continued to run the prison in whichever

Table 4.1 Ratio scale, 1843.

Per week	Without hard labour				With hard labour			
	Class 1	Class 2	Class 3	Class 4	Class 2	Class 3	Class 4	Class 5
	<7 days	>7 days and not >21 days	>21 days and not >4 months	>4 months	>7 days and not >21 days	>21 days and not >6 months	>6 weeks and not >4 months	>4 months
Bread	112	168	140	168	168	140	168	154
Potatoes	–	–	64	32	–	64	32	112
Meat (in ounces)	–	–	6	12	–	6	12	16
Total solid food	112	168	210	212	168	210	212	282
Soup	–	–	2	3	1	2	3	3
Gruel	14	14	14	14	14	14	14	11
Cocoa	–	–	–	–	–	–	–	3
Total liquid food	14	14	16	17	15	16	17	17

way he chose. The House of Lords' Committee of 1862 commented on 'the total absence of uniformity and the irreconcilable inequalities in the nature and amount of the food given' (Du Cane, 1885).

By the mid-nineteenth century it was considered necessary to re-examine prison diets, as the recommended ration scale was not being enforced. They still came in for much criticism, not least of all from a Dr Edward Smith, Licentiate of the Royal College of Physicians and a leading expert of the day, who maintained that the diets of some prisoners remained excessive (Tomlinson, 1978). He argued that it made no sense to give bread and potatoes on three days and meat on the other 4 days, as there was no evidence to show that the body retained nutritive material – therefore meat was required either 7 days a week or not at all. Dr Smith's expertise on the subject of nutrition was not in doubt and, following an inquiry into local prison dietaries, it was decided that meat was not a requirement. This inquiry was commissioned by the Home Secretary Sir George Grey and headed by Dr William Guy, the medical officer of Millbank prison. Guy and his colleagues carried out 'research' – effectively a survey of prison authority opinions – on the cause of diarrhoea and weight loss in prisons. As well as diarrhoea and dysentery, scurvy, scrofula and general weakness were common. Various theories were expounded but poor diet was not one of them (Priestly, 1999). Indeed, Dr Guy's committee was emphatic that there was no link between poor prisoner health and inadequate food. Instead, bad drainage, contaminated water and swallowing hot soup were all proposed as likely explanations (Tomlinson, 1978). The committee may have been influenced by the press and public opinion; whilst prisoners complained that they were hungry or even starving, newspaper articles continued to suggest that prisoners were too well fed, and in the early 1860s an increase in violent robberies left city-dwellers fearful and then angry at the thought of criminals enjoying a hearty meal (Tomlinson, 1978).

Dr Guy considered the earlier scales to be too generous by far and insufficiently penal. He argued for food to be less appealing but to stop short at being 'positively repulsive' (Johnston, 1985). Indeed, Guy had no objections to the standard of food being less than would maintain health and argued that it was unreasonable to provide a diet that would maintain a prisoner '... *in the highest possible stage of health and vigour*' (Johnston, 1985). A new ration scale was devised to replace the earlier one (Table 4.2).

The Guy committee proposed a diet consisting of bread and gruel for breakfast and supper every day. Dinner (the midday meal) incorporated an element of variety and consisted of one of the following: bread and cheese; potatoes; bread; soup; suet pudding. Suet pudding – which together with Indian meal became standard fare – was considered a suitable replacement for meat. Cocoa was removed altogether because it was considered a luxury item. Potatoes were included because the committee acknowledged that they contained a 'vegetable acid' which prevented scurvy (Priestly, 1999). Women were to receive the same food as men but smaller portions.

The committee maintained that a diet must, of necessity, 'be penal' (Priestly, 1999). The home secretary was of the opinion that although the prison diet

Table 4.2 Ration scale, 1864 (without hard labour).

Meals	Days of the week	Articles of food	Class 1 1 week or less		Class 2 After 1 week and up to 1 month		Class 3 After 1 month and up to 3 months		Class 4 After 3 months and up to 6 months		Class 5 After 6 months		Ingredients of soup, etc.
			M	F	M	F	M	F	M	F	M	F	
Breakfast	Every day	Bread (ounces)	6	6	6	5	8	6	8	6	8	6	*In every pint of soup:* the meat and liquor from 6 oz of neck, legs and shins of beef weighed with the bone; 1 oz of onions or leaks; 1 oz of Scotch barley, 2 oz carrots, parsnips, turnips or other cheap vegetables with pepper and salt. On Tuesdays and Saturdays, the meat liquor of previous day to be added.
		Gruel (pints)	–	–	1	1	1	1	1	1	1	1	
Supper	Every day	Bread	6	5	6	5	6	6	8	6	8	6	*Ingredients of suet pudding:* 1½ oz suet; 6½ oz flour and about 8 oz water to make 1 lb.
		Gruel	–	–	–	–	1	1	1	1	1	1	*Ingredients of Indian meal pudding:* To consist of ½ pint of skimmed milk to every 6 oz of meal.
	Sunday	Bread	8	6	8	6	10	8	10	8	12	10	
		Cheese	–	–	1	1	2	2	3	2	3	2	

(Continued)

Table 4.2 Continued

Meals	Days of the week	Articles of food	Class 1 1 week or less		Class 2 After 1 week and up to 1 month		Class 3 After 1 month and up to 3 months		Class 4 After 3 months and up to 6 months		Class 5 After 6 months		Ingredients of soup, etc.
			M	F	M	F	M	F	M	F	M	F	
Dinner	Monday, Wednesday and Friday	Bread	6	5	6	5	4	4	4	4	4	4	*Ingredients of gruel:* To every pint, 2 oz coarse Scotch oatmeal with salt.
		Potatoes	–	–	–	–	12	8	16	12	16	12	
		Suet pudding	–	–	–	–	8	6	12	8	12	8	
		Indian meal pudding	6	4	8	6	–	–	–	–	–	–	
	Tuesday, Thursday and Saturday	Bread	6	5	6	5	8	6	8	6	8	8	The gruel for breakfast on Sundays in Class 4 and for breakfast and supper in Class 5 to contain 1 oz molasses.
		Potatoes	8	6	12	8	8	6	8	6	16	12	
		Soup	–	–	–	–	¾	¾	1	1	1	1	

Additions for prisoners with hard labour.

Male prisoners at hard labour and women employed in the Laundry or other laborious occupations to have the following additions and substitutions: In Class 2: 1 oz extra of cheese on Sundays and 1 pint gruel daily for supper.

In Classes 2–5: 1 oz extra of cheese on Sundays.

In lieu of pudding on Mondays and Fridays: 3 oz beef in Class 3; 4 oz in Classes 4 and 5 for men; 2 oz in Class 3; 3 oz in Classes 4 and 5 for women.

Meat liquor on Mondays and Fridays to form part of soup on Tuesdays and Saturdays. Soup to contain in each pint 2 oz split peas in lieu of 1 oz barley.

should not contrast favourably with that of the honest labourer, it should not be so penal as to endanger health (Johnston, 1985). Although all involved claimed that the ration scale was based on the science of the time and was nutritionally sound, it was in reality more an expression of their moralising stance. The policy was now that:

'prison dietaries should be sufficient, and not more than sufficient, in amount and quality to maintain the health and strength of the prisoners, and ... ought not to be in more favourable contrast to the ordinary food of free labourers, or the inmates of workhouses, than sanitary conditions render necessary'. (Report of the Committee on Dietaries of County and Borough Prisons 1864, quoted in Johnston, 1985)

The Prison Act of 1865 formally amalgamated the jail and the house of correction into what was known as the local prison, which was run by county and borough magistrates. Under the 1877 Prison Act a new prison service was established and control of all prisons was removed from local authorities and vested in central government. The Prison Commission (1925) was established and was tasked with the administration and inspection of prisons in England and Wales. Annual reports had to be submitted to the home secretary for presentation to Parliament. Its chairman was General Sir Edmund Du Cane.

Sir Edmund Du Cane (1830–1903) overhauled much of the penal system, introducing order, efficiency and uniformity. He promised 'hard labour, hard fare and hard board' for prisoners. Hard labour meant the treadwheel and oakum picking. Other forms of occupation including mat making and stone breaking. Hard board was literally what the prisoners had to sleep on and replaced the hammocks they had previously been accustomed to. Each prisoner had a separate cell and women had separate accommodation. All communication between prisoners was forbidden.

Hard fare entailed a meagre and monotonous diet. In 1878 a committee was appointed to 'Consider and Report upon Dietaries of Local Prisons' as a further attempt to enforce uniformity and recommend diets suitable for men, women and children. The committee was also asked to consider whether or not those doing hard labour required a separate diet. *'In framing or recommending the dietaries for the several classes of male and female prisoners, the Committee are requested to avoid any approach either to indulgence or to excess, but to arrange that the diet shall be sufficient and not more than sufficient to maintain health and strength'* (Du Cane, 1885). The committee clearly had no time for earlier, reforming sentiments that the prison diet should not be made 'an instrument of punishment'. Instead, it reaffirmed that prison food was to be of subsistence standard only – in other words, form part of the penal strategy (Du Cane, 1885). The committee reported:

'It appears to us to be a self-evident proposition that imprisonment should be rendered as deterrent as is consistent with the maintenance of health and

strength, whatever may be the sentence, and we think that the shorter the term of imprisonment the more strongly should the penal element be manifested in the diet. It is a matter of universal experience that partial abstinence from food for a limited period is not only safe under ordinary circumstances, but frequently beneficial, and we think that a spare diet is all that is necessary for a prisoner undergoing a sentence of a few days or weeks. To give such a prisoner a diet necessary for the maintenance of health during the longer terms would, in our opinion, be to forego an opportunity for the infliction of salutary punishment; it would constitute an encouragement to the commission of petty crimes; and, by thus paving the way to indulgence in the more serious class of offences, would assist in the manufacture of the habitual criminal'. (Du Cane, 1885)

The committee also inquired into whether or not depression of mind resulting from imprisonment could be prevented by increasing the diet. In view of its hardline position on the importance of a severely restrictive diet, it is hardly surprising that the committee came to the conclusion that '*In a large number of cases, imprisonment, as now conducted, is a condition more or less akin to that of physiological rest. . . of freedom of much worry and anxiety*' (Du Cane, 1885). It also made it clear that it did not believe that giving extra food to improve the health of a prisoner who had lost weight had any beneficial effect. On the contrary, the committee was not convinced that weight loss was associated with reductions in food quantity, despite the fact that those doing hard labour – many of whom were already ill and malnourished when they entered prison – were expected to daily ascend 8640 feet on the treadwheel on their frugal diet (McConville, 1995).

As a result of the committee's deliberations, a uniform, national prison diet was introduced after 1878 (Johnston, 1985). It was based on the previous dietary scales and consisted of bread, soup, gruel, Indian meal pudding, suet pudding, and potatoes. A small amount of meat was however reintroduced to the diet but it was minute – three-quarters of an ounce of bacon (Priestly, 1999). Any prisoner not working hard enough was to be punished with further food restrictions: '*. . . if he should be idle and not execute the work, then the amount of his food is reduced*' (Du Cane, 1882). For good measure, Du Cane's scientific advisers went so far as to issue instructions on the preparation of food in such a way as to make it repulsive to the prisoner and cause nausea and even diarrhoea (McConville, 1995).

It was inevitable that such a harsh regime would precipitate an escalation in death and disease rates, to the extent that by the end of the nineteenth century there was a softening of attitudes. The Report of the Prison Commissioners of 1899 stated that the diet should consist of '*the plainest food, but good and wholesome and adequate in amount and kind to maintain health*', but with the proviso that it should have '*regard to the grave dangers which would accrue should the lowest scale be unduly attractive*' (Pratt, 1999). At least this marked a return to the previous doctrine that prison food should be sufficiently adequate to maintain health. The prison rules even made provision for prisoners to complain, though to do so might have been a challenge in itself. Prison rule 9 stated: *'If any prisoner has any complaint to make regarding the diet, it must be made immediately after a meal is served, and before any portion of it is eaten'* (Priestly, 1999).

The nineteenth century diet stayed much the same until the First World War, with few variations.

4.3.3 Twentieth century

'Our first and most important recommendation relates to fresh vegetables. We desire to urge, as a matter of paramount importance, that every inch of available ground should be cultivated and used for the production of vegetables (more particularly of green vegetables) and of herbs for flavouring'.   (Prison Commission, 1925)

Twentieth century prison life is characterised by overcrowding and under investment, alongside a dramatic increase in crime. Even so, the quality of food in prisons underwent a massive transformation, especially after the First World War. The beginning of the twentieth century became known as the 'golden age of nutrition' as one by one vitamins were discovered in plant foods. As knowledge of health and diet grew, so too did enthusiasm to put that knowledge into practice. In prisons, small amounts of fresh vegetables and beans were introduced into the ration scale. A Departmental Committee on Diets was commissioned to examine the adequacy of prison food, and published its report in 1925. The committee noted that vegetables had been introduced after 1917, albeit only twice a week and in rather small amounts. There was also more variety, and cocoa had made a surprise comeback. The committee reported that although food was of sufficient calorific value, it was low in fat and fresh green foods (Prison Commission, 1925) (Tables 4.3–4.5). The average daily energy value of food given to men in local prisons was calculated to be 3030. After 28 days of incarceration, prisoners had the option to replace half a pint of porridge at breakfast with a pint of tea. This reduced the daily average energy value to 2978. This still compared well with today's recommended dietary reference values for energy:

Men aged 19–50	2550 kcal
Women aged 19–50	1940 kcal
Boys aged 15–18	2755 kcal
Girls aged 15–18	2110 kcal

Source: DH, 1991.

Men in convict prisons were provided with, on average, 3633 calories a day. Their diet was more varied, containing pork soup and beef once a week. Women in local prisons were provided with food containing on average 2456 calories a day. Other than slightly smaller portions, their diet was identical to that of their male counterparts, with the exception that they all received a pint of tea a day, from the beginning of their sentence. The daily diet of boys in borstals contained a daily average of 3775 calories and that of girls 2669 calories.

Table 4.3   Weekly diet of men in local prisons, 1925.

	Breakfast[a]	Mid-day meal	Evening meal	Calorific value
Monday	Bread (8 oz) Porridge (1 pt)	Bread (3 oz) Potatoes (12 oz) Beans (12 oz) Bacon (2 oz) Fresh vegetables (4 oz)	Bread (8 oz) Cocoa (1 pt) Margarine (½ oz)	3296
Tuesday	Bread (8 oz) Porridge (1 pt)	Bread (3 oz) Potatoes (12 oz) Soup (1 pt)	Bread (8 oz) Cocoa (1 pt) Margarine (½ oz)	2842
Wednesday	Bread (8 oz) Porridge (1 pt)	Bread (3 oz) Potatoes (12 oz) Suet pudding (12 oz)	Bread (8 oz) Cocoa (1 pt) Margarine (½ oz)	3294
Thursday	Bread (8 oz) Porridge (1 pt)	Bread (3 oz) Potatoes (12 oz) Beef (5 oz) Fresh vegetables (4 oz)	Bread (8 oz) Cocoa (1 pt) Margarine (½ oz)	3059
Friday	Bread (8 oz) Porridge (1 pt)	Bread (3 oz) Potatoes (12 oz) Soup (1 pt)	Bread (8 oz) Cocoa (1 pt) Margarine (½ oz)	2842
Saturday	Bread (8 oz) Porridge (1 pt)	Bread (3 oz) Potatoes (12 oz) Suet pudding (12 oz)	Bread (8 oz) Cocoa (1 pt) Margarine (½ oz)	3294
Sunday	Bread (8 oz) Porridge (1 pt)	Bread (3 oz) Potatoes (12 oz) Preserved meat (5 oz)	Bread (8 oz) Cocoa (1 pt) Margarine (½ oz)	2582

[a] After serving 28 days, prisoners could choose to replace half a pint of porridge with a pint of tea.

If the committee's calculations and observations were correct, prisoners' energy requirements were indeed being met and even exceeded. These findings were substantiated by an analysis of the weights of prisoners, as part of the report, which found that in general prisoners gained weight during their incarceration. This finding led the committee to conclude that prisoners were released from prison in better physical condition than when they entered. They might not have had sufficient plant food but at least they were receiving three meals a day, a luxury which for many would have been ordinarily beyond their means. Troublemakers were less likely to be so well nourished: punishment diets were still in operation, for 'bad conduct or idleness'. There were two types: one which lasted three days or less and consisted of bread and water and the other which lasted for twenty-one days or less and consisted of bread, water, potatoes and porridge (Prison Commission, 1925).

The quantity of food supplied may have been more than adequate (wastage was common) but the quality still left something to be desired. The committee was particularly critical of suet – 'stodgy and heavy' – and bacon which often consisted of a lump of solid fat and which prisoners would put to better use such as greasing hair or softening leather shoes.

Table 4.4   Weekly diet of women in local prisons, 1925.

	Breakfast	Mid-day meal	Evening meal	Calorific value
Monday	Bread (6 oz) Porridge (½ pt) Tea (1 pt)	Bread (2 oz) Potatoes (8 oz) Beans (10 oz) Bacon (2 oz) Fresh vegetables (4 oz)	Bread (6 oz) Cocoa (1 pt) Margarine (½ oz)	2721
Tuesday	Bread (6 oz) Porridge (½ pt) Tea (1 pt)	Bread (2 oz) Potatoes (8 oz) Soup (1 pt)	Bread (6 oz) Cocoa (1 pt) Margarine (½ oz)	2364
Wednesday	Bread (6 oz) Porridge (½ pt) Tea (1 pt)	Bread (2 oz) Potatoes (8 oz) Suet pudding (10 oz)	Bread (6 oz) Cocoa (1 pt) Margarine (½ oz)	2644
Thursday	Bread (6 oz) Porridge (½ pt) Tea (1 pt)	Bread (2 oz) Potatoes (8 oz) Beef (4 oz) Fresh vegetables (4 oz)	Bread (6 oz) Cocoa (1 pt) Margarine (½ oz)	2414
Friday	Bread (6 oz) Porridge (½ pt) Tea (1 pt)	Bread (2 oz) Potatoes (8 oz) Soup (1 pt)	Bread (6 oz) Cocoa (1 pt) Margarine (½ oz)	2364
Saturday	Bread (6 oz) Porridge (½ pt) Tea (1 pt)	Bread (2 oz) Potatoes (8 oz) Suet pudding (10 oz)	Bread (6 oz) Cocoa (1 pt) Margarine (½ oz)	2644
Sunday	Bread (6 oz) Porridge (½ pt) Tea (1 pt)	Bread (2 oz) Potatoes (8 oz) Preserved meat (4 oz)	Bread (6 oz) Cocoa (1 pt) Margarine (½ oz)	2040

The will to provide a nutritious diet which enabled prisoners at the end of their sentences to '*re-enter the world in as good a physical condition as possible*' (Prison Commission, 1925) had finally been established. The committee was keen to make further improvements, mainly by introducing more variety and more vegetables. It advised that the amount of vegetables supplied should be limited only by the growing capacity of the prison lands. In-house agriculture was seen as a way of significantly increasing the amount of fresh produce in the diet at little cost. Any surplus could be passed on to other prisons. Suggested vegetables for cultivation included potatoes, spinach, kale, cabbage, watercress, carrots, onions, parsnips and swedes. The committee certainly appear to have been enlightened on the subject of nutrition: '*We think, however, that where grown, lettuce, onions and watercress should be issued raw when in season, as an addition to the diet. All these contain valuable food accessory factors, which are partly destroyed in the process of cooking*'.

They also advised that those doing hard labour required more energy – 3400 calories for men in convict prisons doing light labour and 4000 for those doing hard labour. They proposed 3000 calories a day for men in local prisons engaged in sedentary occupations. Women should receive 4/5 of the amount given to men.

Table 4.5 Weekly diet of men in convict prisons, 1925.

	Breakfast	Mid-day meal	Evening meal	Calorific value
Monday	Bread (8 oz) Porridge (1 pt) Tea (1 pt)	Bread (4 oz) Potatoes (12 oz) Beans (12 oz) Bacon (2 oz)	Bread (12 oz) Cocoa (1 pt) Margarine (½ oz) Cheese (1 oz)	3804
Tuesday	Bread (8 oz) Porridge (1 pt) Tea (1 pt)	Bread (4 oz) Potatoes (12 oz) Mutton (5 oz) Fresh vegetables (4 oz)	Bread (12 oz) Cocoa (1 pt) Margarine (½ oz) Cheese (1 oz)	3980
Wednesday	Bread (8 oz) Porridge (1 pt) Tea (1 pt)	Bread (4 oz) Potatoes (12 oz) Pork soup (1 pt)	Bread (12 oz) Cocoa (1 pt) Margarine (½ oz) Cheese (1 oz)	3657
Thursday	Bread (8 oz) Porridge (1 pt) Tea (1 pt)	Bread (4 oz) Potatoes (12 oz) Beef (5 oz) Fresh vegetables (4 oz)	Bread (12 oz) Cocoa (1 pt) Margarine (½ oz) Cheese (1 oz)	3615
Friday	Bread (8 oz) Porridge (1 pt) Tea (1 pt)	Bread (4 oz) Potatoes (12 oz) Soup (1 pt)	Bread (12 oz) Cocoa (1 pt) Margarine (½ oz) Cheese (1 oz)	3336
Saturday	Bread (8 oz) Porridge (1 pt) Tea (1 pt)	Bread (4 oz) Potatoes (12 oz) Suet pudding (12 oz)	Bread (12 oz) Cocoa (1 pt) Margarine (½ oz) Cheese (1 oz)	3850
Sunday	Bread (8 oz) Porridge (1 pt) Tea (1 pt)	Bread (4 oz) Potatoes (12 oz) Preserved meat (5 oz) Fresh vegetables (4 oz)	Bread (12 oz) Cocoa (1 pt) Margarine (½ oz) Cheese (1 oz)	3186

Unfortunately, the committee's dietary expertise fell short when it came to other foodstuffs. It was thought that wholemeal bread contained too much bran, which might be an irritant and be poorly assimilated. However, rather than recommending an entirely white, refined loaf they suggested bread made from half white, half brown flour. Fish too fell foul of the committee's recommendations. They claimed that it was 'inadvisable' to include fish in the diet as they believed it to be of 'small food value'. However providing fish was also impractical because of the limited variety available and spoilage issues.

In 1940, when wartime rationing was introduced nationwide, the opportunity was taken to review prison diet. A ration scale was drawn up for each prisoner, strictly along the lines of the civilian scale. The set meals were abolished and the cook was tasked with serving the rations in the most suitable manner he could devise (Bradley, 1979).

Despite the best intentions of the 1925 committee, by 1944 prison diet was still considered a problem (Home Office, 1946). In that year the Prison

Commission asked the Ministry of Food for assistance in studying the *'problem of prison diets'* (Home Office, 1946). The scientist Magnus Pyke was appointed to examine the nutritional adequacy of the average diet of seven prisons. His overall view was that the diet was satisfactory: levels of protein, calcium, iron, vitamin B1, riboflavin and nicotinic acid were found to be adequate. However the diets were consistently low in vitamin C, and occasionally deficient in vitamin A. Dr Pyke recommended at least 10 oz carrots as part of the weekly ration to remedy the vitamin A deficiency (carrots are rich in beta carotene which is converted into vitamin A). To prevent vitamin C deficiency he suggested increasing the ration of green vegetables and recommended investigating the possibility that losses were occurring through poor cooking and storage methods.

According to the 1949 Prison Rules (Home Office, 1949) the diet was to be of a *'nutritional value adequate for health and of a wholesome quality, well prepared and served and reasonably varied'*. The Commissioners Report for the year 1953 noted that the quality of the cooking and variety of meals had steadily improved and that high standards had been attained (Home Office, 1954). Three years later the Commissioners Report refers to other improvements to the diet, such as additional sausage and gravy or bacon and fried bread for breakfast. By 1958 fresh meat was in use and there was an increase in potato and fresh fruit allowances. By 1963 the milk ration had been increased by half a pint a week and eggs were part of the regular weekly dietary allowance.

The food may have continued to improve in terms of variety and nutritional adequacy but not apparently in terms of taste. Food was cooked, weighed and measured in tins to ensure that each prisoner got his entitlement, although there was no guarantee that this was indeed the case. As a result the meal was cooked long before it was served, and a constant complaint was that it all tasted the same (Bradley, 1979). Still, prison catering was heading in the right direction. By 1963, some prisons offered as many as four choices as the main meal. By 1973 it was reported that there was a greater variety of food with more fresh fruit and vegetables, and poultry was on the menu for the first time (Home Office, 1974). By 1974 a vegetarian diet had been introduced. An article on prison diet published in 1978 in the *Journal of Consumer Studies and Home Economics* (Tomlinson, 1978) noted that in Oxford prison breakfast porridge was followed by sausage, scrambled egg or grilled bacon – a menu which would be the envy of many prisoners today.

Until the 1990s the ration scale (as described in Table 4.6) was still in place, but was gradually being fazed out. After benefiting from the *golden age of nutrition* for nearly a hundred years, the prison service throughout the UK was about to undergo a major transformation.

4.4   Food today

Unlike people in other institutions, those held in prisons in the UK are only permitted to eat what is provided to them by that institution. In England and

Table 4.6 Ration scale prior to the pre-select system.

Food item	Daily or weekly	Local prisons and remand centres		Prisons other than local		Young offenders locations	
		Male	Female	Male	Female	Male	Female
Cheese (g)	Weekly	105	105	105	105	105	105
Chicken, oven-ready (g)	Weekly	220	220	220	220	220	220
Coffee, instant (g)	Weekly	5	5	5	5	5	5
Cornflakes (g)	Weekly	75	75	75	75	75	75
Cornflour/custard powder (g)	Weekly	60	60	60	60	60	60
Eggs, grade 4	Weekly	3	3	3	3	3	3
Fish, fresh	Weekly	Weekly cash allowance as notified by Supply Group					
Flour – bread (g)	Weekly	1575	1140	1750	1140	1750	1140
Flour – wholemeal (g)	Weekly	390	285	440	265	440	285
Flour – culinary (g)	Weekly	655	475	750	475	750	475
Fruit, fresh	Weekly	Two pieces purchased from cash allowance notified by Catering Group					
Fruit, dried (g)	Weekly	100	100	100	100	100	100
Jam/marmalade (g)	Weekly	130	130	130	130	130	130
Margarine – table (g)	Weekly	400	350	400	350	400	350
Meat, fresh	Weekly	Weekly cash allowance as notified by Supply Group					
Meat – corned beef, chopped pork, pork luncheon meat (g)	Weekly	60	60	60	60	60	60
Milk, fresh (ml)	Weekly	2070	2070	2070	2070	2070	2070
Milk, dried (g)	Weekly	35	35	35	35	35	35
Oats – rolled (g)	Weekly	100	100	100	100	100	100
Oil, vegetable cooking (ml)	Weekly	195	150	195	150	235	150
Pasta (g)	Weekly	30	30	30	30	30	30

Pork (g)	Weekly	80	80	80	80	80	80	80
Pork, cured (bacon) (g)	Weekly	385	385	385	385	385	385	385
(choice of) Sago, semolina, tapioca, ground rice, pudding rice, long grain & brown rice – within total ration (g)	Weekly	120	120	120	120	120	120	120
Sausage meat (g)	Weekly	160	160	160	160	160	160	160
Sugar (g)	Weekly	400	400	400	400	400	400	400
Tea (g)	Weekly	50	50	50	50	50	50	50
Tomato puree (g)	Weekly	10	10	10	10	10	10	10
Vegetables								
Beans in tomato sauce (g)	Weekly	170	170	170	170	170	170	170
Carrots (g)	Weekly	450	450	450	450	450	450	450
Other root vegetables (g)	Weekly	225	225	225	225	225	225	225
Cabbage (g)	Weekly	450	450	450	450	450	450	450
Cauliflower/broccoli/ Brussels sprouts (g)	Weekly	225	225	225	225	225	225	225
Onions (g)	Weekly	150	150	150	150	150	150	150
Peas, marrowfat/split (g)	Weekly	100	100	100	100	100	100	100
Potatoes, fresh (g)	Daily	480	450	450	540	450	540	450
Or								
Potatoes, fresh (g)	Daily	385	360	435	435	360	435	360
and								
Potatoes, dried (g)	Daily	17	15	18	18	15	18	15

Source: Prison Department Manual V. Supply and Transport Branch Volume 4.

Box 4.1   Catering responsibilities.

Catering manager
Compiles recipes, compiles menu cycles, identifies purchasing requirements, ensures budget targets are met and generates the correct number of meals.

Procurement clerk
Places the orders stipulated by the catering manager, sources for local purchases, processes goods received and deals with the practical issues of delivery, stocktaking, etc.

Medical officer
Prescribes medical dietary requirements.

Caterer/storeman
Receives goods, documents and transfers goods, assists in stock takes, ensures standard recipes are adhered to.

Finance manager
Authorises payment of invoices.

Source: HM Prison Service (1999).

Wales the rules stipulate that '*... No prisoner shall be allowed, except as authorised by a health professional ... to have any food other than that ordinarily provided*' (HMPS, 2006). This also includes drinks (alcoholic beverages are prohibited). The only exception to this rule is food which is integral to religious festivals. Prisoners may purchase snacks from the prison shop to supplement their diet, but access is limited.

The responsibility for providing food in prisons lies with the prison governor who also sets the budget. The prison kitchen is run by the prison catering manager who is in charge of implementation of standards, staff training and budget control. Other responsibilities are outlined in Box 4.1.

4.4.1   The pre-select system

Until 1996 the ration scale system was still widely in place. This was based on the prisoner's 'allowance' of raw ingredients. By 1997 around half of all prisons had adopted a pre-select system whereby prisoners select their meals in advance. By September 2005 all prisons, including privately run establishments, had adopted a pre-select, multi-choice, cyclical menu for both lunch and dinner. According to the requirements of the Prison Service Catering Manual (page 302) there must be a minimum two-week and maximum five-week menu cycle in operation (HMPS, 1999). Prisoners usually select meals between three and five days in advance. A similar system is also in operation in Scotland and Northern Ireland.

The pre-select system has a number of advantages. Caterers are better able to plan meal requirements and reduce excessive waste (Edwards *et al.*, 2001). Where cafeteria-style dining environments still exist, prisoners at the back of the queue have some guarantee that they will get what they want, without having to accept leftovers. This means reduced risk of conflict and confrontation at the serving point (NAO, 1997; Edwards *et al.*, 2001).

Prisoners can choose from a range of meal categories, including 'normal', vegetarian, vegan, halal and 'healthy'. The Prison Service caters for eleven different religious and cultural diets, which require special preparation.

Each prisoner receives three meals a day. Breakfast is usually in the form of a pack which includes a cereal, UHT milk, bread, spread, conserve, tea bag and a sachet of whitener and sugar. Lunch and dinner tend to be similar meals, with a choice of around five main dishes plus potatoes and vegetables. Portion sizes are strictly controlled, although potatoes, vegetables and bread are less rigidly monitored. (Edwards *et al.*, 2007). Table 4.7 outlines a typical pre-select menu served in England and Wales.

4.4.2   Northern Ireland

The catering service in Northern Ireland prisons was, until 1999, largely directed by its political history. For thirty years consideration was made not for ethnic, religious or other requirements but for the demands of two warring factions. Food was provided on a 'take it or leave it basis' – suppliers to the prisons were at considerable risk of attack from paramilitary groups and those few suppliers who did provide the prisons with commodities did so at a premium (private email correspondence, 23/08/07). As a result there was no choice and little ceremony.

The signing of the Good Friday Agreement in 1998 transformed prison catering in Northern Ireland. A pre-select system, similar to that in place in England and Wales, was introduced. Prisoners now pre-select their meals from a multi-choice menu with four main meal choices and three light meal choices, which include vegetarian, healthy (low-fat) and ethnic options. See Table 4.8 for a sample Northern Ireland menu.

4.4.3   Dining environment

Although some prisons do still have a central dining hall, in the style of a cafeteria, most male prisoners now eat their meals in their cells. The removal of the dining hall came about following the Woolf report into prison disturbances (see page 302). Food is delivered to each cell on heated trolleys. In overcrowded prisons where inmates share cells, it is not uncommon for meals to be consumed sitting on the bed, or even on the toilet. In women's prisons, most prisoners still eat in communal dining halls.

4.5   Catering standards

Under current Prison Rules, food provided *'shall be wholesome, nutritious, well prepared and served, reasonably varied and sufficient in quantity'* (HMPS, 2006).

Table 4.7 Example of a pre-select menu in England and Wales.

Day	Breakfast	Lunch choice	Evening meal
Monday	Cornflakes, milk, bread, jam/marmalade	Vegetable casserole/stir fried rice/turkey casserole (halal)/gammon & pineapple/Mexican chicken leg *with* Boiled potatoes, mixed vegetables, gravy Eves pudding & custard or pear	Rice salad/jacket potato & pilchard salad/battered sausage (halal)/farmhouse pasty/egg mayo sandwich/turkey sandwich *with* mashed potato, spaghetti Biscuits
Tuesday	Malt crunchies, milk, bread, jam/marmalade	Soya steak & kidney pudding/vegetable curry & rice/curried chicken leg (halal)/steak & kidney pudding/braised sausages *with* Boiled potatoes, peas, gravy Yoghurt or orange	Battered vegetarian sausages/jacket potato & beans/fish fingers/beef burger/chicken roll sandwich/spicy crab sandwich/beef sandwich *with* Roast potatoes, beans supper bun
Wednesday	Shredded wheat, milk, bread, jam/marmalade	Pasta in tomato sauce/fish curry & rice/chicken tandoori (halal)/roast beef/Lancashire hotpot *with* Boiled potatoes, carrots, gravy Fruit crumble & custard or pear	Tomato & mushroom bake/jacket potato & cheese salad/savoury mince (halal)/spam fritter/BBQ chicken sandwich/savoury cheese sandwich/cheese & onion *with* Boiled potatoes, peas, gravy Ice cream or apple
Thursday	Rice krispies, milk, bread, jam/marmalade	Soya curry & rice/broccoli and cheese sauce/Beef chow mein (halal)/chicken & mushroom pie/fish in breadcrumbs *with* Boiled potatoes, green beans & gravy Rice pudding or apple	Stuffed tomatoes/jacket potato & chilli beans/sausage Lyonnaise (halal)/curried pasty/egg & bacon sandwich/cheese & spring onion sandwich/ham sandwich *with* Boiled potatoes, mixed veg, gravy supper bun

Friday	Honeynut cornflakes, milk, bread, jam/marmalade	Stuffed peppers/vegetarian chilli & rice/battered fish/hot & spicy chicken leg/savoury mince & yorkshire pudding *with* Boiled potatoes, cabbage & gravy Apple pie & custard or orange	Vegan pizza/curried eggs/lamb & onion pie (halal)/cold sliced ham/chinese chicken sandwich/Savoury corned beef sandwich/chicken sandwich *with* Chips, mushy peas Apple
Saturday	Frosties, milk, bread, jam/marmalade	Vegan brunch/vegetarian brunch/Muslim brunch/healthy option brunch/scrambled egg & beans *with* Fried bread & tomatoes Yogurt or pear	Nasi goreng pattie/bacon & egg sandwich/fish fingers/pork pie *with* Chips, spaghetti Supper bun
Sunday	Weetabix, milk, bread, jam/marmalade	Carrot & nut cluster/mushroom vol au vent/roast beef (halal)/roast chicken/roast beef *with* Roast potatoes, cauliflower & gravy Torte or banana	Grated cheese/ cheese slice/spicy tuna sandwich/ham slice/corned beef slice *with* Chips & pickle Supper bun

Source: National Offender Management Service (2007).

Table 4.8 Sample pre-select menu in Northern Ireland.

Day	Breakfast	Lunch choices	Lunch vegetables/accompaniment	Dinner choices	Dinner vegetables/accompaniment	Sweet choices	Supper
Monday	Cornflakes	A. Steak sausages B. Vegetarian hotpot (V) (L) C. Corn beef baguette & Cupasoup (HO)	Creamed potatoes & Pea & onion gravy	A. Chicken breast & sweet chilli sauce (L) B. Lambs liver & onion gravy (L) C. Vegetarian curry (V) (HO) D. 5-inch floury bap (tuna & onion) (HO)	Chips & peas	A. Ice lolly B. Fresh fruit	Chocolate biscuit
Tuesday	Weetabix	A. Fish burger B. Cheese & tomato toastie (V) C. Ham salad (L) (HO)	Croquette potatoes & spaghetti hoops	A. Beef casserole (L) B. Chicken leg & gravy (L) C. Vegetable pie (V) C. Ham salad (L) (HO)	Boiled potatoes & cabbage	A. Apple crumble & custard B. Fresh fruit	Plain scone
Wednesday	Alpen	A. Pork sausage fry B. Cheese & onion pasty & baked potato (V) C. Tuna salad (L) (HO)		A. Chicken olive & gravy B. Lemon & pepper haddock (L) (HO) C. Vegetarian cottage pie (V) D. Tuna salad (L) (HO)	Chips & sweetcorn	A. Ice cream cornet B. Fresh fruit	Shortbread
Thursday	Weetabix	A. Sausage rolls × 2 B. Macaroni cheese (V) C. Quiche salad (L) (HO)	Baked beans	A. 8oz Aberdeen Angus burger & gravy B. Chicken & mushroom slice (L) C. Vegetable lasagne (V) D. Quiche salad (L) (HO)	Roast potatoes & carrots	A. Chocolate frozen yoghurt B. Fresh fruit	Filled roll

Day	Breakfast	Lunch		Dinner		Dessert	Snack
Friday	Cornflakes	A. Chicken curry (L) B. Egg & onion baguette & Cupasoup (V) C. Chopped ham/pork salad (L) (HO)	Boiled rice	A. Battered fish B. Beef sausages C. Battered vegetables (V) D. Chopped ham/pork salad (L) (HO)	Creamed potatoes & m/fat peas	A. Jam sponge & custard B. Fresh fruit	Banana
Saturday	Boiled egg	A. Mince & onion pie B. Grilled gammon steak & pineapple (L) C. Leek & pasta bake (V) D. Corned beef salad (HO)	Roast potatoes & green beans	A. Beef stew (L) B. Vegetarian stir fry & rice (L)		A. Jelly fruit & cream B. Fresh fruit	Pancake
Sunday	Pork sausages	A. Chicken breast & Chinese gravy (L) B. Chinese style pork chops (L) C. Vegetarian slice in puff pastry (V) D. Cheese salad (L) (HO)	Creamed potatoes, carrots & parsnips	A. Hamburger with roll & onions B. Veg. burger with roll & onions C. Cheese salad (L) (HO)	Chips	A. Fruit split ice lolly B. Fresh fruit	Mini packet biscuits

L = low fat, HO = healthy option, V = vegetarian.

Source: NIPS, 2007.

Prisons are run in accordance with guidelines laid down in Prison Service Orders (PSOs) and Prison Service Instructions (PSIs). A PSO is a long-term, mandatory rule. A PSI is an instruction which is often used to amend existing PSOs. In 1999, Prison Service Order 5000 – the *Prison Service Catering Manual* – was introduced, in order to deliver good catering practice, food safety and menu management.

Catering standards came about largely as a result of an inquiry into the 1990 prison riots which began at Strangeways in April that year and were followed by protests and disturbances in prisons throughout the country. These riots were the most serious to occur in British penal history and led to an inquiry, headed by Lord Justice Woolf, into the causes of the disturbances and the wider implications for the prison system (Prison Reform Trust, 1991).

The Woolf report found that poor quality food – said to be monotonous, inedible, cold and insufficient – was the most common complaint from prisoners. Other complaints included shortage of clothing and oppressive behaviour on the part of some officers. Both the quality and timing of meals were criticised in the report, as were standards of hygiene. The timing of meals meant that prisoners had to endure very long periods between the evening meal and breakfast, and the Woolf report recommended that the Prison Service review its staffing arrangements to ensure that meals were served at reasonable times. The report also recommended that the dietary scales then in place should be reviewed and that catering officers should have greater control over the food budget. Prisoners should be given the choice of eating in their cells or communally (Prison Reform Trust, 1991).

The manual covers all aspects of prison catering and food provision, from food hygiene to the nutritional value of meals provided. It was produced by HMPS Catering Services and agreed by the Prison Service Management Board. Although private sector prisons work to individual contract terms and conditions, they are still required to comply with the mandated requirements laid down in the manual.

The manual is designed to enable catering managers to compile menus in accordance with prison regulations, and plan a multi-choice, pre-select menu. This menu must allow for special dietary requirements and be produced within budget. It must include healthy options and at the same time reflect prisoners' preferences. There are five sections, or chapters. Chapter 1 is an introduction and overview; chapters 2, 4 and 5 concern food safety management. Chapter 3 is dedicated to menu management.

4.5.1   Caterers as healthy eating providers

'Establishment catering departments will continue in their endeavour to promote the concept of healthy eating by ensuring that nutritious balanced meals are made available'.   (HMPS, 1999 §3.2.3)

'It is an objective of Prison Catering Services to encourage establishments to offer a range of foods which enable consumers to make a healthy eating choice'.   (HMPS, 1999 §3.4.2)

The Prison Service is expected to encourage action in the following key areas:

- reduction of fat, especially saturated fats
- promotion of starchy, fibre-rich foods and fruits and vegetables
- reduction of sugar intake
- avoidance of excessive salt

In devising recipes, caterers are advised to:

- replace saturated fats with margarine and plant oils such as rape and other seed oils, nut and olive oils
- include fish, both white and oily
- use the leanest possible cuts of meat
- use reduced, skimmed fat products wherever possible, particularly in the case of dairy
- increase fibre by incorporating more wholemeal flour in recipes
- use more fruit-based desserts to help reduce sugar levels

Specific cooking advice includes:

- restrict deep fat frying
- bake, grill, poach roast or steam
- steam vegetables to maintain vitamins and minerals

With regard to food service/counter presentation, caterers are advised that:

- alternatives should be offered next to each other, for example, butter and spreads
- vegetables and sauces can be offered separately
- reduced fat salad dressings can be served separately from undressed salads
- fresh meat and fish can be offered alongside tinned varieties and pastry items
- bread on offer can include whole grain varieties and high fibre biscuits
- a wide variety of 'interesting' fresh fruits, vegetables and salads can be offered.

All menus should include a healthy option which must be clearly marked as such. Each establishment must offer at least one lower fat/high fibre/lower sugar or lower salt item on each menu. Staff should be provided with the training, information and skills required to produce healthy food. A specific member of staff should be charged with responsibility for healthy eating.

With regard to genetically modified food, all prison menus must contain the following statement:

'Items on this menu marked with an asterisk (*) contain ingredients produced from genetically modified maize or soya'. (HMPS, 1999 §3.11)

Each dish must carry a symbol identifying its category – for example, ♥ denotes healthy eating, vegetarian = V and Halal = H. A descriptive menu outlining the ingredients of each dish must be provided.

4.5.2   Specific nutrient standards

'Caterers must be aware of current nutritional guidelines and recommendations. They must use up-to-date information and advice from reliable sources such as HMP Catering Services, environmental health officers, dieticians, health education officers'.   (§3.9.1)

Guidelines for specific, mandatory nutrient standards are, as yet, not in place, but the prison catering manual states that, *It is essential in order to maintain budgetary control that portion sizes are controlled in line with consumer needs.* These needs (reference nutrient intakes for individual vitamins and minerals) and energy requirements are outlined in annexes 20 and 21 of the manual and are based on the standards set in *Dietary Reference Values for Food Energy and Nutrients for the UK* (DH, 1991). The possibility of setting nutrient guidelines specifically for prison food is one which has been considered from time to time and is still under consideration by the Prison Service and Food Standards Agency (private email correspondence, 29/08/07).

4.5.3   Menu planning

There must be a minimum two-week maximum five-week menu cycle in operation.

Catering managers are expected to take account of the following when compiling their menus:

- category and locality of the establishment
- type of consumer (male, female, mixed, adult, YOI)
- religion
- cultural background
- medical diets
- time of year (seasonality)
- time of day (breakfast, lunch, dinner)
- cost of commodities (ingredients)
- repetition of commodities (e.g., cheese in cauliflower cheese, Welsh rarebit, lasagne)
- repetition of texture of dishes (e.g., using too many soft textures: mashed potatoes, creamed swede, rice pudding)
- repetition of flavours
- repetition of colour
- nutritional value
- number of courses

- meat or non-meat preferences
- equipment available
- staff skills

4.5.4   Minimum frequency of provision

Meat	daily
Vegetables	daily
Poultry	twice weekly
Fresh fruit	daily
Fish	twice weekly
Drinks (hot or cold)	each meal service

4.5.5   Portion sizes

Portion sizes must be controlled in order to meet budgetary restrictions, and must be consistent, *'without bias to any individual'* (§3.16.4). Specific weights and measures are given for main ingredients and components, for example:

Cheddar cheese	60 g
Rasher grilled bacon	40 g
Slice tomato	17 g
Medium portion chips	165 g
Medium sized apple	112 g
Instant coffee	2 g

4.5.6   Variations in diet

The catering manual gives basic guidance for vegetarian, vegan, medical, Buddhist, Church of Jesus Christ of Latter-day Saints ('Mormons'), Ethiopian Orthodox, Greek Orthodox, Hindu, Jain, Jewish and Islamic diets, including storage and preparation requirements. Basic terms such as halal are explained.

4.5.7   Scotland

The Governor shall ensure that every prisoner is provided with sufficient wholesome and nutritious food and drink, well prepared and presented, which takes into account the prisoner's age, health, and, so far as reasonably practicable, his religious, cultural or other requirements.   (SPS Prison Rules)

There is a clear need for improved dietary practice within the Scottish Prison Service and the other public services as well. The Scottish Prison Service is particularly well placed to influence diet. Unlike most other institutions, the Service provides the total food intake of substantial numbers of mainly young men for long periods of time. Most prisoners are drawn from that section of the population with the least healthy eating habits and the highest rate of coronary heart disease in middle age.   (Scottish Office, 1996)

In 1996 the Scottish Office (now the Scottish Government) drew up plans to improve the diet of its people. The *Scottish Diet Action Plan* (Scottish Office, 1996) made 71 recommendations which included plans for a model contract for catering specifications for wide use in institutions and the public sector. Recommendation 52 states that '*The Scottish Office should ensure that the catering services of the Scottish Prison Service and other public services in Scotland reflect the guidance in the* Model Nutritional Guidelines for Catering Specifications for the Public Sector in Scotland'. The general principles of the *Model Nutritional Guidelines* include:

- availability of healthy choices (including fresh fruit and vegetables) in sufficient quantity and quality to enable clients to meet their daily needs
- choice of basic commodities available, for example types of bread and milk.
- healthy food production methods and ingredients, for example content of salads and dressing.
- the use of standard recipes based on healthy catering practices.
- menu planning, including the frequency of food items, such as fried foods, on menus.
- advice that nutrient targets may be included in the form of dietary reference values but that food-based targets are also essential (Scottish Office, 1996).

As far as prisons are concerned, these guidelines were largely ignored. Instead, more plans were drawn up. The Scottish Prison Service (SPS) in its document *The health promoting prison: A framework for promoting health* (2002) identified four core health topics as starting points for action. These were: *eating for health, active living, tobacco use and mental health wellbeing*. Under *Eating for health*, the SPS put forward ten changes for prisons with a target to fully meet all these changes by 2005. These were:

(1)   change to low sugar preserves
(2)   change to low sugar/salt tinned vegetables
(3)   change to tinned fruit in fruit juice
(4)   offer fruit juice at meal times
(5)   increase vegetable uptake to 400 g per day
(6)   provide sugar substitutes for beverages, and so on
(7)   reduce fried dishes (puddings, (sic) chips, etc.) to 3 per week
(8)   increase uptake of wholemeal foods by 100%
(9)   increase availability of salad meals by 50%
(10) advertising on vending machines should be for diet varieties (sic)

The SPS made a number of further recommendations, which included:

- the introduction of a healthy eating policy
- ensuring availability of fruit at meals and as a snack
- competitive pricing policy to encourage fruit uptake

- involving staff and prisoners in healthy eating special events
- providing information on healthy eating
- encouraging prisoners to learn cooking skills
- encouraging the use of alternatives to salt and ways to cut down on sugar
- monitoring targets against the uptake of healthier meal options or of fruit and vegetables (SPS, 2002).

By 2005 these targets had not been met. Instead, in that year, the Scottish Executive established The Good Food Group, with members from key stakeholders including local authorities and the Food Standards Agency Scotland (FSAS). The remit of the Good Food Group was to improve and monitor the safety and nutritional standards of food in prisons.

In the meantime, by 2004 the Scottish Prison Service was in the early stages of developing nutritional standards for prison food. The purpose of introducing these standards was to ensure that food provided met the majority of the prison population's energy and nutrient requirements and that menus met government guidelines for intakes of fruit and vegetables and fish in the Scottish population. In 2006 the FSAS published the draft document *'Nutrient and Food Standards for the Scottish Prison Service'*. This draft is no more than a recommendation that food provided in prisons meets the recommendations published in the Department of Health's (1991) report *Dietary Reference Values for Food Energy and Nutrients in the United Kingdom* (DH, 1991). Despite there being nothing new about these standards, by August 2007 the FSAS was still working with the SPS, the Good Food Group and a private consultancy firm – FM Specific – towards their full implementation. According to the SPS, the role of this private company is *'to work in conjunction with the Good Food Group and Prisons' Directorate to review our current catering operations and provide recommendations for improvements'* (private email correspondence, 23/10/07). The Good Food Group, in conjunction with FM Specific, has produced more targets, to be met over three years (from 2008) to replace previous, unmet targets (private email correspondence, 21/11/07).

4.5.8 Northern Ireland

The sophistication of prisoners is not usually sufficient to ensure that the menus reflect healthy eating or the guidelines applied to good menu planning. Because of this there may well be conflict between consumer requirements and the balanced diet. (NIPS, 2006a)

Under Northern Ireland prison rules, prison catering departments (Northern Ireland Prison Service, 1995) are required to provide every prisoner 'with sufficient food which is wholesome, nutritious, palatable, adequately presented and well prepared and which takes into account age, health and work and, as far as practicable, religious or cultural requirements'. (NIPS, 1995)

The *Northern Ireland Prison Service Food Safety and Catering Manual* (NIPS, 2006a) provides mandatory guidelines on a number of catering issues including contracts, procurement, monitoring, menu management and catering quality. It is mandatory for caterers to provide a multi-choice, pre-selection menu which includes healthy options. The manual states that *'There must be a facility within the menu for the consumer to be given a choice to eat not only in the way they are accustomed to, but also variations of ethnic/cultural dishes and healthy foods'*. The NI manual is similar to the one governing prisons in England and Wales: advice on healthy eating, healthy cooking methods and menu structure is more or less identical. One interesting difference is that Northern Ireland clarifies the meaning of five portions of fruit and vegetables and gives examples of portion sizes as well as indicating that which does not constitute a portion, for example, ketchup or fruit cake.

4.6   Expenditure, procurement and staffing

In 2004–2005 the Prison Service spent £94 million on catering (NAO, 2006a). How much each prison spends on food is determined by the governor (known as the director in privately run prisons) of that establishment.

In England and Wales the average daily spend on prisoners' food (known as the daily food allowance) is £1.87. In Young Offenders' Institutes that figure is £3.81. Such disparity in expenditure can be partially explained by the differing requirements of institutions: YOIs usually have higher daily allowances because juveniles tend to eat more, and they receive extra money for food from the Youth Justice Board. Those held in open prisons (where expenditure can be as low as £1.21) often only require two meals a day (NAO, 2006a). However, wide variations in expenditure occur not only among different types of establishment but also among similar ones and these are less easily explained. In 2004–2005 the cost of food per prisoner, per day, varied by over 180% between the cheapest and the most expensive. The cost of food at male YOIs varied by 95% between the cheapest and most expensive (NAO, 2006a).

In Scotland, the budget is, as in England and Wales, the responsibility of the governor, and the catering manager determines how it is spent. Average daily expenditure by the Scottish Prison Service is £1.57, 30p less than the average spent on prisoners in England and Wales. This includes all food and drink consumed by each prisoner every day. The Scottish expenditure figure has not increased since 1996 and according to the Chief Inspector of Prisons for Scotland, not enough food is provided for young men, particularly fresh fruit and vegetables (NAO, 2006a).

The Northern Ireland prison food budget is surprisingly high at £2.43 per prisoner per day. The prison catering manager is accountable and responsible for the provision of food within the catering budget.

Any institution which has to procure food on a large scale is aware that efficiency is paramount if the best value is to be obtained with available financial resources. However, efficiency has not always been central to the modus operandi of prison catering. By 1997 caterers were preparing over 60 million meals a year at a cost of about £3 per prisoner per day. That same year, the National Audit Office published a report on the quality and cost of prison catering (NAO, 1997). Among the prisons visited, the NAO found that poor organisation meant that there were no procedures in place for economic ordering and stock control, with the result that there were large variations in the amount of stock held and in food and staff costs. The NAO also found that the Prison Service did not hold comprehensive financial information on its catering expenditure. The conclusion was that there was plenty of scope for improvement and for making very extensive savings if catering expenditure were organised more efficiently. The NAO recommended that the Prison Service review its options for suppliers, reduce stock holding and make better use of systems already in place to generate information on costs of catering and to compare costs with similar establishments.

None of this would have come as a surprise to the Prison Service at the time: in 1998 an internal review of procurement within the Prison Service also found it to be fragmented and inefficient according to an NAO report published in 2003 (NAO, 2003). Large numbers of staff were involved in procurement with duplication of decision making, a high volume of stock holding and no overall corporate strategy covering purchasing, stock holding and distribution.

The Prison Service already knew that its procurement and expenditure systems were in need of a major overhaul and indeed improvements were under way before the NAO report was published. One of the recommendations of the Woolf report into the prison riots of 1990 was the adoption of a cash catering system, and this was introduced across the prison estate in 1996 and is still in place today. This means that prison caterers are given a budget, as set by the governor, and discretion to buy the food they need. They are not allowed to change any aspect of the prison catering system without authorisation from HM Prison Catering Services (HMPS, 1999). The catering manager compiles standardised recipes which are costed by the computer system. Any changes in the cost of ingredients will automatically adjust the cost of the recipe, in order to ensure that every menu falls within the budget. All food purchases have to be recorded accurately and linked to planed menus. The introduction of this system has led to considerable progress in prison catering.

When it came to making financial savings, the Prison Service was swift to act. By 1999 numerous local purchasing food supply contracts and national contracts had been replaced by a greatly reduced number of central and regional contracts (NAO, 2006a). In 2000–2001 the Prison Service was able to report savings of £1 250 000 in the procurement of food (NAO, 2003). By 2005 there were only eight national and 14 regional contracts for fresh produce. All contracts are now let competitively every two to three years. Prisons can choose from a number of contractors for fresh and frozen goods but there is only one contractor supplying non-perishable foods (NAO, 2006a).

In Scotland the SPS oversees the procurement of food and drink which is also now arranged on a centralised basis. There are five contracts in place and total expenditure under these contracts in 2003/04 was £3.5 million (Scottish Government, 2005). All three prisons in Northern Ireland operate on centralised contracts for non-perishable stock. Frozen food and vegetables are sourced by the catering personnel of each establishment.

Since 2005 savings of up to £2.5 million, or around 6%, have been made on expenditure on food in England and Wales, largely as a result of introducing national mandatory contracts (NAO, 2006a). The NAO in its 2006 report *Serving time: Prisoner diet and exercise* acknowledged that the Prison Service had made significant financial savings from both its food and catering staff budgets but claimed that there was still scope for more savings. The NAO recommended that the Prison Service further improve its purchasing power by adopting joint purchasing arrangements with other public sector bodies such as local schools and hospitals and setting up joint local storage and distribution facilities (NAO, 2006a). The NAO also recommended that high spending prisons should reduce their spend on daily allowance to make it closer to average spend. It remains to be seen in future reports whether or not these recommendations have been adopted.

4.6.1 Staffing

As well as making financial savings on the cost of food, the NAO also reported in *Serving time* that the Prison Service was saving £1.7 million a year on catering staff (NAO, 2006a). These savings were attributed to the replacement of officers in the kitchen by civilians. The Prison Service in its 2000 PSO document 5010 *Prison Service Catering: Staffing of Prison Kitchens* set targets to increase the proportion of non-prison officer staff by 31 December 2002. These targets were:

High security establishment:	not less than 33%
Adult male category B:	not less than 50%
All other establishments:	100% (HMPS, 2000a)

By November 2004 the proportion of civilian staff had risen to 85%, from 55% in 2000. Governors – who are still ultimately responsible for the running of prison kitchens – can choose whether to employ civilians, prison officers or supervised prisoners as caterers. They can opt for a combination of all three, or contract out the catering entirely, if they believe it to be cost effective (NAO, 2006a). If contracted out, the service must still adhere to the same standards as in-house catering. Within the private prison estate, most prisons use in-house catering; however, some use outside contractors such as Aramark to provide meals (NAO, 2006b). Some prisons which had previously contracted out services later returned to in-house catering as contracted out services are generally more expensive and do not employ prisoners. Five prisons which until 1998 had used outsourced catering firms had, by 2006, reverted to in-house catering (NAO, 2006b).

The aim of replacing prison officer caterers with civilian caterers was to achieve a more cost-effective operation. In the past, prison officers could choose to specialise in catering and often ran kitchens and worked as chefs. Catering assistants were drawn from volunteer inmates (Crow, 1995). Civilian caterers are cheaper to employ than prisoner officers, although in some areas prisons are not considered attractive career options for civilians, which makes recruitment difficult (NAO, 2006a).

Employing prisoners in the kitchen is an effective way of keeping staffing costs down – wages couldn't come much lower at £7 to £34 a week depending on the level of responsibility and hours worked (NAO, 2006a). Although this is obviously much cheaper than employing civilians, additional costs are incurred through the necessity of providing a safe, secure environment in kitchens where hazards such as knives and boiling liquids are present.

Since November 2000, the assembly of breakfast packs and single portion beverages has been undertaken in prison workshops, replacing the previous system whereby packs were sourced through a central contract. One of the perceived benefits of this new system is 'maximising prisoner employment opportunities' (HMPS, 2000b). All handlers must receive training in basic food hygiene and operational requirements, and all workshop facilities, processes and practices must comply with the requirements of all relevant Health and Safety and Food Hygiene legislation.

4.6.2   Prisoners in the kitchen

The purpose of the training and treatment of convicted prisoners shall be to encourage and assist them to lead a good and useful life.   (HMPS, 2006)

Employing prisoners in the kitchen brings more than financial gain. Prisoners can study a wide range of subjects during their incarceration, leading to vocational qualifications relevant to future employment. Over 80 prison kitchens currently offer national vocational qualifications (NVQ) courses in catering, food hygiene and preparation, as part of a process of rehabilitation and preparation for employment. These courses are run by the Offenders' Learning and Skills Unit, established in 2001 as a partnership with the Department for Education and Skills and as part of the Government's plans to reduce re-offending. For some prisoners, an apprenticeship in the kitchen can provide an introduction to and an interest in a subject which previously may never have been considered a career option. Indeed, for some with chaotic backgrounds and a history of poor diet, food preparation and the pleasure that brings can be a whole new experience. So valuable is this experience believed to be that the House of Commons Committee of Public Accounts (2006) has criticised the Prison Service for the fact that not all prisons offer NVQs in catering. According to the catering manager of Highdown prison in Surrey, Alberto Crisci, who won the 2005 BBC Radio 4 Food and Farming Award, *'The prisoners who work in the kitchen take a real pride in what they produce and constantly strive to improve. It's great to watch them develop their skills and their esteem grow when they gain a qualification'* (HMPS, 2005).

4.6.3   Scotland and Northern Ireland

In Scotland most prisons offer Scottish Vocational Qualifications issued by the Scottish Qualifications Authority in catering and hospitality. Eleven of the sixteen prisons offer SVQs levels 1 and 2 in *food preparation and cooking*. Eight offer SVQ level 1 in *kitchen portering*. In Northern Ireland, prisoners are able to take courses leading to qualifications accredited by the Royal Institute for Public Health and Hygiene and the Chartered Institute of Environmental Health. They may also study for NVQ Levels 1, 2 and 3 in kitchen portering and food preparation and cooking, and catering. Prior to 1999 and the Good Friday Agreement, kitchens provided prisoners with no opportunity for training. Now, the NI catering department works with hospital trusts, a supermarket chain and several employers who take trained prisoners on release.

However, opportunities for training appear to be given to male prisoners only. All women prisoners in Northern Ireland have since June 2004 been held in Hydebank Wood, a medium-security male young offender's centre on the outskirts of Belfast. A study carried out in 2005–2006 into conditions for women prisoners in Northern Ireland found that catering training in the kitchens was confined to the young male prisoners only (Scraton & Moore, 2007).

4.7   Monitoring standards

Conditions within prisons, including the quality of food provided, are monitored on various levels, both externally and internally. Internally, the governor of each establishment has overall responsibility for catering standards. The Prison Service has its own Standards Audit Unit and there are external independent monitoring bodies including Her Majesty's Inspectorate of Prisons.

4.7.1   Internal monitoring

It is the responsibility of each establishment's catering manager to implement standards and oversee the training of staff and prisoners. The Head of Prison Service Catering Services advises headquarters and establishments on all Prison Service catering matters. See Box 4.2 for assignment of duties in accordance with the Prison Service Catering Manual.

In 1999 the Prison Service introduced the Prison Service Standards Manual (PSO 0200) as part of the established framework in place for self-audit. This manual covers all aspects of prison life, and section 4 – *Catering and Food Safety Standards* – states: *'Establishments provide a varied and healthy menu which takes account of prisoners' preferences whilst maintaining compliance with all relevant food safety legislation'* (HMPS, 2002a). There are 21 'key audit baselines', most of which relate to food hygiene matters. Those which are concerned with food quality and serving issues state:

- *The time lapse between the completion of the cooking process and commencement of service does not exceed 45 minutes.*

Box 4.2   Internal monitoring responsibilities.

Governor
On a daily basis, the prison governor or one of his or her assistants inspects the kitchen and tastes the food at the time and point of prisoner feeding. Checks are recorded in the kitchen journal. Inspection criteria include: quantity, appearance, value (regarding cost), colour, temperature, texture, preparation, production, presentation and service crockery.

Head of Prison Catering Services
Advises headquarters and establishments on all Prison Service catering matters.

Area Catering Manager
Monitors HM Prison Service food chain facilities and standards. Inspects contracted food supplies facilities.

Line Manager
Assists with implementation of standards and monitor budgetary responsibility

Catering Manager
Responsible for the implementation of standards, monitoring assessments of local risks and arrangements; training of staff and prisoners; budgetary responsibility; inspection of local suppliers.

Adapted from *HMPS Prison Service Catering Manual* (HMPS, 1999).

- *There is a minimum of 4½ hours between the beginning of one meal and the next and meals are served within the following times:*

Breakfast	07.30 to 09.00
Midday	12.00 to 14.00
Evening	17.00 to 19.00

- *Where prisoners are locked up in the evening, and the time between the evening meal and the next meal exceeds 14 hours, establishments specify and provide an additional snack and hot drink for consumption later than the evening meal.*
- *In establishments holding young people under 18 years and/or serving a Detention and Training Order there is a minimum of 4.5 and a maximum of 5.5 hours between breakfast and lunch and between lunch and tea.*
- *Recorded surveys of prisoners' views concerning food preferences are carried out regularly and the results published at least every six months.*
- *A member of senior management at the time of service makes a daily-recorded survey of food quality.*
- *A member of senior management makes a recorded inspection of the food areas at least once a week.*
- *The menu choices and meal provision reflect the religious and cultural needs of the establishment.*
- *Prisoners are offered opportunities to engage in hotel and catering education and training programmes, or work-related activities leading to accredited qualifications* (HMPS, 2002a).

Table 4.9   Required outcomes for self audit.

1.	Food Facilities, Processes & Practices	All food facilities, processes and practise comply with relevant food safety legislation
2.	Hazard Analysis and Critical Control Points (HACCP)	A fully documented HACCP system showing daily monitoring of time and temperature control is in operation
3.	Management Systems	Catering management systems ensure a high standard of menu is delivered economically
4.	Decency – meal times	Meal times reflect those in the community
5.	Menu options	There is a multi-choice, pre-select menu, which includes healthy options and reflects prisoners' preferences.
6.	Monitoring	There are regular independent inspections of the food production and servery arrangements.
7.	Diversity	Specified religious and cultural dietary needs are met.
8.	Resettlement	NVQ qualifications in the hospitality and leisure industry are provided.

Source: Prison Service Standards Manual (HMPS, 2002a).

Eight 'required outcomes' are stipulated to ensure that these standards are met (Table 4.9). Each establishment has a structured system of self-audit headed by the audit manager. On completion of audits, findings are submitted to the governor who agrees dates for completing action to rectify any non-compliance with standards. If this is not achieved, the matter must be brought to the attention of the area manager.

4.7.2   Prison service monitoring

The catering service of each establishment is monitored by the Prison Service's Catering and Physical Education Service, and this monitoring is carried out by six area catering advisers who also provide technical advice to catering managers. The catering advisers carry out a minimum of four visits annually to each prison to check hygiene, catering standards and staffing. These advisers are credited with playing a key role in the improvement in standards (NAO, 2006a).

In addition, standards are also audited at each public prison by the Prison Service's Standards Audit Unit every two years. The Standards Audit Unit monitors a wide range of standards, not just those relating to catering, and reports directly to the relevant heads of Prison Service Directorates. The unit measures the performance of prisons by examining whether they are compliant with 29 key standards (Figure 4.1) and scores them on a scale from zero (non-compliant) to four (fully compliant).

4.7.3   External monitoring

There are two external bodies responsible for monitoring all aspects of prison life, including the provision of food. These are Her Majesty's Inspectorate of Prisons (HMIP) and the Independent Monitoring Board (IMB).

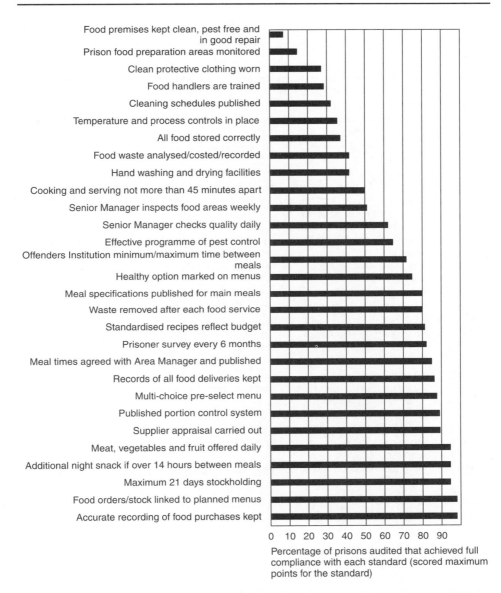

Figure 4.1 Although most prisons are fully compliant with catering standards, compliance with some standards in low. Prison Service Standards Unit 2004/05. (Reproduced from: NAO, 2006a. © The National Audit Office.)

HMIP is an independent inspectorate reporting directly to the home secretary on the treatment and conditions of prisoners, including those held in private prisons, young offender institutions and immigration removal centres. HM Chief Inspector of Prisons also inspects prisons in Northern Ireland, the Channel Islands, the Isle of Man and some Commonwealth territories. The Chief Inspectorate

Box 4.3   HMIP expectations for assessing catering standards.

1   All areas where food is stored, prepared or served conform to the relevant food safety and hygiene regulations.

2   Religious, cultural or other special dietary requirements relating to food procurement, storage, preparation, distribution and serving are fully observed and communicated to prisoners.

3   All areas where food is stored, prepared or served are properly equipped and well managed.

4   Prisoners and staff who work with food are health screened and trained, wear proper clothing and prisoners are able to gain relevant qualifications.

5   Prisoners' meals are healthy, varied and balanced and always include one substantial meal each day.

6   Prisoners have a choice of meals including an option for vegetarian, vegan, religious, cultural and medical diets. All menu choices are provided to the same standard.

7   Prisoners are consulted about the menu and can make comments about the food.

8   The breakfast meal is served on the morning it is eaten.

9   Lunch is served between noon and 1.30 p.m. and dinner between 5 p.m. and 6.30 p.m.

10   Prisoners have access to drinking water (including at night time), and the means of making a hot drink after evening lock-up.

11   Prisoners are able to dine in association (except in exceptional circumstances).

12   Staff supervise the serving of food in order to prevent tampering with food and other forms of bullying.

13   Where prisoners are required to eat their meals in their cells, they are able to sit at a table with the cell toilet fully screened off.

14   Pregnant prisoners and nursing mothers receive appropriate extra food supplies.

15   All prisoners in training prisons are given the opportunity to cater for themselves.

Source: HMIP (2008).

inspects private prisons in the same as public sector prisons. The HMIP produces a document entitled *Expectations*, which sets out detailed inspection criteria for assessing every area of prison life. *Expectations* lists 15 criteria relating to catering standards (Box 4.3).

Every establishment in England and Wales (including private prisons) is required, under the Prisons Act 1952 and the Immigration and Asylum Act 1999, to have its own Independent Monitoring Board (formerly the Board of Visitors) made up of watchdogs from the local community. Appointed by the home secretary to monitor the welfare of staff and prisoners, members of the Board are unpaid members of the public who have unrestricted access to their local prison or immigration removal centre at any time and can talk to any prisoner or detainee they wish, out of sight and hearing of a member of staff if necessary.

Each Board member is charged with monitoring the rights and wellbeing of all prisoners. This includes prisoner satisfaction with food provided. They are expected to be familiar with the standards which the establishment is obliged to meet and make frequent visits, often without notice. Members are required to attend monthly board meetings. Concerns are taken up first with the prison authorities, and if they are not resolved they are then taken up with a higher authority, possibly even the home secretary.

4.7.4 Scotland

4.7.4.1 *Internal monitoring*

As in England and Wales, the governor must taste the food prepared in the kitchen on a daily basis. According to SPS prison rules the governor shall ensure that:

(a) *he tastes some food and drink prepared for prisoners for the purpose of checking its quality and condition;*
(b) *he checks that the quantity of food and drink prepared for prisoners is adequate and*
(c) *the conditions under which such food and drink are prepared and served (or re-heated prior to serving) are inspected by an officer.*

4.7.4.2 *External monitoring*

Standards are monitored by HM Inspectorate of Prisons, headed by HM Chief Inspector of Prisons. The Chief Inspector is independent of both the Scottish Prison Service and of the Scottish Government and reports to the secretary of state. The main statutory responsibility of HMCIP is the regular inspection of individual establishments. Matters that are inspected and reported on include physical conditions, quality of prisoner regimes, morale of staff and prisoners, facilities and amenities, questions of safety and decency, and the establishment's contribution to preventing re-offending.

It is the aim of the Inspectorate to carry out a full inspection of each of these establishments once every 3 years. Each full inspection normally lasts between one and two weeks, depending on the size and complexity of the establishment. Following each inspection a report is prepared, which is submitted to Scottish ministers and published. In addition to the programme of full inspections, follow-up inspections – which normally last one or two days – are undertaken on each establishment not subject to a full inspection.

The Inspectorate determines its own programme for the year. During any inspection the inspectors have free access to any part of the establishment or to any individual therein. During all full inspections and on most follow-up inspections, arrangements are made to meet groups of prisoners and staff. Arrangements are also made on full inspections to give prisoners' visitors an opportunity to meet members of the inspection team. All reports are submitted to Scottish ministers and published in full. In addition to publishing a report of each inspection, there is a statutory requirement to publish an annual report.

HMCIP publishes the document *Standards used in the inspection of prisons in Scotland* (HMCIPS, 2006a). A total of nine outcomes are defined, including:

Prisoners are held in conditions that provide the basic necessities of life and health, including adequate air, light, water, exercise in the fresh air, food, bedding and clothing.

The standard set for the 'food' aspect of this outcome is *Food is adequate for health, varied and religiously and culturally appropriate.*

4.7.4.3   Prison Visiting Committee

The Scottish equivalent of the Independent Monitoring Board is known as the Prison Visiting Committee. Committee members visit the prison fortnightly to ensure that the prison is being properly run and that prisoners are treated well. Members hear complaints or requests from individual prisoners on matters relating to prison life.

4.7.5   Northern Ireland

Internally, it is the governor's responsibility (or that of a member of senior management) to ensure that the condition, quality and quantity of food and conditions under which it is prepared are inspected frequently (on a daily basis) and that appropriate action is taken as soon as possible where deemed necessary (NIPS, 1995). It is also the duty of the medical officer to ascertain that the nature, quality and quantity of food is appropriate to the prisoners' health. Prisoners are surveyed bi-annually for their views on catering standards and complaints considered by the governor.

Each prison has an Independent Monitoring Board (formally known as the Board of Visitors) drawn from the general public and appointed by the secretary of state. The board works in a similar way to the IMB in England and Wales and the Prison Visiting Committee in Scotland.

4.8   Nutritional adequacy and meeting standards

'*Generally, the sophistication of prisoners is not sufficient to ensure that the menus reflect healthy eating or the guidelines usually applied to good menu planning. Because of this there may well be conflict between consumer requirements and the balanced diet*'.   (HMPS, 1999)

Just how good (or bad) is the food served up in UK prisons? Food in schools and hospitals has only really become a focus of national interest in recent years, whereas prison fare has frequently been a subject of debate – usually because of concerns that it was too good for its undeserving recipients. Prison authorities have been, historically, at pains to ensure that provisions were neither too good nor too plentiful, for fear of incurring press and public wrath. Yet public perception has usually been at variance with the truth – history shows us that in reality prisoners were frequently left to starve on meagre, repugnant rations. Is prison diet today still frugal and unpalatable? The answer is most definitely no. Indeed, some prisoners eat better when incarcerated than when living in the community. Prison life offers a guarantee of three meals a day, at no cost to the prisoner, with a varied selection of menus for lunch and dinner. For people in prisons, most of whom come from marginalised sections of society and chaotic backgrounds, the enforced routine of daily life offers the opportunity to establish regular eating habits. It is clear, from recent studies, that prison food is better today than it has ever been. Many of the Woolf report recommendations (page 302) were indeed enacted and it is believed that the introduction of Prison Service standards contributed to the overall improvement in the quality of catering which has taken place since 1998 (NAO, 2006a). Prisoners' comments on food quality have, since then, also been generally favourable (NAO, 2006a). The question now is: with all the mandatory standards in place, and monitoring systems designed to enforce their compliance, does the food served up meet all standards in all establishments?

Probably more effort to analyse the quality of prison food in England and Wales has been made by the National Audit Office than any other organisation in recent years, perhaps because the NAO is charged with making sure that public money is well spent. The NAO audits the accounts of all central government departments and reports to Parliament on the efficiency and effectiveness with which public money is spent. In 1997, after the adoption of the pre-select system by around half of prisons but before the introduction of mandatory catering standards, the NAO examined prison catering in twelve prisons, focusing on:

- quality of catering
- specifications and procedures
- quality, diversity and timing of meals
- cost of catering (NAO, 1997)

The NAO reported that the Prison Service 'did well' in what it described as 'difficult conditions'. Although the quality of catering overall was described as acceptable, it was found to vary considerably from one establishment to another. The NAO identified a number of general problems, including:

- food was cooked too far in advance, and then left on heated trolleys for prolonged periods
- there were problems with delivery times, lack of wastage, monitoring and limited information on food quality
- no prison examined fully met the Prison Service's ruling on the timing of meals – for example, most prisoners received their last meal of the day at around 4.30 p.m. This meant that there was often a long interval – over 14 hours – between evening meal and breakfast.

The NAO recommended that the Prison Service:

- needed more specification and guidance for catering
- should improve monitoring of catering processes and quality of food served
- should review options for supplies (NAO, 1997).

In 1998 the Committee of Public Accounts made its own recommendations, based on these findings. The committee advised that the Prison Service improve the provision of food by developing standards and effective quality control arrangements. It also recommended that the Prison Service make greater use of the role of area catering advisers. In response, HM Prison Service gave a number of undertakings to the Committee of Public Accounts, including:

- To put in place catering standards by 31 July 1998. (Standards were put in place, but not until May 1999.) These standards set out legal and practical requirements designed to allow auditors to test compliance as part of their audit routine when visiting prisons.
- To make better use of area catering advisers by producing reports of their visits within 10 days of the visit and to review the role of these advisers. As a result, area catering advisers now provide technical advice to prison caterers and make up to four visits annually to each prison.
- To work with governors to achieve more reasonable intervals between meals (HMPS, 2004).

Nine years later the National Audit Office examined prison food again and findings were published in its report *Serving Time – Prisoner diet and exercise* in March 2006 (NAO, 2006a). The NAO considered whether prison diet and exercise regimes allowed prisoners to follow a healthy lifestyle. A total of 16 prisons were visited for the purposes of the report. The NAO investigated:

- whether the Prison Service was providing a cost-effective meal service
- whether the above Committee of Public Accounts recommendations had been adopted
- whether food provided met nutritional requirements. To determine this, the NAO commissioned primary research by Bournemouth University into the nutritional composition of a day's menu in eight prisons in England.

The NAO concluded that there had been significant improvements to the Prison Service's catering arrangements since its 1997 report, resulting in financial savings and improved quality of service (NAO, 2006a). On the whole, the NAO believed that the Prison Service now provided '*a well managed and professional catering service*'.

However, some previous concerns had not been addressed and some standards had still not been met. The main concerns now expressed by the NAO were:

- Meals were often still served at irregular times, such as lunch at 11.15 a.m and the evening meal at 4 p.m. at weekends. Serving of meals was timetabled around staff shifts and breaks, as well as prison education and work regimes. This could result in long periods – over 14 hours – between meals. In addition to causing discontent among prisoners, it was thought that this schedule might also result in behavioural problems as a consequence of low blood sugar levels (NAO, 2006a). The problem was compounded by the fact that in 60% of the prisons visited, a cooked or morning breakfast service had been replaced by breakfast packs which were given to the prisoners in the evening. Many prisoners consumed these in the evening and then had to wait until lunchtime the next day before eating again, although most do have a kettle for making hot drinks and can receive extra bread in the evening. These packs (see page 297), introduced to reduce staff duties, were found to be unpopular with prisoners because they were perceived to be frugal (NAO, 2006a).

- Although standards for religious and ethnic requirements were being met, the equipment for the production of halal food (such as knives, cutting boards, pots and pans) was not always separately labelled. There were suspicions among Muslim prisoners that food was not meeting standards for their requirements.
- Although area catering advisers provided advice on kitchen catering to the catering managers at prisons, one third of those managers claimed that the advice was not helpful.

The research carried out on behalf of the NAO by Bournemouth University into the nutritional adequacy of meals provided found that:

- On the whole, nutrient levels met Department of Health recommendations (DH, 1991). There were some exceptions: levels of selenium, iodine and vitamin D were found to be below recommended levels in all meals. Although vitamin D can be made by the body, it does so in the presence of sunlight. Therefore there is a strong possibility that most prisoners are at risk of vitamin D deficiency. Vitamin E was found to be low in some meals for male prisoners and all meals for female prisoners. Vitamin B12 was found to be low in vegan meals. Despite the apparently encouraging findings that most nutrient levels met DH recommendations, the researchers pointed out that actual vitamin consumption was likely to be lower than the results suggested, because their estimation of nutritional content was based on the assumption that standard cooking methods were used. It was also based on the assumption that food was consumed immediately after preparation, but in reality most food is kept warm on heated trolleys for up to 45 minutes, which would result in substantial reduction of some vitamin levels.
- Salt levels were found to be up to 93% higher than the government's recommended daily limit for adults (6 g). This was ascribed to the use of processed and ready-made meals and high consumption of bread.
- Dietary fibre was found to be low in all meals – between 29% and 68% below the recommended level of 18 g daily. This shortfall was attributed to lack of wholegrain bread and cereals.

- The total amount of fruit and vegetables on offer amounted to less than five portions a day; prisoners were found to eat around three portions daily. Fresh fruit was offered once a day, in all prisons, but always as an alternative to dessert. Although vegetables were offered daily they were often tinned or frozen. Salad as a main meal was offered, on average, three out of four days.
- Although fish was available most days there was found to be little in the way of oily fish – it usually came supplied as breaded, filleted fish, fish cakes and pies or poached fish.
- The calorific value of some meals exceeded recommendations (especially in women's prisons) with the exception of meals labelled as healthy and vegetarian at adult men's prisons (see Figure 4.2). It was found that meals offered to women provided similar energy levels to meals offered to male prisoners (other than meals labelled as healthy). This was attributed to the high availability of fried food, especially chips. On the whole, meals were in line with recommendations for proportions of macronutrients, measured as a percentage of dietary energy (carbohydrates at least 50%, fat less than 35% and protein making up the balance) (NAO, 2006a).

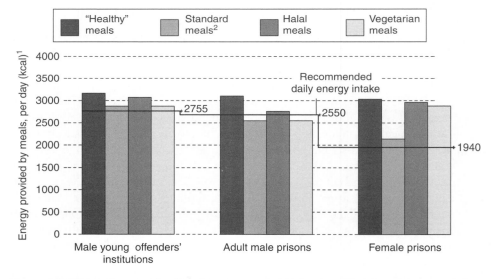

Figure 4.2 Most prison meals offered to prisoners are higher in energy than recommendations set by the government especially in women's prisons.

Notes:
1 Energy content is based on meals offered to prisoners. Any plate waste (food thrown away by prisoners) will reduce the energy content of the food consumed. Prisoners can also supplement their food with items that they purchase from prison shops which is likely to increase their energy intake.
2 Standard meals are the most frequently chosen meal options.

Source: Bournemouth University data in NAO, 2006a. © The National Audit Office.

- All kitchens visited provided a choice of at least four options at each meal time, including vegetarian, vegan and religious dietary options and at least one meal labelled as healthy. 'Normal' meals were the most popular. Although all sixteen prisons were found to offer at least one meal option labelled as healthy, meals high in salt, and salads high in fat were found to be incorrectly labelled as healthy, which would add to any existing confusion. This would suggest that caterers do not always understand what constitutes a healthy meal.
- There was found to be heavy reliance on processed, tinned and convenience foods, which was considered to be a concern. There was little use made of seasonal produce.
- In most cases prisoners did not actually know what constituted a healthy diet.

To address these concerns the NAO recommended:

- that governors should enforce compliance with standards
- that equipment should be labelled appropriately so that prisoners, especially minorities, have confidence that food is stored, prepared and served in the appropriate manner
- reducing the high-energy content of some meals to take into account the different requirements of prisoners (i.e. age and gender)
- providing specifications for suppliers for healthier products
- offering fried food less frequently
- offering more wholegrains, fruits and vegetables
- offering more fish, especially oily fish
- increasing dietary fibre
- that the Prison Service offer practical guidance and training to all prison caterers on healthy catering practices and nutrition
- that the Prison Service should raise awareness of healthy eating among the prison population, through, for example, the use of posters.

The results of the NAO study were similar to those found by the Prison Service Standards Audit Unit in its most recent audit. In 2004–2005 the Unit visited 65 prisons and found that, on the whole, standards were being met, but a large minority of prisons were still not meeting many standards (Figure 4.1). Overall they were fully compliant with 66% of standards, partially compliant with 32% of standards and non-compliant with 2% (NAO, 2006a). One of the most repeated failings however had only been addressed by half of the prisons: cooked food taking longer than 45 minutes to be delivered to prisoners.

Food that is served and food that is consumed are two separate issues so it makes more sense to analyse the food selected and eaten by prisoners rather than all the food available at the counter. An earlier effort to do this was carried out as part of a wider study into the effects of dietary supplements on the behaviour of offenders at Aylesbury Young Offenders' Institution (page 344) (Eves & Gesch, 2003). During 1996/1997, a total of 159 prisoners (96 in 1996 and 63 in 1997) took part in the study which assessed their diets over a one-week period. Table 4.10 shows

Table 4.10 A typical week's food provision within a young offenders institution.

Meal	Monday	Tuesday	Wednesday	Thursday	Friday	Saturday	Sunday
Breakfast	Porridge Sausage Beans on toast Bread Margarine	Cereal (choice) Milk Croissant Jam Margarine Toast	Porridge Boiled egg Toast Bread Margarine	Cereal (choice) Milk Jam Croissant Toast Margarine	Porridge Sausage Toast Margarine	Alpen Milk Jam Toast Croissant Margarine	Cereal Boiled egg Toast Bread Margarine Milk
Lunch	Chicken fingers Veg sausage roll Boiled potato Spaghetti Melon	Sausage roll Chicken sandwich Cheese & onion pie Chips Beans Apple Orange	Egg & bacon flan Vegeburger Boiled potatoes Mixed veg Jelly	Fish fingers Chicken sandwich Fried egg Chips Apple Orange Spaghetti rings	Chicken & mushroom slice Pasta/sweetcorn Peas Doughnut	Ham pizza Cheese pizza Chips Spaghetti Lemon torte	Jerk chicken Roast pork & gravy Pancake roll & rice Sauté potatoes Cauliflower cheese Carrots & peas Yogurt
Tea	Sausage roll Beef lasagne Veg hot pot Mash potatoes Cabbage Carrots Gravy Rice pudding Bread Margarine	Turkey escalopes Steak & kidney pie Pommes au gratin Mash potatoes Green beans Carrots Yogurt Bread Margarine	Chicken pie Fisherman's pie Noodle patti Mash potatoes Cabbage Sponge Custard Bread Margarine	Meat & potato pie Lamb hot pot Veg pasty Green beans Mash potatoes Yogurt Bread Margarine	Pork chop Shepherds pie Veg curry & rice Boiled potatoes Cabbage Gravy Rice pudding Bread Margarine	Beef & onion pie Vegetable pie Mash potatoes Mixed veg Gravy Yogurt Bread Margarine	Beef pie Vegeburger Salad Coleslaw Ice cream Bread Margarine
Supper	Biscuits	Biscuits	Biscuits	Biscuits	Biscuits	Biscuits	Apple/orange

a typical week's food provision. Dietary assessment also included snacks bought from the prison shop. Analysis was crude rather than specific, as it was based on the food diaries provided by the participants.

Like the NAO a decade later, the Aylesbury researchers found that the food provided was broadly in line with government dietary recommendations, with most vitamin values actually exceeding recommendations. However:

- a number of minerals fell below recommended levels, most notably selenium which was low in all meals, especially the vegetarian option in 1997
- fat intake exceed the recommended 35% (as a proportion of energy) in 82% of diets in 1996 and 64% of diets in 1997. This was largely due to items consumed from the prison shop
- vitamin D intake was low in both years. This is of particular concern because most prisoners have very limited exposure to sunlight
- zinc levels were below the RNI in menus prepared for Muslims and vegetarians
- sodium levels were well in excess of recommended levels, and this finding did not take into consideration salt added at the table

Vitamin values may have been over estimated because the findings did not take into account the effects of delays between cooking and delivery. Nor did they take into consideration losses which may have been incurred during pre-cook storage.

The food items which contributed most to the fat component of the diet were chips, meat products (especially sausage rolls and lamb curry), milk and margarine. Other significant contributors included ice cream, pizza, coleslaw and sponge pudding. However, it was found that most of the dietary fat consumed came not from meals provided but from snacks bought in the prison shop, most notably biscuits, cakes and savoury snacks. Carbohydrate levels were close to recommended levels, but protein content was, in both years, in excess of recommendations. On average, fibre intake compared well with the recommendation of 18 g of non-starch polysaccharides per day.

The transition from ration scale to a multi-choice, pre-select system has been shown, in one study on eight prisons published in 2001, to have had no detrimental effect on prisoner diet. This study, a visual estimate, produced similar results to others: mean nutrient intake from food provided by HM Prisons fell within current recommendations, but half of those prisons were found to provide a number of micronutrients (vitamins A, B2, C, D and calcium), as well as energy, at levels below recommendations. Most notably, vitamin D was found to be below recommendations in all prisons (Edwards et al., 2001).

Whatever the nutritional adequacy of meals provided, there is no doubt that, in terms of quantity, taste and popularity, standards continue to be raised. The Independent Monitoring Board produced annual reports on 21 prisons in 2007. Of these, 17 made specific reference to the quality of food produced. Comments made by the respective board members are outlined in Table 4.11. Only four prisons (Ford, Littlehey, Pentonville, Rye Hill) received overall negative feedback and several received rather glowing reports.

Table 4.11 Observations on food made by the IMB in 17 annual reports published in 2007.

Prison/type	Comments
Ford Cat D Open	'Poor … . One of our members declined to sample the meal due to the general hygiene on that occasion'
Leicester Local; adult male	'The organisation, standards of food, and hygiene have been consistently high throughout the year. The results of the internal survey carried out in November were very positive, and there have been few relevant complaints from prisoners via the comments book'.
Lincoln Local; adult male	'The catering team conducted a prisoner food survey. The results show more than satisfactory comments for most of the items surveyed'.
Lindholme Cat C & Immigration Removal Centre	'The Board feels that generally there is a reasonable choice of menu and the dishes are appetising'
Littlehey Cat C adult male	'Throughout the year, the facility for prisoners to give written feedback and comment (on) both positive and negative issues relating to their food through comment books at the wing food serveries throughout the year has frequently not been readily available and this should be addressed'.
Morton Hall Semi Open; women	'The Board is pleased to comment that the food provided ensures all prisoners get a balanced and nutritional diet; in fact it is interesting to note that we get few complaints about the quality of food provided, receiving more about the quantity and size of portions – which is monitored and felt to be more than sufficient'.
New Hall Female; young offenders & juveniles	'The kitchens continue to supply a wide and nutritious variety of food which takes into account the ethnic mix of the prison population. The quality is of a high standard demonstrated by the very few complaints received by the Board'.
North Sea Camp Cat D open male	'With regard to the food supplied to the prisoners, this continues to be one of the best in the Prison Service and is a credit to the kitchen staff'.
Onley Cat C adult/YOI	'The kitchen faced significant staff shortages during the year … . There has been concern throughout the year about the general state of repair … Despite all the difficulties, the general quality and variety of meals was commendably high and sometimes showed great imagination'.

Parc
Adult; YOI

'The kitchen, equipped to provide meals for an average population of 820 prisoners, is stretched to the limit to cope with the current size of the population ... Despite the fact that the kitchens produced over 1.1 million meals during the year, only eight applications concerning food were received by the Board during the current reporting period'.

Pentonville
Adult male

'Local sourcing has been stopped resulting, we are advised, in a rise in costs for providing fresh fruit and vegetables. This means there is an overall lack of vegetables in the prison diet ... The kitchen struggles to meet dietary requirements ...'

Reading
Remand & YOI

'Catering is very good ... The lunch menu is more basic and some processed food is used, whilst the evening meal is freshly made using raw ingredients. Fresh fruit and vegetables are always on offer. ... Menus reflect all dietary needs ... The Board rarely receive complaints from prisoners regarding cooked food'.

Risley
Adult male

'The quality of food prepared by the kitchens is of a consistently high standard. Very few complaints are made to the Board so it has become practice to ask prisoners their views about food. The general view is that it is better than other establishments'.

Rye Hill
Adult male

The quality of meals is variable and not always acceptable. Some substantiated complaints concern mistakes that should not have happened'.

Send
Cat C adult male

'The catering manager and his staff, including at any one time 20 prisoners, have once again maintained high food preparation and service standards this year ... Whist it is pleasing to note that this level of service has been officially recognised by a number of official audits .... the Board take specific notice of the prisoners comments book; the majority of comments are appreciative of the food'.

Shepton Mallet
Cat C adult male

The food provided remains at a very good quality with few complaints. Indeed, many prisoners make regular comments that they have not tasted any better food during their time in prison! The catering staff endeavour to cater for all national occasions, within their budgetary constraints, by producing a menu suitable for the day; something which the prisoners appreciate'.

Thorn Cross
Open YOI

'Food is generally good .... Food is transported from the main kitchen in heated trolleys but sometimes food cannot be kept hot enough using the old, ineffective serveries ... Chips are excellent when they leave the kitchen but a bit soggy on arrival at the units'.

4.8.1 Scotland

Scotland does not fare so well in inspection reports. Its inadequacies appear to have more to do with lack of quantity than quality, resulting from low funding. The Chief Inspector of Prisons for Scotland has stated that prison food is insufficient for young men. For the year 2004–2005, the Chief Inspector reported that:

- there was not enough food provided for young men
- expenditure on food had not risen since 1996
- most prisoners do not receive as much as half of the Scottish Executive minimum recommendations (five portions) for fruit and vegetables.
- there was not a prison in Scotland where a prisoner could possibly eat five portions of fruit and vegetables every day, and the average across all establishments was found to be less than three portions per day (HMCIP, 2005).

The following year there was little improvement. Much of the problem remains with the budget which in 2006 had still not been increased. As the Chief Inspector stated in his 2005–2006 annual report, '*It is difficult to see how the budget can continue to be met without reducing quantity and/or quality*' (HMCIP, 2006b).

4.8.2 Northern Ireland

The three prisons in Northern Ireland are subject to separate annual reports from the Independent Monitoring Board. In its 2005–2006 annual report for Hydebank prison, the IMB highlights the fact that the food budget had not increased in over six years, despite inflation, and recommended a review with a view to increasing expenditure. The IMB did, however, observe that the kitchen staff provided a varied and balanced meal for inmates (IMBNI, 2006a).

Women prisoners (who have been held at Hydebank male young offenders unit since 2004) appear to be worse off than their male counterparts. A study into the prison conditions of women prisoners in Northern Ireland reported that because food was prepared in the main young offenders' centre kitchen and then brought to the women's unit, it was sometimes not sufficiently hot on arrival and meals were sometimes missing (Scraton & Moore, 2007). Contrary to the IMB annual report for Hydebank, the researchers of this study claimed it was difficult for the kitchen manager to provide nutritious food for prisoners on a 'normal' diet; the budget created even greater challenges for those on special diets such as diabetics or vegetarians. Little fruit was provided: unless it was ordered as a dessert it had to be bought from the tuck shop and for many women this was not a priority compared to spending money on telephone calls or cigarettes.

The IMB is considerably more critical of the catering facilities at Maghaberry. It noted that the catering unit was purchasing more 'high-risk' ready-to-eat foods. It highlighted under-capacity as a concern: the kitchen, which was built for 400 prisoners had to serve over 700 daily, and the structure of the kitchen itself *'continues to deteriorate'* (IMBNI, 2006b). The Board recommended – for the fourth year running, as it pointed out – that the timing of meals be reasonably spaced and that *'service times should reflect a normal day'*.

Magilligan Prison fares better. The IMB reported that kitchen equipment was constantly updated, the quality of food was good and spot checks with inmates revealed no complaints. In the tuckshop, tinned tuna was a best seller and demand for cranberry juice increasing (IMBNI, 2006c).

4.8.3 Prisoners' views on food in prisons

Complaining about food in prisons is as traditional as complaining about food in schools. In prison, a place where people in the main do not want to be, grumbling about meals can be a means of letting off steam about the system in general. Even as recently as the early 1990s, the level of complaints about prison food was high (NAO, 1997). But changes in the provision of food, and the introduction of standards, have undoubtedly brought about considerable improvements and this has now been reflected in feedback from the consumers themselves. The 2006 NAO study *Serving time* observed that it was a widespread view among governors that complaints about the quality of prison food had diminished in recent years. As well as researching the quality and value of the food served, the NAO also sought the view of prisoners which were, overall, favourable – see Box 4.4.

Studies based on qualitative research can vary widely in their findings and it may be inappropriate to draw overall conclusions. An earlier report published in 2004 by HM Inspectorate of Prisons described opinions which differed somewhat to those reported by the NAO. When the views of over 1200 young offenders held in 30 establishments were sought, it was found that food provided came in for criticism in most establishments, with only 15% of respondents reporting that it was 'good'. Those who did think it good were most likely to cite the choice of menu as the main reason for their response, and those who thought the food 'bad' were most likely to cite the quality of food as their main reason (Challen & Walton, 2004).

4.8.3.1 *Scotland*

In 1990, the SPS introduced The Prison Survey (now the Prisoner Survey), a yearly census created in order to inform and support the SPS's business planning process. This annual survey is undertaken in each prison in Scotland and solicits the views of all prisoners on the basic elements of prison life, such as living conditions and food and issues such as health, drug use and bullying. The objectives of the survey include allowing the SPS to track progress, providing prisoners

---

Box 4.4   Prisoners talk about food.

'The food has got better. Considering how it used to be, it's improved hell of a lot.'

'We used to only have two menus a week. Right, one week something and then the next week something different and then you go back to the same and it was the same for two or three years.'

'Personally, we don't have any problem whatsoever with eating healthily and getting as much, if not more than we need really but that's just my perspective'.

'The food here has changed. It has dramatically changed. It's not bad, it's not bad, I'm in prison, I'm not going to moan because at the end of the day I'm in prison – what do I want? Yeah, sometimes you get something and you say yeah that was nice, I want some more but then the next day it might not be so good and that's how it is'.

'You get salad and fruit – not lots but certainly a couple of times a week and there's always a vegetable... that's the one thing we look forward to in prison and if we didn't get that we'd be on the roof!'

Source: National Audit Office, 2006a. © National Audit Office.

Table 4.12   Percentage of prisoners who gave a positive response to questions about food in Scottish prisons.

	2003	2004	2005	2006
How would you describe the following in THIS prison?				
The choice of menu	53	54	53	55
The size of portions	49	50	51	54
The temperature of the food	n/a	56	58	60
The way in which food is served	58	62	66	69
The timing of meals	70	74	82	79

Source: SPS, 2006.

with an opportunity to air their views and shaping and informing best practice (SPS, 2006). Even in Scotland there has been a discernible reduction in criticism of prison food. Table 4.12 illustrates that in 2006, responses to five key questions showed that there had been a more or less year-on-year improvement since 2003 in prisoners' perception of food. However, despite these positive results, only 25% of prisoners reported that they were satisfied, that is, felt full, after a meal. When asked what they would like to see more of on the menu, prisoners showed a surprising inclination for healthier options, such as fruit (Table 4.13).

4.8.3.2   *Commonalities of studies*

The emerging picture of food in prisons today is one of steady improvement, albeit not in all areas. The introduction of mandatory standards has clearly played a

Table 4.13 What Scottish prisoners would like to see more of on the menu (%).

Fish	49
Fresh fruit	47
Chicken	45
Salad	42
Red meat	39
Healthy option	35
Pasta	34
Puddings	29
Tinned fruit	29
Vegetables	25
Chips	22
Baked potatoes	20
Burgers	19
Vegetarian option	8

Source: SPS, 2006.

major contributory role in enhancing quality, but even the Department of Health admits that due to 'juggling of priorities', the nutritional value of food served can vary in quality (DH, 2004). Of the 15 'expectations' for assessing catering standards, as laid down by HM Inspectorate of Prisons (Box 4.3), those numbered 8, 9, 11 and 13 are regularly not met across the prison estate. A number of general conclusions can be drawn from the commonalities of the few studies which have in recent years been carried out into the quality, quantity and nutritional adequacy of food provided in prisons. These are:

- there is still an unacceptable interval of over 14 hours between the evening meal and breakfast in many prisons
- food is still cooked too far in advance and left on heated trolleys for over 45 minutes in many prisons
- meals continue to contain low levels of certain micronutrients, especially selenium and vitamin D
- it is very difficult, if not impossible, to eat a minimum of five portions of fruit and vegetables every day
- meals contain too much salt and it is very difficult to avoid excessive consumption
- meals are often too calorific, mainly because of too many high fat options
- prisoners in Scotland do not receive enough food, probably due to an insufficient budget.

4.9 Good practice

Advancements in Prison Service catering are evidenced by awards made in recognition of the high standards now being attained. In 2005 the catering manager of Highdown, Alberto Crisci, won the annual BBC Radio 4 Food and Farming Award for meals served to inmates every day in that establishment. According to Crisci, using fresh, cheap ingredients to create meals from scratch may be time consuming but it allows him to work within tight budgets, especially as much of the fresh produce is home-grown or delivered from another prison (Standford Hill). It is not just the catering which makes High Down exemplary; there is a strong focus on training prisoners to achieve NVQs in food preparation, cooking and basic hygiene. As a result of this focus, prisoners are able to secure jobs in the catering industry on their release.

A year later, the Public Sector Caterer of the Year award went to Alan Tuckwood, the head of catering and physical education services for HM Prison Services. Tuckwood took over the catering position in 1997, a time of much upheaval in the catering department. He is credited with much of the vast improvement in the meals service since then and oversaw the switch to devolved budgets, the arrival of government auditing and the introduction of catering standards.

4.9.1   Northern Ireland

Much changed after the signing of the Good Friday Agreement in 1998. A catering manager (later to become the catering adviser) with responsibility for all three prisons was appointed, and catering requirements were provided by an in-house team of officers and civilians who provided meals for staff and prisoners in accordance with a Service Level Agreement which was achieved in 1999. Various training schemes leading to catering qualifications for prisoners were introduced. Northern Ireland prisons were the first in the British Isles to achieve the quality standards award ISO 9000:2000.[1] With a central 'driver' in place, the catering service enjoyed a period when rapidly improving catering standards were recognised by a series of awards. In 2006 the Northern Ireland Prison Service Catering Department was presented with The Butler Trust Group Award *'in recognition of the exceptional work undertaken to improve catering standards and training and employment opportunities for prisoners in Northern Ireland'* (NIPS, 2006b).

Having come so far, Northern Ireland Prison Service catering suffered a setback in 2005 when, in an effort to cut costs, the position of catering adviser was withdrawn, along with the Service Level Agreement. It remains to be seen what effect this will have on the quality of the catering service.

4.10   What prisoners choose to eat, and what they know about healthy eating

Do prisoners think constantly about food – like C-list celebs in make-believe jails apparently do? I imagine the young ones spend more time dreaming about sex, but food would run a decent second, I guess.   (Allison, 2004)

Dr Johnson once said that when two Englishmen meet the first thing they do is to talk about the weather; when two prisoners meet, the first thing they do is talk about the food.   (Probation officer, Bradley, 1979)

Having a choice of menus means, inevitably, the option to make unhealthy choices. It is not surprising, in view of the eating habits of people generally, including those in other institutions, that people in prisons do not on the whole tend to make healthy dietary choices. A number of studies have made this observation. They have also observed that on the whole prisoners (with the exception of female prisoners, as we shall see below) do not have a basic understanding of the meaning of healthy eating. When Gesch *et al.* (2002) examined the effect of nutrient supplementation on the antisocial behaviour of young adult prisoners, they found that, when questioned, some prisoners did not possess the most basic knowledge of a healthy diet, with some not having heard of vitamins.

The pre-select menu may offer nutritionally adequate meals, in terms of government nutrient recommendations, but prisoners have been found to select meals low in nutrients and with higher than recommended levels of fat. Favourites include chips, meat pies, sausage rolls and sponge pudding. This diet is then finished off with more high fat, high sugar foods such as biscuits, cakes and savoury snacks purchased from the prison shop (Eves & Gesch, 2003).

The National Audit Office 2006 report, *Serving time*, also noted that although prisoners did have access to a nutritionally balanced diet, because they were able to select meals from a multi-choice menu, they often made poor food choices. Nor did they, in most cases, have an understanding of what constitutes a healthy balanced diet. Chips were often chosen instead of vegetables, and wholemeal bread rejected for white. Younger prisoners were found to be more likely to request high fat dishes than older prisoners, who were more likely to request salad items and fruit. Research on the dietary habits of 133 inmates at HMP Cardiff found that although the menu provided allowed for at least five daily portions of fruits and vegetables, most respondents (83.6%) reported eating less than three (Lester *et al.*, 2003). Combined with the fact that, of these prisoners, 33% reported using illegal drugs in prison, 84% smoked and 68% never took vigorous exercise, it could be assumed that the prisoners were at considerable risk of health deterioration.

In Scotland, when questioned about their consumption of fruit and vegetables, half of the prisoners responding to the 2006 *Prisoner Survey* reported that they ate 1–2 portions of fruit and 1–2 portions of vegetables daily (SPS, 2006). This was roughly the same quantity they consumed when not in prison. However, a worrying 41% reported that they ate no fruit at all in prison, and 30% reported that they ate no vegetables. Yet only 1% reported that they did not like fruit, and 4% reported that they did not like vegetables.

It is clear that although poor food choices mean that prisoners are at risk of micronutrient deficiency, they are also at risk of consuming too many high-fat, high sugar and high-energy foods. Prisoners in the NAO study were found to receive very little education on the subject of healthy eating. Lack of nutrition education was not helped by unreliable and in many cases misleading labelling of dishes. The NAO researchers were critical of the poor guidance, verbal and visual, at the service counter to help prisoners select healthier meals. Lack of guidance suggests that healthy food is provided because it is a mandatory requirement, but that there is very little interest in promoting it, or motivation to do so. One of the NAO's recommendations in its report was that the Prison Service should raise the level of awareness of healthy eating among the prison population.

Despite what is known about prisoners' food choices, it would be naive to assume that if they were just educated on the value of a healthy diet, they would adjust their flawed dietary habits accordingly. If education were this effective the vast majority of people in the UK would be eating exemplary diets and nobody would be smoking. Food may be inordinately important to prisoners, but healthy food is not usually considered a priority. All the same, people still have a right to be educated on the subject, and have access to information which is in the public domain, before making their choices. A major obstacle to education is illiteracy. The NAO in its report makes recommendations that the Prison Service promote healthy eating by using posters and leaflets, and so on, but these would be of little consequence in view of the fact that half of all prisoners are at or below the level expected of an 11-year-old in reading (PRT, 2008).

Women are often regarded as the main or sole food providers for their families. Most female prisoners come from socially disadvantaged backgrounds and cannot afford a healthy diet on their incomes when not in prison. Therefore, educational programmes may actually make women feel guilty that they cannot meet what might be regarded as their health responsibilities (Smith, 2002). Although studies which have examined prisoners' knowledge of healthy eating have focussed on male prisons, one study carried out into the meaning of food to women prisoners found that they had an awareness of the link between diet and health, and described being healthy as having a good diet, with *'plenty of fresh food, especially fruit and vegetables'*. They were also aware of the risks associated with an unhealthy diet (Smith, 2002). They were highly critical not only of the quality of food produced but of standards of cooking and hygiene, although they did acknowledge that their attitude could be seen as an emotional response to imprisonment (Smith, 2002).

Food choices are attributable not so much to the effect of education as to the influence of deeply rooted psychological and social factors. Within prison, food can bring solace to what might otherwise be a pleasureless day. Meal times are awaited with anticipation, even if they often bring a sense of disappointment. As in the armed forces, food in prison can also lift morale. Prisoners often choose what is familiar and recognised – they tend to eat the same sort of foods as they would at home (NAO, 2006a). In that sense, food, whatever its nutritional value, can taste good and wholesome, if it serves as a reminder of life on the outside and familiar pleasures.

Food can also be powerfully symbolic of the prison experience, as revealed by the women prisoner study. When a total of 50 female prisoners were interviewed at depth over a period of two years about their feelings on the subject, it was observed that food was seen as part of the 'disciplinary machinery' and was a *'powerful source of pleasure, resistance and rebellion'* (Smith, 2002). Complaints about prison food are often really complaints about conditions in prison more generally. As one woman stated, *'But at the end of the day, steak or Spam, prison food is prison food. I think it's the fact that we're in here that makes it seem bad, it's having to be here, rather than the food itself'*. Paradoxically, women often chose 'bad' food to make themselves feel better, and maintain a sense of control. Women prisoners who were allowed to cook for themselves and have some choice over eating habits described the experience as an 'intense pleasure' (Smith, 2002).

Food therefore may be experienced as punitive. It also serves as a constant reminder of loss of freedom: prisoners will avoid television commercials that remind them of what is not available to them (Godderis, 2006a). It can also erode their sense of ethnic identity: although meals are provided to meet religious or moral requirements, such as halal and vegetarian, they are not culturally sensitive. (Godderis, 2006a). Personal identity is also diminished, as there is no possibility of making personal decisions about what, where and when to eat, or how the food should be prepared (Godderis, 2006b).

Power struggles occur repeatedly inside a prison (Godderis, 2006a), and food can be used to bully others or assert independence (NAO, 2006a). Constrained choices about what can be eaten and where is a constant reminder of lack of control and a reminder of the institution's power over the prison population (Godderis, 2006a). A study using semi-structured interviews with prisoners in the US revealed the use of food as a display of institutional power to be a real source of frustration to prisoners. They felt that certain actions which were ostensibly imposed as a measure to handle certain safety concerns were really a demonstration of institutional control. An example given was the prohibition of fruit purchases in case it was used to make alcohol (Godderis, 2006b).

4.11   The prison shop

Prisoners' choices are not entirely restricted to the pre-select menu: they are allowed access to the prison shop, also known as the canteen (tuck shop, in Northern Ireland) at least once a week. This provides an opportunity to supplement the diet with additional items. The shop is, these days, more of a 'virtual' entity; most prisons throughout the UK have moved towards an ordering system, also known as the 'bag and tag' system, whereby a prisoner places an order for goods which are later delivered to his cell in a clear, sealed plastic bag. The range of products available can vary considerably from one establishment to another, but generally, throughout the UK, the shop stocks confectionery, biscuits, groceries (including fresh fruit), batteries, stationery, tobacco, toiletries and 'hobby' items. Prisons are expected to regularly consult prisoners about their needs and the product range is expected to reflect this.

The shop service provides an approved range of products, at prices which are supposed to be in line with the Catering Price Index[2] or at a level no more than the recommended selling price, although inspections have shown that this is not always the case. In prisons run by the Prison Service and which still manage their shops in-house, it is the responsibility of the head of finance to ensure that prices are set at the manufacturer's recommended retail price and that goods on sale reflect the ethnic and diverse needs of the prison population (HMPS, 2003a). Only a minority of prisons still run their shops in-house, the majority have privatised the service. The contractor (most commonly the US company Aramark) has full responsibility for the administration of the service (HMPS, 2003a).

Prisoners pay for goods with their earnings – the average rate of pay for employed prisoners is £8 per week – plus an authorised amount of private cash. They are therefore limited in their choices, which, it may be argued, is not necessarily a bad thing. However, in many cases it is the healthy options which are most restricted. HM Inspectorate of Prisons (HMIP), which carries out inspections of prisons (including privately run establishments) at least once every five years, also inspects the shop, including the range of goods available, efficiency of service and prices. Lack of consistency between establishments is evident from the reports published by HMIP on individual prisons. Some shops are commended for their wide range of products, but the HMIP frequently highlights the limited choice of foods available, especially those of a more healthy nature, such as fresh fruit. Some shops have been found to provide fresh fruit but others none at all. Some prisons have been found to ban tinned foods for security reasons – which HMIP considers unnecessary because tinned foods can provide valuable nutrition. Another frequent complaint is lack of consultation with prisoners about their needs, despite the fact that prisons are supposed to regularly consult inmates on their needs and preferences. Black and ethnic minority groups have been frequently found to be disadvantaged because their particular needs are not met by the shop product range.

Despite Prison Service guidelines on the cost of items, high prices are a regular complaint from prisoners. HMIP frequently agrees that prices are too high and on occasion describes contractors as employing a pricing policy more akin to that of a corner shop than a supermarket. Prices are sometimes described as reasonable, but can vary considerably between establishments. Table 4.14 shows items typically available in Scottish prison shops, and their retail prices. Fresh foods such as fruit are ordered separately. A glance at the price list is sufficient to see that prices are, on the whole, considerably higher than supermarket prices (as of September 2007). There is little on the grocery list which might be considered healthy, with the exception of a few items such as some cereals and tinned fruit – also at comparatively high prices.

Like prison meals, the prison shop can be a source of comfort and shopping itself an activity which unites the prisoner with the outside world, serving as a reminder of life at liberty. It is a place where earnings can be spent on treats, even if that place is a major source of high-fat snacks (Eves & Gesch, 2003). Among women prisoners, the shop may be considered a source of comfort food which may be favoured over normal prison food (Smith, 2002). These snacks can also help bridge the long gap which is commonly experienced between the evening meal and breakfast.

4.12   The health of people in prison

'*Good health is central to successful rehabilitation and resettlement, and in turn requires an environment in each prison that is supportive of health*'.   (DH, 2002)

Table 4.14 Convicted prisoners canteen requisition (Scotland) (September 2007).

Item	Price	Item	Price
Groceries		**Cereals**	
All day breakfast	1.06	Alpen 350 g	1.36
Ambrosia rice pudding	0.71	Crunchy nut cornflakes 370 g	1.88
Cheesy pasta	0.90		
Chopped pork & ham	0.72	Scotts porridge oats 500g	1.04
Corned beef	0.91		
Cup-a soup chicken	1.18	Kellogs coco pops 375 g	1.95
Cup-a soup chicken noodle	1.00		
Cup-a-soup variety	1.29	**Confectionery**	
Custard	0.85	Bounty	0.31
Farmlea rice pudding	0.41	Campino strawb/cream	0.80
Heinz tomato sauce	1.28	Caramel wafer	0.15
Hot dogs	0.48	Chewits	0.21
HP brown sauce	1.38	Chomp	0.15
Macaroni cheese	1.07	Crisps	0.22
Mace beans	0.28	Crunchie	0.33
Mace beans/sausages	0.59	Dairy milk	0.32
Mace drink chocolate	0.91	Double decker	0.31
Mace honey	1.73	Drifter	0.31
Mace instant coffee	1.09	Extra strong mints	0.26
Mace peanut butter	0.81	Fizzy cola bottles	0.10
Mace spaghetti tomato	0.26	Fruit & nut	0.33
Mace sweetcorn	0.38	Kit kat (4 fingers)	0.29
Mackerel fillets	0.73	Kp nuts salted	0.32
Marvel milk powder	1.62	Maltesers	0.34
Nescafe	2.01	Mars bar	0.30
Noodles	0.17	Milky bar chunky	0.38
Nutri grain bar	0.29	Milky way	0.15
Pasta 'n' sauce	0.85	Nik naks	0.16
Pot noodles	0.76	Onion rings	0.10
Salad cream	1.52	Polo mints	0.23
Sardines in tomato sauce	0.48	Ripple	0.33
Savoury rice	0.52	Rolo	0.34
Smash original	0.50	Snickers	0.30
Spaghetti bolognaise	1.07	Space raiders	0.10
Sugar	0.73	Sweet packets	0.59
Sweetex	0.99	Topic	0.30
Tea bags best buy	0.52	Tunnocks logs	0.15
Tea bags tetley	0.87	Twix	0.28
Tinned fruit cocktail	0.51	Wine gums	0.26
Tinned milk (carnation)	0.66	Yorkie	0.48
Tinned peaches	0.88		
Tinned pears	0.64	**Boxed sweets**	
Tinned pineapple chunks	0.74	Milk tray 227 g	2.44
Tinned soup	0.73	Roses 275 g	2.22
Tuna	0.92		

(Continued)

Table 4.14   Continued

Item	Price	Item	Price
Biscuits		Barrs cans[a]	0.41
Blue Riband	0.69	Coca cola	1.37
Breakaway 6 pack	0.71	Just juice apple[a]	0.33
Cream crackers	0.57	Jucee	1.00
Fox's classic 6 pack	0.88	Mace 2 litre	0.50
Hobnobs	0.69	Mace pure orange	
Jaffa cake	0.91	juice[a]	0.22
McVities rich tea	0.71	Vimto can[a]	0.37
McVities digestives	0.60	Volvic touch of fruit	
		water peach 50 cl[a]	0.52
Drinks		Volvic touch of fruit	
Barrs 2 litre Tizer	1.25	water straw 50 cl[a]	0.52
Barrs 2 litre	1.38		

[a] A maximum of six large bottles of juice can be purchased.

On arrival at prison, healthcare needs of the individual are assessed on a triage system. First the prisoner is seen by a member of the healthcare team to identify significant or immediate healthcare needs. If the screening identifies an immediate need further assessment is carried out. A second general health assessment is carried out a week later (Hek *et al.*, 2005).

The need for nutritionally adequate prison food becomes all the more evident when viewed in the context of prisoner health. Most prisoners are in poor health. They tend to have poorer physical, mental and social health than the general population and have lifestyles more likely to put them at risk (DH, 2002; Smith, 2002). A high proportion come from socially excluded sections of the community and around 90% of those who enter prison have a mental health or substance misuse problem (DH, 2003). Seventy two per cent of male and 70% of female prisoners suffer from two or more mental health disorders (PRT, 2008). Of the 24% of prisoners who report that they have injected drugs, 20% are infected with hepatitis B and 30% with hepatitis C (DH, 2002). Over 80% of prisoners smoke (DH, 2002). Nearly two-thirds of male prisoners and two-fifths of female prisoners admit to hazardous alcohol drinking, and of these around half have a severe alcohol dependency (PRT, 2008). Prevalence of HIV infection in prisons is 15 times higher than in the community (PRT & National Aids Trust, 2005). In addition to communicable diseases, mental health disorders and addiction, the most prevalent health problems among prisoners include diabetes and asthma (Hek *et al.*, 2005).

The number of older people (aged 60 or over) in prison has risen by over 149% in the last ten years (to 2006) (PRT, 2008). The female prison population has nearly doubled. A review of the health needs of prisoners in England and

Wales found that there were high levels of drug misuse and alcohol consumption amongst women prisoners. Women were more like than their male counterparts to be heavy smokers and there was little evidence that women's health needs were being met (Harris *et al.*, 2006). Limited evidence suggests that female prisoners have more long-standing physical problems than male prisoners (Harris *et al.*, 2006).

The number of children in prison has nearly doubled over the last decade (PRT, 2008). Lifestyle behaviour and health abuse are considered a major concern for younger prisoners, with high levels of smoking, alcohol and drugs use (Harris *et al.*, 2006).

The first analysis of the health status of male prisoners in England and Wales was published by the Office of Population Censuses & Surveys in 1995 (Bridgwood & Malbon, 1995). The survey reported that 48% of prisoners had a long-standing illness or disability, compared to 29% of the general population. The most commonly reported health problems were musculoskeletal and respiratory conditions. Although a significant number of people who arrive in prison are already obese, few prisoners develop the condition during their stay in prison (Wheatley, 2006). Male prisoners have also been found to have lower blood pressure than men in general. However, because of significantly higher levels of smoking and an increasingly ageing prison population, the risk of cardiovascular disease is likely to be increased (Hek *et al.*, 2005). Poor dietary choices and lack of exercise (NAO, 2006a) exacerbate that risk. Imprisonment is known to worsen both mental and physical health; a number of studies have shown that prisoners perceive their health to worsen by imprisonment, with stress being a major concern (Hek *et al.*, 2005).

4.12.1 Exercise

According to the prison rules, adult prisoners should have the opportunity to exercise at least one hour a week, and young offenders at least two hours a week. Because prisoners are given time in the open air each day, they can use this time to exercise if they wish (NAO, 2006a). Prisons also offer physical education activities which prisoners can choose to attend. Around 43% of prisoners engage in organised physical education activities, but there is considerable variation among prisons in the range of activities available, as well as variations in facilities provided, emphasis given by individual prisons to some activities and limitations on staff availability (NAO, 2006a).

4.12.2 Diabetes

Type 2 diabetes is a major health concern in the UK. The number of people diagnosed with diabetes is expected to exceed 3 million by 2010 and around half of those will be from disadvantaged communities (Diabetes UK, 2006).

The most deprived people in the UK are 2.5 times more likely to have the disease. The prison population is largely drawn from lower socioeconomic groups, yet it has been found that prison officers may fail to understand the needs of diabetics and may confuse hypoglycaemia with 'acting up' (Diabetes UK, 2006). Diabetic prisoners have expressed concerns that their condition is not taken seriously and that meals do not correspond with insulin doses, in content or in timing, and that procedures for obtaining medication are laborious, conflict with medical confidentiality and are often unsuccessful. Despite the transfer of prison healthcare services to the NHS in 2000, and the issue of *The National Service Framework for Diabetes* (DH, 2001) to every prison in 2002, over half of primary care trusts have been found to have no strategies in place for treating diabetes in prisons (Diabetes UK, 2006).

4.12.3 Healthcare provision

Although 80% of prisoners are incarcerated for a period of six months or less, good healthcare during that time can make a significant contribution to the health of the individual. Because so many prisoners come from chaotic and socially excluded backgrounds, the prison in theory provides an excellent opportunity to meet the health needs of those who are otherwise hard to reach – half of those sentenced are not registered with a GP (PRT, 2008). When incarcerated, prisoners use the health services on offer more frequently than an equivalent general population. However there is only limited research as to whether a prisoner's health improves whilst in prison (Hek *et al.*, 2005). Addressing inmates' needs presents a formidable challenge: imprisonment can lead to boredom and damaged self-esteem (DH, 2002) and as a result, healthcare and a healthy diet may not be a priority for the individual who cannot see a bright future ahead.

Until very recently, most healthcare was delivered by the Prison Service rather than the NHS. This system came in for much criticism and it was generally recognised that prisoners did not receive healthcare standards equivalent to those provided by the NHS; the gulf between prison care and NHS standards was described, by the Department of Health, as 'very disturbing' (DH *et al.*, 2003). In 1996, the then Chief Inspector of Prisons, Sir David Ramsbotham, published *Patient or Prisoner? A New Strategy for Heath Care in Prisons* (HMCIP, 1996) – a highly critical review of the state of healthcare in prisons which described a health care service in crisis. Before health care was transferred to the NHS, the level of service varied across the prison estate, with staff often found to be inadequately qualified and/or trained, with low morale and poor communication among doctors and nurses. Nurses working in prison had few links with the NHS (Hek *et al.*, 2005). Healthcare providers had little incentive to provide quality care and doctors and nurses had to seek approval to request tests and surgical procedures, which was sometimes very slow to arrive (Awofeso, 2005).

In order to tackle such health inequalities, the Department of Health, the National Assembly for Wales and the Home Office agreed to establish a formal partnership between the Prison Service and the NHS. This officially began on 1 April 2000 and was led by two organisations: the Prison Health Policy Unit (PHPU) whose task was to review and develop policies for prison health services and the Prison Health Task Force (PHTF) whose task was to provide prisons and their NHS partners with operational support and guidance. These two organisations later merged into one single unit, now known as Prison Health. Prison Health is responsible directly to the Prison Service and the Department of Health. The aim of Prison Health is to provide prisoners with access to the same standards and range of health care services as those provided to the general public by the NHS. By April 2006, full budgetary and healthcare administration had been transferred from HM Prison Service to the Department of Health.

Also in 2002, and as part of an agenda to tackle health inequalities, the government launched a new health promotion strategy called *Health promoting prisons – a shared approach* (DH, 2002). The three dominant issues were mental health, drug dependency and communicable diseases such as hepatitis B and C and sexually transmitted infections. With this publication, health promotion was placed on the prison agenda. The issue of *Prison Service Order 3200 – health promotion* (HMPS, 2003b) meant that each prison now has to demonstrate that health promotion is integral to its management. PSO 3200 states that:

'*The Prison Service in partnership with the NHS has a responsibility to ensure that prisoners have access to health services that are broadly equivalent to those the general public receives from the NHS*'.

Both governors of the Prison Service and directors of contracted-out prisons are required to ensure that efforts are made to:
- *Build the physical, mental and social health of prisoners (and where appropriate staff) as part of a whole prison approach.*
- *Help prevent the deterioration of prisoners' health during or because of custody, especially by building on the concept of decency in our prisons.*
- *Help prisoners adopt healthy behaviours that can be taken back into the community upon release.*

Health promotion is to specifically address five major areas:

- Mental health promotion and well-being
- Smoking
- Healthy eating and nutrition
- Healthy lifestyles
- Drug and other substance misuse

Efforts to improve health care provision are hindered by the difficulty of recruiting staff to work in prisons (HMCIPS, 2007). In 2004 the *British Medical Association* warned of a crisis in general practitioner recruitment and retention in the Prison Service, a service '*consistently starved of adequate funding to meet this clinical and social care agenda*' (Keavney, 2004). The BMA also blamed the Prison Service itself and the agenda set for governors who, the BMA claimed, have a lack of understanding of clinical governance.

Despite these difficulties, there does appear to be early, limited evidence that since reform was introduced, standards of care and patient outcomes have improved (Hayton & Boyington, 2006). Extra funding from the Department of Health has led to around 300 NHS mental health nurses being recruited to provide primary mental health services to prisoners (Hayton & Boyington, 2006). The main improvements in health care services have been enhanced GP availability and out-of-hours cover and better staffing, particularly nursing (McLeod, 2006).

Although these initial, positive observations were confirmed by the Chief Inspector for Prisons in her 2005/2006 annual report, she also warned that '*There are considerable pressures on primary care trusts, and it will be important to ensure that prison healthcare does not once again slip out of sight and down the list of priorities*' (HMCIP, 2007).

Improvements may have been made but that does not necessarily mean the system is adequate. Prisons are notoriously overcrowded, and overcrowding makes good health care provision all the harder to deliver. In July 2006 the Ministry of Justice introduced emergency measures designed to alleviate the overcrowding crisis in England and Wales. It was believed that these measures – mainly the early release of more than a thousand low category prisoners – would lead to better conditions across the service. According to the British Medical Association, however, these measures had '*failed to solve the crisis that is undermining prison healthcare and prison rehabilitation programmes*' (BMA, 2007).

4.12.4 Health in private prisons

The 11 privately run prisons in England and Wales are excluded from NHS regulations and health care is provided by a company called Primecare Forensic Medical. Primecare supplies doctors, nurses and other support staff. However, the Government has decided that after 2005 any new contractually-managed prison will have NHS commissioned care from the outset. At the time of writing (July 2007) the Government was said to be looking at the role of the Healthcare Commission in privately managed prisons, with a view to ensuring that their health services are subject to the same scrutiny as public sector prisons (private email correspondence, 13/07/07). At the moment they are not. Although both public sector and privately run prisons are inspected by HM Chief Inspector of Prisons, health care does not fall under the remit of the Inspectorate. In its 2005–2006 annual report HMCIP (2007) expresses concerns about private sector provision, in both prisons and immigration removal centres: *'Health services there are separately commissioned, without the supporting framework of accountability in the public sector, and there is a danger of inconsistency, less supervision and procedures that drift away from best practice'.*

4.12.5 Scotland

What makes the task (of reporting on health care provision in prisons) peculiarly difficult is the great difference – far bigger than in any other aspect of prison life – between the service which professionals say prisoners are getting and the service which prisoners feel they are getting. (HMCIPS 2006b)

In Scotland

- over 80% of prisoners smoke
- over 80% of prisoners have mental health problems, and as many as 7% have psychotic illness
- over 80% have drug-related problems (HMCIPS, 2006b)

In 1998 the Scottish Prison Service published *Standards for the health care of prisoners* which set out the need for the SPS to provide services to prisoners which prevent illness, promote health and enable prisoners to make healthier lifestyle choices (SPS, 2002). The SPS then went on to develop a formal 'Framework for Promoting Health' in order to achieve these aims, which concentrated on four main topic areas:

- healthy eating
- active living
- tobacco use
- promotion of mental well-being (SPS, 2002)

Health care in Scottish prisons is overseen by the Health and Care Directorate. According to the Chief Inspector of Prisons in Scotland, those working in health care in Scottish prisons do not have *'anything like'* the resources of the NHS at their disposal (HMCIPS, 2006b). According to the CIPS, there are three main obstacles to providing an efficient health care service in Scotland:

- the difficulty in recruiting staff to work in prisons
- the fragmentation of provision: GP services are provided by a private company, nursing services are provided by the Scottish Prison Service and other services (e.g. hospital care) are provided by the National Health Service.
- the extant poor physical, mental and dental health of those who enter prison.

According to the Chief Inspectorate, the time has come to examine the possibility of the provision of healthcare in prisons by the National Health Service (AR, 2005–2006).

4.12.6 Northern Ireland

Since the Good Friday Agreement of 1998, when large numbers of prisoners were released, the character of the Northern Ireland prison population has undergone significant changes and now more closely resembles that of the rest of the United Kingdom. Chronic disease, mental illness (as many as 90% of prisoners have a mental health or personality disorder problem) and drug addiction are serious concerns. High levels of chronic disease are said to be an 'issue' (NIPS & HPA, 2006). In 2005 the Director-General of the NI Prison Service announced that lead responsibility for health care in prisons would be transferred, in April 2007, to the Department of Health, Social Services and Public Safety.

4.13 Diet, nutrition and criminal behaviour

It is well established and accepted that physical health and wellbeing are largely dependent upon diet. The World Health Organization has stated that '*Nutrition is coming to the fore as a major modifiable determinant of chronic disease, with scientific evidence increasingly supporting the view that alterations in diet have strong effects, both positive and negative, on health throughout life*' (WHO, 2003).

Twenty or thirty years ago the suggestion that diet could influence mental health and behaviour, to the extent that it could even engender criminal behaviour, would have been dismissed outright by the wider scientific community. Now, many accept that there is a potential link, and that that link is indeed worth investigating. In January 2006, the Mental Health Foundation published findings of a review of literature relating to nutrition and mental health. One of the Foundation's conclusions was that '*There is a plethora of anecdotal, clinical and controlled studies that point to the importance of diet as one part of the jigsaw in the prevention of poor mental health and the promotion of good mental health*' (MHF, 2006). In Autumn 2007 the Food Standards Agency announced the results of commissioned research which confirmed that artificial additives in food could trigger hyperactive behaviour in some children (McCann, 2007). The hypothesis that some adults might behave aggressively or violently because of what they've eaten had already moved out of the realm of the absurd, thanks largely to a major study reported in the *British Journal of Psychiatry* in 2002 (Gesch *et al.*, 2002).

In order to examine possible links between nutrition and behaviour, research was carried out on 231 young adult prisoners (between the ages of 18 and 21) at Aylesbury Young Offenders' Institution. The lead researcher was Bernard Gesch, director of the research charity Natural Justice and senior research scientist at the University Laboratory of Physiology, University of Oxford. The aim of the Aylesbury study was to observe changes in behaviour when prisoners' intake of vitamins, minerals and essential fatty acids was brought up to government dietary reference values (DH, 1991). Dietary analysis of the food available for selection, carried out prior to the trial, had shown that it provided close to the current UK dietary recommendations. However, because prisoners often made poor food choices, this meant that in reality their diets were low in many minerals, including selenium, magnesium, potassium and zinc (Eves & Gesch, 2003).

Half the subjects were given nutritional supplements containing 28 vitamins, minerals and fatty acids (both omega-6 and omega-3), in a double-blind, placebo-controlled, randomised trial. The other half were given placebos. The researchers found that, compared with the placebo-controlled group, prisoners whose diets were supplemented for four consecutive months committed an average of 26.3% fewer offences. Of particular note was the finding that, for serious breaches of conduct such as the use of violence, the number of violations decreased by 37%. These results were remarkable, and all the more so because those on placebos showed no notable change in behaviour. Furthermore, when the trial ended, levels of violence returned to pre-trial status. The researchers concluded that anti-social behaviour in prison, including violence, was significantly reduced by supplementation with vitamins, minerals and fatty acids.

The results of the trial were well received by the scientific community and widely publicised in the media. Despite this, government response was slow and the Home Office was rebuked for not acting on the results and accused by the former chief inspector of prisons Lord Ramsbotham of delaying further research. The government originally ruled out establishing a nutritional regime for prisoners until the results were known of a pilot scheme in Dutch jails. The Netherlands was the first country to act on the results of the Aylesbury study, and the pilot, involving nutritional supplements in 11 institutions was underway at the time of writing (autumn 2007).

Following pressure from various quarters, in January 2006 the Home Office asked Natural Justice to carry out further, more detailed research into the relationship between diet and prisoners' behaviour. Scientists from Oxford University, the Medical Research Council, the Institute of Psychiatry and Imperial College are aiming to replicate the Aylesbury findings at three establishments: Warren Hill, Stoke Heath Young Offenders' Institution and Polmont Young Offenders' Institution in Scotland. This project, which began in 2008, will go further than the original in that it will aim to examine the exact relationship between different levels of nutrients and a range of specific behaviours. These include violence, self-harm, impulse control, drug offences and how individual prisoners relate to others.

According to the former chief inspector of prisons, Lord Ramsbotham, better nutrition would have a 'huge impact' on prison life, dramatically reducing offending behaviour in jails (Lawrence, 2006a). The Aylesbury trial was built largely on the work of Dr Stephen Schoenthaler, a criminologist at California State University in Long Beach who has studied the effect of nutrition on behaviour in numerous juvenile and adult penal institutions for over twenty years, completing three trials. In 1997 Schoenthaler published results of a randomised, double-blind placebo-controlled trial on delinquent offenders in a correctional facility. Subjects who were given vitamin and mineral supplementation were found to commit significantly fewer violent and non-violent antisocial behaviour offences (Schoenthaler *et al.*, 1997). In 2000, Schoenthaler published another study which set out to determine whether schoolchildren aged 6–12 who were given low dose vitamin–mineral supplements demonstrated significantly less violent and antisocial behaviour in school than fellow students given placebos. This randomised, double-blind, placebo-controlled trial found that the 40 children who received the active tablets were disciplined, on average, once each. This represented a 47% lower mean rate of antisocial behaviour than the 40 children who received placebos and who were disciplined on average 1.875 times each (Schoenthaler & Bier, 2000).

Suspicions of a causal link between poor diet and antisocial behaviour have long been bruited. According to Gesch, the Quakers had referred to the significance of a good diet in addressing criminal behaviour as far back as the 1820s (Gesch, 2007). In 1984, the International Clinical Nutrition Review published an article outlining numerous small studies, carried out in the US during the 1970s and 1980s, which suggested a causal link between poor nutrition and antisocial behaviour (Schauss, 1984). In the 1970s, a growing number of scientists had started to question the belief that criminal behaviour was exclusively a function of socio-economic, psychological or environmental factors and started to examine diet as a variable worthy of scrutiny (Schauss & Simonsen, 1979).

Since the Aylesbury trial, the Department of Health has acknowledged that '*poor diet may be associated with anti-social behaviour*' (DH, 2004). HM Chief Inspector of Prisons for Scotland states that '*It is possible that encouraging prisoners to eat nutritious food might be a contribution not only to healthier living but also to less destructive behaviour*' (HMCIPS, 2005). Lord Ramsbotham has said that he is now '*absolutely convinced that there is a direct link between diet and antisocial behaviour, both that bad diet causes bad behaviour and that good diet prevents it*' (Lawrence, 2006b).

Studies are continuing. More evidence is emerging of a link between omega-3 fatty acid deficiency and aggressive behaviour which suggests that optimal levels of this fatty acid may prevent aggressive behaviour (Hibbeln *et al.*, 2006). In 2003 American researchers found that children given good nutrition (including lots of fish), as well as increased exercise and better education were significantly less prone to conduct disorder and criminal behaviour at ages 17 and 23 than a control group. (Raine *et al.*, 2003). However it is not clear whether nutrition was solely or at all responsible for this result.

If indeed improved nutrition has such positive effects on behaviour, both prisoners and the Prison Service stand to benefit. So too does the whole of society, if dietary modifications are maintained beyond the prison environment. According to Natural Justice, the dietary causes of antisocial and criminal behaviour are largely ignored by the criminal justice system. The human diet has undergone massive transformations in a relatively short period of time and there has been little examination of the potential impact of these changes on brain function or behaviour (Gesch, 2007). The classic criminal justice model has always assumed that antisocial behaviour is a matter of free will; Natural Justice argues that free will must engage the brain and the brain does not work without an adequate nutrient supply (Gesch, 2007).

4.14   Prisons worldwide

The January 2007 edition of the International Centre for Prison Studies *World Prison Population List* claims that more than 9.25 million people are currently held in penal institutions throughout the world – an increase of a quarter of a million since previous figures were published 18 months earlier.

Life in prisons in many countries can be particularly grim, especially in the developing world. Human rights abuses are often horrific, and well documented by various human rights organisations. Food deprivation is just one means of abuse and it is widely employed. In some parts of the world, violence characterises the prison system. Latin America is one such area. Self-appointed prison leaders control access to common areas such as the canteen; access may be limited to those who can pay. In the worst prisons, inmates have to pay these 'leaders' to get access to food (Coyle, 2002a). It is not unusual in many prisons in the world where corruption is institutionalised for prisoners to have to pay for food, as well as clothing and the use of a bed. Where once prisoners in England routinely paid their jailers a garnish (page 278), that is still the norm in many poor countries, where almost every aspect of prison life is subject to corruption. Staff can demand payment for food, medicine or contact with family, operating on the basis of a 'price-list' for various levels of basic essentials and facilities (ICPS, 2004a).

The first step towards eradicating abuses is the setting of standards and the creation of instruments. Human rights standards have been established mainly through the United Nations. Standards for the treatment of prisoners worldwide derive from Article 10 of the United Nations International Covenant on Civil and Political Rights, which states: '*All persons deprived of their liberty shall be treated with humanity and with respect for the inherent dignity of the human person*'.

There is a number of international instruments which deal specifically with prisons and prisoners' rights, including the *Standard Minimum Rules for the Treatment of Prisoners,* adopted by the First United Nations Congress on the Prevention of Crime and the Treatment of Offenders, on 30 August 1955 (UN, 1955). These standards are not legally binding, but they set out guidelines for good practice in the treatment of prisoners and management of institutions. They represent minimum conditions accepted as suitable by the United Nation. With regard to food and drink, these standards stipulate:

- *Every prisoner shall be provided by the administration at the usual hours with food of nutritional value adequate for health and strength, of wholesome quality and well prepared and served.*
- *Drinking water shall be available to every prisoner whenever he needs it.*

These standards are supplemented by regional human rights instruments such as the *European Prison Rules,* originally published in 1987 and revised in 2006. (Council of Europe, 2006). These are laid down by the Council of Europe, which currently has 47 member states.

The European Prison Rules state that:

- *Prisoners shall be provided with a nutritious diet that takes into account their age, health, physical condition, religion, culture and the nature of their work.*
- *The requirements of a nutritious diet, including its minimum energy and protein content, shall be prescribed in national law.*
- *Food shall be prepared and served hygienically.*
- *There shall be three meals a day with reasonable intervals between them.*
- *Clean drinking water shall be available to prisoners at all times.*
- *The medical practitioner or a qualified nurse shall order a change in diet for a particular prisoner when it is needed on medical grounds.*

In 2002 the International Centre for Prison Studies (ICPS), part of the School of Law of King's College, University of London, published a handbook outlining internationally agreed standards on the use of imprisonment and conditions of detention (Coyle, 2002b). Its advice on prison management is intended for those who actually work in prisons and deal with prisoners on a daily basis, in every prison system in the world. It is based on the international human rights standards agreed by the member states of the United Nations.

International standards are clear that when a person is sent to prison, the punishment imposed should be solely deprivation of liberty (Coyle, 2002b). This means that food cannot be used to form part of the punishment, in terms of deprivation or the deliberate provision of low-quality food. The state is obliged to fulfil its duty of care, which includes adequate provision of accommodation, hygienic conditions, clothing, bedding, food, drink and exercise. Box 4.5 outlines the basic international standards concerning the provision of food (Coyle, 2002b).

According to the ICPS handbook, providing adequate food and drink to prisoners, to ensure that they do not suffer from hunger or an illness associated with under-nourishment, is one of the most basic obligations of care in prison. Even prisons in countries where the general population does not get enough to eat cannot overrule their obligations, because by depriving people of their liberty, the state assumes the obligation to care for them properly (Coyle, 2002b). In very poor countries, prisoners usually rely on food and medicines brought in by relatives (Coyle, 2007). If the country is in a post-conflict situation, relying on humanitarian aid, so too will be the prison system. The ICPS states that it is advisable for prisons to start with the assumption that feeding prisoners will be a problem, else wise they may find they cannot survive without aid. For many countries, where ordinary citizens are unable to obtain enough food to feed themselves, this presents a real dilemma. It is not one without solutions, however. One way to overcome

---

Box 4.5   Basic international standards concerning the provision of food.

One of the most basic obligations of care is that prison administrations should provide all prisoners with sufficient food and drink to ensure that they do not suffer from hunger or an illness associated with under-nourishment.

Meals should be provided at regularly spaced intervals throughout each 24-hour period. In many countries it is not acceptable to have the last meal of the day served in mid-afternoon with no more food provided until the following morning.

Arrangements should also be made for prisoners to eat their meals in circumstances that are appropriate. They should be given individual utensils and the opportunity to keep these clean. They should not normally have to eat in the same room where they sleep. If this is necessary, a special area should be provided for eating.

It is essential that prisoners should have regular access to clean water. Such water supplies should be separate from any provided for sanitary needs.

Source: Coyle, A. (2002b). Reproduced with kind permission from the ICPS.

---

this challenge is to explore the use of available land within or belonging to prisons for the cultivation of food (Coyle, 2002b). This has already happened in Malawi where the prison administration has developed a project to increase productivity on prison farms in order to move towards self-sufficiency in food production in order to feed prisoners, staff and their families and train prisoners in agriculture (Coyle, 2002b).

It is important to establish agriculture as soon as possible, in order to meet the daily needs of prison life (Coyle, 2007). Another benefit of maximising self-sufficiency is that it decreases dependency on purchases which are usually made centrally from private contractors, and which provide considerable scope for corruption and distribution problems (ICPS, 2004b). If well run, prison farms can help solve these problems, alleviate the inadequacy of the diet and improve health. Many prisoners may have been subsistence farmers before imprisonment, so require little training, whereas others would benefit from acquiring the agricultural skills which would help them survive, once released (ICPS, 2004b). This has worked in Rwanda, where the organisation Penal Reform International organised agricultural development and training for around 12 000 prisoners awaiting trial following the genocide in 1994 (ICPS, 2004b).

4.14.1   Health

In all countries of the world, it is the poorest and most marginalised members of society who make up the bulk of the prison population (WHO Europe, 2003a). Many of these people have communicable diseases such as tuberculosis, HIV/AIDS and mental health disorders, often diagnosed at a late stage (WHO Europe, 2003a). According to the WHO, *'no country can afford to ignore widespread precursors of disease in prisons such as overcrowding, inadequate nutrition and unsatisfactory conditions'* (WHO Europe, 2003a). Poor conditions in prison represent a real public health concern, because many prisoners become infected during their incarceration, and are then released back into society where they risk spreading infection. Yet the living conditions in most prisons of the world are unhealthy with overcrowding, violence, lack of light, fresh air, clean water and food and these conditions only serve to exacerbate communicable diseases (WHO Europe, 2003a).

Many of these prisons do not offer even the most basic healthcare, providing neither doctors nor medicines. Health may not be considered a matter of importance and nursing is often provided by unqualified guards (WHO Europe, 2003b). In 1995 the WHO established the Health in Prisons Project (HIPP), with the aim of supporting member states in improving public health by addressing health care in prisons. It also aims to facilitate links between prison health and the public health system at both national and international levels. When HIPP was established, it was agreed uniformly that the public health importance of prisoner health was neglected throughout Europe (Gatherer *et al.*, 2005). The prison is seen as a setting in which to promote health and tackle health inequalities. The WHO has called for member governments to work to improve prison conditions so that the minimum health requirements for light, air, space, water and nutrition are met (WHO Europe, 2003a). Twenty-eight countries in the European Region of the WHO have joined the HIPP. England and Wales are part of the HIPP and information about the reforms to the healthcare service in HM Prison Service is considered significant enough to be shared with other member states who could benefit from the Prison Service's experiences (Gatherer *et al.*, 2005).

The priority health problems in prisons throughout Europe have been identified as communicable diseases, mental health and drugs. In 1997 a meeting between the HIPP and the Joint United Nations Program on HIV/AIDS (UNAIDS) identified specific factors that applied in prisons and acted as a barrier to progress. It was stated that *'Overcrowding, malnutrition and poor hygiene conditions in prison must be overcome in the interests of public health in all societies'* (WHO/ UNAIDS, 1998).

Malnutrition is a major cause of morbidity and mortality in prisons, along with HIV, mental health and violence. There is a higher prevalence of conditions such as HIV/AIDS and communicable diseases such as TB in prisons in Europe than in the wider community (Gatherer *et al.*, 2005). Overcrowding, poor nutrition and poor hygiene conditions encourage the spread of infections, including TB (Lindkvist, 2000). If treatment of a prisoner is interrupted, when he or she is released, this can contribute to the development and spread of resistant tuberculosis in the general population. One of the ways to deal with the alarming increase of TB in prisons is to provide healthcare in prisons which mirrors that provided in civil society (Lindkvist, 2000).

Case history – Norway

In 2007, Norway announced that it had created 'the world's first ecological prison'. The inmates of Bastoey Island low security prison, located about 50 miles south of Oslo, are involved in the daily running of the prison which includes producing most of its own food. It is able to sell any surplus food produced. Food is produced organically, without the use of pesticides. Chickens, sheep and cows are reared to produce meat, and fish are caught from the waters of the Skagerrak Sea. The prison also uses solar panels for energy and recycles as much as it can. The idea behind the system is to develop a sense of responsibility among prisoners. Bastoey has a relaxed prison policy which is intended to reduce re-offending rates.

Case history – India

In 2007 it was reported that prisoners at the Parappana Agrahara prison in Bangalore, southern India (an overcrowded prison containing more than twice its capacity) are so well fed they do not want to leave, and are refusing to apply for bail. Food is supplied by the International Society for Krishna Consciousness, a Hindu evangelist organisation commonly known as the Hare Krishna movement. The all-vegetarian dishes include hot rice with two vegetables and spicy lentils with buttermilk. One of the prisoners is quoted as saying: '*When we are getting tasty, nutritious food three times a day here, why should we go out and commit crimes*' (Guardian, 23/06/07).

Case history – Republic of Equatorial Guinea

Prisoners in Black Beach prison were at risk of starvation, particularly those without families to support them. Food rations, reduced to one or two bread rolls a day in late 2004, were cut again in late February, with prisoners receiving no food at all for days at a time.

Source: Amnesty International (2006).

4.15   Discussion and conclusion

'*The sustained damage to health from a prison diet based on cheap carbohydrates and insufficient fresh fruit and vegetables, combined with a lack of exercise in fresh air and no opportunity to learn about healthy living, will compound the existing poor diet and health found amongst prisoners*'.   (Howard League, 2006)

In some regards prisoners can be more vulnerable than people in other institutions. Their stay can be very long or indefinite and they may receive no supplementary or alternative food from other sources. In hospitals and care homes patients and residents are often able to draw on the support of family members and friends to compensate for the failings of the catering service of that establishment. The prison population is sicker, less educated and more disadvantaged than the general population, making good nutrition in prisons all the more pivotal in the elimination of inequalities in health. Because a large proportion of prisoners come from socially excluded sections of the community, often living chaotic, unstable lives, prison may be the first opportunity they have to improve their health through diet. This is especially true where health has not been a priority during life in the community.

There can be no doubt that prison food is better now than it has ever been, thanks to recent reforms and the determination of those in charge of Prison Service catering. Their achievements are all the more remarkable because of the broad expectations they have to meet. They are required to work within very tight budgets, produce very large numbers of meals and reduce waste to a minimum. They cannot stop prisoners making unhealthy choices, yet the responsibility to do so has somehow been delegated to them, by both the government and the Prison Service. Caterers – who are notoriously low paid – are expected to be nutrition experts: the Prison Service catering manual includes, as annexes, recommended dietary reference values for nutrients. It is not clear how caterers are expected to transform this information into meals. The Prison Service is quite aware that prisoners reject the healthy options in favour of less healthy ones; it is likely that providing appealing but unhealthy meals will result in much less wastage. To be fair, the Prison Service has been (and continues to be) put under a great deal of pressure by the government to continue to make savings on expenditure on food. It has also shown that it can move swiftly when motivated to save money. Whilst it is true that the Prison Service has not in the past always operated on the most efficient basis, there is now the risk that its cost-cutting skills may take priority over the drive to produce quality, nutritious food.

How well prisoners are fed is difficult to determine on a broad basis as each prison sets its own budget which is dependent on the priorities of the governor. A devolved cash catering system means that variations in standards across the prison estate are likely and indeed this has been the case (Hansard, 1998). In Scotland where the budget has remained low for years, such parsimony has resulted in prisoners being underfed and quite probably malnourished. Whilst documents are regularly published outlining plans to improve catering services in Scottish prisons, action remains elusive.

In prison, as in other institutions, the provision of food is a human rights issue. Prisoners have a right to be treated with dignity, but this is not always the case. Food can be used to humiliate and degrade. Martin Narey, ex-director General of the Prison Service of England and Wales commented to staff at the Prison Service Conference in February 2000:

> I visited a prison just a few days ago and saw a notice on a door which said: No Entry While Feeding in Progress. What does that convey about our attitude to prisoners? (Coyle, 2003)

Clearly, the attitude it conveys suggests a desire to dehumanise the prisoner and set him further apart from the rest of society. The issue of providing food is always tinged by an undercurrent of sentiment that prisoners somehow do not deserve to enjoy their food, or eat food of any decent quality. It is the principle of less-eligibility (see page 281) which endures, as if enjoyment of food is tantamount to a travesty of social justice. As recently as 1997 the NAO stated in its report on prison catering that *'whilst prison food must be decent, nourishing and hygienically prepared, provision reflects the fact that the meals are for prison inmates, most of whom are convicted criminals'* (NAO, 1997). Most of them are in fact mentally ill and/or drug/alcohol dependent, from marginalised sections of society with little experience of gourmet dining. The Prison Service's statement that it is *dedicated to treating prisoners with decency* is undermined by the fact that two prisoners often share a cell meant for one, with a common toilet in full view – and this toilet often providing the only place where one of them can sit to eat (Coyle, 2003). Eating in a cell may be a good way of avoiding disturbances – the dining area can be a battleground where prisoners and the authorities clash (Godderis, 2006a) – but it is a lonely and isolating experience. Sitting on a toilet in an overcrowded cell makes it an unpleasant experience, and does a disservice to the catering skills of those involved in the production of the meal. Food is at its best when it is served directly from the kitchen to the dining room and is considered at its worse when it is transported on heated trolleys to cells. The positioning of kitchen facilities and the way in which food is served can make a critical difference to prisoner satisfaction.

Overcrowding diminishes the value and enjoyment of eating meals in prisons. It is defined by the Prison Service as the percentage of prisoners who are held two to a single cell (Solomon, 2004). Overcrowding is at an all-time high – in 2003–2004, 21.7% of prisoners (an average of 16 500 prisoners) were being held two to a single cell. These figures do not take into account prisoners held three to a double cell or held in overcrowded dormitories (Solomon, 2004). On Friday 30 March, 2007 there were a total of 80 303 prisoners being held in jails in England and Wales, an all-time high. The more people in a prison at any one time, the greater the strain is put on that prison's catering service, as kitchens – many of which were built in the mid-Victorian era – have to cope with larger populations than they were designed for. They are also catering for a different sort of population: no longer mainly of British, or of British descent but a variety of ethnicities and religions, whose dictates concerning food have to be respected. The introduction of new facilities is an onerous task – when prisons were built, food quality and standards were not considered a priority. It is to a large extent this inheritance which has hindered the building of new and adequate facilities.

As we have seen, food in prisons is highly symbolic. Prisoners often speak disparagingly of the food they are given, but perhaps that is because it is representative of the system which they despise. According to reformed criminal John McVicar who spent many years in different prisons, those in high-security wings get the best food because the authorities are keen to avoid riots (Gould, 2000). Religion-based meals are perceived as better, resulting in religious conversions (Gould, 2000).

Diet is an important determinant of health, yet it has not, historically, been a priority in prisons, despite the deplorable health status of those in the care of the Prison Service. However there has been an exception to this historical constant: we have seen how the beginning of the twentieth century was known as the 'golden age of nutrition', when micronutrients were discovered. This golden age prompted a sense of urgency that led the Prison Departmental Committee of Diets to report in 1925: *'Our first and most important recommendation relates to fresh vegetables. We desire to urge, as a matter of paramount importance, that every inch of available ground should be cultivated and used for the production of vegetables (more particularly of green vegetables) and of herbs for flavouring'*. It is somewhat ironic that prison farms have now virtually all been phased out and sold off. The reason for this is that it is thought that they do not offer the experience and training prisoners need to help them find work on release (NAO, 2006a). Whilst developing countries are turning to agriculture to improve nutrition and provide food for inmates, the UK is switching to horticultural training, with the focus on providing the skills and qualifications most likely to lead to employment. It is true that the number of people working in agriculture in the UK has declined. But it is also true that there has been a marked upward trend in the production of home-grown vegetables and the cultivation of allotments. It is odd that the assembly of breakfast packs in prison workshops is considered more useful in terms of employment than the acquisition of agricultural skills.

Although the prison services of the UK must ensure that they provide for the religious and ethical requirements of their diverse populations, anyone whose health beliefs prompt them to consume minimum five portions a day of fruit and vegetables would be hard pushed to do so. The role of fruit and vegetables in maintaining health and reducing the risk of developing chronic diseases such as cancer, diabetes and heart disease has been scientifically proven and a low intake of fruit and vegetables means that prisoners are likely to be deficient in micronutrients. It could be argued that denying a prisoner the opportunity to consume at least five portions of fruit and vegetables a day constitutes a human rights violation.

This potential violation can be extended: not only is it impossible to attain the five-a-day goal, it is at the same time difficult not to over consume salt. Whether they like it or not, salt is present in much of the food prisoners eat, putting them at risk of cardiovascular disease. A possible antidote to this risk is the consumption of oily fish. Although fish is available most days there is little in the way of oily fish, yet the benefits of oily fish have been well documented and the Food Standards Agency recommends that adults consume at least one portion a week. In reality, only a small percentage of inmates are likely to be concerned about the quantity of fresh fruit, vegetables and oily fish they consume on a weekly basis. Nutrition is just not a priority for most. It has been found that 30% of people released from prison will have nowhere to live, and two thirds have no employment (PRT, 2008). These people are not likely to be so much concerned about nutritional matters as a roof over their heads. But other minorities have to be catered for, and the health conscious have as good a claim as anyone.

There are only three opportunities in the day to consume fruits and vegetables: breakfast, lunch and evening meal. The breakfast currently provided by the prison services of the UK represents a missed opportunity. Fruit, or tomatoes or mushrooms, for example, could easily be provided. The current provision is poor and it is well known that prisoners will eat their breakfast pack in the evening, partly out of boredom and partly because of the need for sustenance during the long gap between evening meal and breakfast. It has been argued that a return to serving porridge would greatly improve the prison diet. Some prisons do still offer porridge, usually at weekends (Committee of Public Accounts, 2006). Porridge is hardly expensive and if it were accompanied by a banana or other piece of fruit prisoners would get a helping of both soluble fibre and complex carbohydrate plus a portion of fruit.

The prison shop is another area of missed opportunities. We have seen that food consumed from prison shops makes a major contribution to dietary fat intake (Eves & Gesch, 2003). Fresh fruit and other healthy options should certainly not be charged at excessive prices and there is even a case for subsidising fresh fruit. However because the shop is run primarily as a commercial operation there are many more unhealthy snacks than healthy and little incentive for contractors to review their stock.

As in other institutions, there is that contentious matter of choice. Time and again it has been shown that when provided with choice, people tend to select less healthy items. There is no reason to expect people in prisons to behave any differently. Should prisoners be offered a choice, or instead be restricted to healthy options only? This becomes a moral dilemma: is it ethical to force prisoners to eat healthy food only? Do prisoners have a right to choose, and should they be forced to eat healthily when much of the rest of the nation does not? Limiting choice would certainly make life easier for juggling caterers, but it would make the Prison Service more than a little nervous about keeping a roof over its establishments.

The Natural Justice trials at Aylesbury have added a whole new dimension to this conundrum. If Bernard Gesch and his colleagues are correct, what prisoners eat affects us all. Furthermore, if they leave prison in as poor health as when they entered, they will continue to be a burden on National Health services. Allowing prisoners to eat food low in nutrients, especially fatty acids, and high in sugar, refined carbohydrates and saturated fat could in the future be deemed irresponsible. The eighteenth century reformer John Howard was perhaps remarkably prescient when he wrote: '*I am sensible that persons confined, whose minds are depressed, need more nourishment than such as are at liberty*' (Carpenter, 2006). No one would suggest that criminal behaviour is entirely attributable to poor diet. But if the government's determination to be '*tough on crime, tough on the causes of crime*' is genuine, then poor diet has to be included with other known causes of crime, and addressed accordingly.

Notes

1 ISO – International Standardization Organization – a network of 156 national standards bodies, based in Geneva.
2 Catering Price Index – the CPI is an independent company that benchmarks the catering prices of over 24 000 products each month.

References

Allison, E. (2004) Crime and nourishment. *The Guardian,* 11 February.

Amnesty International (2006) *Amnesty International Report 2006 – Equatorial Guinea, 23 May 2006.* www.unhcr.org.

Awofeso, N. (2005) Making prison health care more efficient. *British Medical Journal,* **331**:248–249.

Bradley, D. (1979) The kitchen. *Catering News,* **1**(5):12–13.

Bridgwood, A. & Malbon, G. (1995) *Survey of the Physical Health of Prisoners 1994.* London: Office of Population Censuses & Surveys.

British Medical Association (BMA) (2007) Crisis in the Cells: Prison healthcare continues to fail the public and prisoners despite emergency measures, warns BMA. eGov monitor press release. www.egovmonitor.com.

Brown, A. (2007) The amazing mutiny at the Dartmoor convict prison. *British Journal of Criminology,* **47**:276–292.

Carpenter, K.J. (2006) Nutritional studies in Victorian prisons. *Journal of Nutrition,* **136**:1–8.

Challen, M. & Walton, T. (2004) *Juveniles in Custody.* HMIP: TSO.

Committee of Public Accounts (2006) Fifty-sixth Report of Session 2005–2006. *"Serving time" prisoner diet and exercise.* House of Commons.

Council of Europe (2006) *European Prison Rules.* Strasbourg: Council of Europe.

Coyle, A. (2002a) *Managing Prisons in a Time of Change.* London: International Centre for Prison Studies.

Coyle, A. (2002b) *A Human Rights Approach to Prison Management. Handbook for Prison Staff.* London: International Centre for Prison Studies.

Coyle, A. (2003) *Humanity in Prison. Questions of Definition and Audit.* London: International Centre for Prison Studies.

Coyle, A. (2005) *Understanding Prisons. Key Issues in Policy and Practice.* Maidenhead: Open University Press.

Coyle, A. (2007) *Development of human rights standards in post conflict penal systems.* A presentation to the Swedish UN Prison and Probation Officer Course. London: ICPS.

Crow, N. (1995) Improving catering quality and value for money in HM Prison Service. *Facilities,* **13**(12):21–25.

Department of Health (DH) (1991) *Dietary reference values for food energy and nutrients for the United Kingdom.* Report of the panel on dietary reference values of the Committee on Medical Aspects of Food Policy. London: HMSO.

Department of Health (DH) (2001) *National Service Framework for Diabetes: Standards.* London: DH.

Department of Health (DH) HM Prison Service & Welsh Assembly Government (2003) *Prison Health Handbook.* London: DH.

Department of Health (DH) (2002) *Health Promoting Prisons: A Shared Approach.* London: Department of Health.

Department of Health (DH) (2004) *Choosing Health: Making Healthy Choices Easier.* London: TSO.

Diabetes UK (2006) *Diabetes and the disadvantaged: Reducing health inequalities in the UK.* A report by the All Parliamentary Group for Diabetes and Diabetes UK. www.diabetes.org.uk

Drummond, J.C. & Wilbraham, A. (1957) *The Englishman's Food.* Oxford: Alden.

Du Cane, E. (1885) *The Punishment and Prevention of Crime.* London: MacMillan & Co.

Du Cane, E.F. (1882) *An Account of the Manner in which Sentences or Penal Servitude are Carried Out in England.* London: HM convict Prison, Millbank.

Edwards, J.S.A., Edwards, A. & Reeve, W.G. (2001) The nutritional content of male prisoners diet in the UK. *Food Service Technology,* **1**:25–33.

Edwards, J.S.A., Hartwell, H.J., Reeve, W.G. & Schafheitle, J. (2007) The diet of prisoners in England. *British Food Journal,* **109**(3):216–232.

Eves, A. & Gesch, B. (2003) Food provision and the nutritional implications of food choices made by young adult males, in a young offenders' institution. *Journal of Human Nutrition and Dietetics,* **16**(3):167–179.

Food Standards Agency Scotland (2006) *Nutrient standards for the Scottish Prison Service.* Draft, April 2006. FSAS & SPS.

Gatherer, A., Moller, L. & Hayton, P. (2005) The World Health Organization European Health in Prisons Project after 10 years: Persistent barriers and achievements. *American Journal of Public Health,* **95**(10):1696–1700.

Gesch, B., Hammond, S., Hampson, S. *et al.* (2002) Influence of supplementary vitamins, minerals and essential fatty acids on the antisocial behaviour of young adult prisoners. *British Journal of Psychiatry,* **181**:22–28.

Gesch, B. (2007) The links between diet and behaviour. *Associate Parliamentary Food & Health Forum.* Minutes 25 April 2007.

Godderis, R. (2006a) Dining in: The symbolic power of food in prison. *The Howard Journal,* **45**(3):255–267.

Godderis, R. (2006b) Food for thought: An analysis of power and identity in prison food narratives. *Berkeley Journal of Sociology,* **50**:61–75.

Gould, K. (2000) Slops and Robbers. *Waitrose Food Illustrated.* www.waitrose.com

Griffiths, A. (1884) *Memorials of Millbank.* London: (s.n.), 1875.

Guardian 23 June 2007 (page 2). News from Bangalore.

Hansard (1998) House of Commons written answers, 9 January 2007. In: *Prison Reform Trust. Bromley Briefings.* Prison Factfile May 2007.

Harris, F., Hek, G. and Condon, L. (2006). Health needs of prisoners in England and Wales: the implications for prison healthcare of gender, age and ethnicity. *Health and Social Care in the Community,* **15**(1):56–66.

House of Commons Select Committee on Public Accounts (1998) *The Prison Service: Prison Catering.* 30 March 1998. Hansard Archives.

House of Commons Select Committee on Public Accounts (2006) *Serving time: prisoner diet and exercise.* The United Kingdom Parliament. Fifty-Sixty Report of Session 2005–06.

Hayton, P. & Boyington, J. (2006) Prisons and health reforms in England and Wales. *American Journal of Public Health,* **96**(10):1730–1733.

Hek, G., Condon, L. & Harris, F. (2005) *Primary Care Nursing in Prisons: A Systematic Overview of Policy and Research Literature.* Bristol: The University of West England.

Hibbeln, J.R., Ferguson, T.A. & Blasbalg, T.L. (2006). Omega-3 fatty acid deficiencies in neurodevelopment, aggression and autonomic dysregulation: Opportunities for intervention. *International Review of Psychiatry,* **18**(2):107–118.

Hinde, R.S.E. (1951) *The British Penal System 1773–1950.* London: Gerald Duckworth & Co Ltd.

HM Chief Inspector of Prisons for Scotland (HMCIPS) (2005) *Annual Report for 2004–2005.* Edinburgh: TSO.

HM Chief Inspector of Prisons for Scotland (HMCIPS) (2006a) *Standards Used in the Inspection of Prisons in Scotland.* Edinburgh: TSO.

HM Chief Inspector of Prisons for Scotland (HMCIPS) (2006b) *Annual Report for 2005–2006.* Edinburgh: TSO.

HM Chief Inspector of Prisons (1996). *Patient or Prisoner? A New Strategy for Health Care in Prisons.* London: DH.

HM Chief Inspector of Prisons (2007) *Annual Report for 2005/2006.* London: The Stationery Office.

HM Inspectorate of Prisons (2008) *Expectations. Criteria for assessing the conditions in prisons and the treatment of prisoners.* April 2008. www.inspectorates.homeoffice.gov.uk

HM Prison Service (1999) *Prison Service Catering Manual.* Prison Service Order 5000 www.hmprisonservice.gov.uk

HM Prison Service (2000a) *Prison Service Catering: Staffing of Prison Kitchens.* Prison Service Order 5010. Issued 06/07/2000.

HM Prison Service (2000b) *Single Portions*. Prison Service Order 5005. Issued 23/10/2000.

HM Prison Service (2002a) (1st edition issued 1999) *Prison Service Standards Manual*. Prison Service Order 0200. Issued July 2002.

HM Prison Service (2002b) *National Service Framework for Diabetes: Standards*. Prison Service Order 3500. Issued 19/02/2007.

HM Prison Service (2003a) (revised) *Finance*. Prison Service Order 7500. Revised July 2003.

HM Prison Service (2003b) *Health Promotion*. Prison Service Order 3200. Issued 23/10/2003.

HM Prison Service (2004) *Prison Service Performance Standards*. Prison Service Order 0200. Issued October 2004.

HM Prison Service (2005) A recipe for success. *Prison Service News*, 242.

HM Prison Service (2006) The Prison Rules 1999 (consolidated January 2006) Statutory instrument no.728. www.hmprisonservice.gov.uk

HM Prison Service (2007) *Prison Service Self-audit*. Prison Service Order 0250 Issued 13/09/2007.

Home Office (1946) *Report of the Commissioners of Prisons and Directors of Convict Prisons for the Years 1942–1944*. London: HMSO.

Home Office (1949) *Prison Rules*. London: HMSO.

Home Office (1954) *Report of the Commissioners of Prisons for the Year 1953*. London: HMSO.

Home Office (1974) *Report on the Work of the Prison Department 1973*. London: HMSO.

Home Secretary's Circular, January 24th 1843. In: Drummond, J.C. & Wilbraham, A. (1957) *The Englishman's Food*. Oxford: Alden.

Howard, J. (1929) *The State of the Prisons*. London: J M Dent & Sons.

Howard League for Penal Reform (2006) Memorandum submitted by the Howard league for the Committee of Public Accounts fifty-sixth Report of Session 2005–06, published on 19 July 2006.

Independent Monitoring Board for Northern Ireland (2006a) Hydebank Wood Young Offenders' Centre and Prison. Annual report to the Secretary of State for Northern Ireland 2005/2006.

Independent Monitoring Board for Northern Ireland (2006b) Maghaberry Prison Board. Annual report to the Secretary of state for Northern Ireland 2005/2006.

Independent Monitoring Board for Northern Ireland (2006c) Magilligan Prison. Annual report to the Secretary of state for Northern Ireland 2005/2006.

International Centre for Prison Studies (ICPS) (2004a) Guidance Note 6. *Bringing Prisons within the Rule of Law*. London: King's College.

International Centre for Prison Studies (ICPS) (2004b) Guidance Note 9. *Humanising the Treatment of Prisoners*. London: King's College.

Johnston, V.J. (1985) *Diet in Workhouses and Prisons 1835–1895*. New York: Garland Publishing Inc.

Keavney, P.J. (2004) Prison medicine: A crisis waiting to break. *British Medical Association*. www.bma.org.uk

Lawrence, F. (2006a) Delayed: The food study that could cut prison violence by 'up to 40%'. *The Guardian*, 17 October 2006.

Lawrence, F. (2006b). Omega-3, junk food and the link between violence and what we eat. *The Guardian*, 17 October 2006.

Lester, C., Hamilton-Kirkwood, L. & Jones, N.K. (2003) Health indicators in a prison population: Asking prisoners. *Health Education Journal*, 62:341.

Lindkvist, P. (ed) (2000) *Tuberculosis among prisoners – interdisciplinary expert meeting on prevention and control*. Report from an International Meeting, Sigtuna, Sweden, October 4–6, 2000.

McCann, D., Barrett, A. *et al.* (2007) Food additives and hyperactive behaviour in 3-year-old and 8/9-year-old children in the community: a randomised, double-blinded, placebo-controlled trial. *The Lancet*, 370(9598):1560–1567.

McConville, S. (1995) The Victorian Prison. England, 1865–1965. In Morris, N. & Rothman, D.J. (eds) *The Oxford History of the Prison*. Oxford: Oxford University Press.

McGowen, R. (1995) The Well Ordered Prison. England, 1780–1865. In Morris, N. & Rothman, D.J. (eds) *The Oxford History of the Prison*. Oxford: Oxford University Press.

McLeod, H. (2006) *Prison health partnership survey 2006*. Final Report. Health Services Management Centre, University of Birmingham.

Mental Health Foundation (MHF) (2006) *Feeding Minds. The Impact of Food on Mental Health*. London: The Mental Health Foundation.

National Audit Office (NAO) (1997). Press notice. *Prison catering*. Report by the Comptroller and Auditor General. HC 277 Session 1997/1998. 7 November 1997.

National Audit Office (NAO) (2003). *Modernising procurement in the Prison Service*. Report by the Comptroller and Auditor General. HC 562 Session 2002–2003: 4 April 2003.

National Audit Office (NAO) (2006a). *Serving Time: Prisoner Diet and Exercise*. Report by the Comptroller and Auditor General. HC 939 Session 2005–2006. 9 March 2006. London: TSO.

National Audit Office (NAO) (2006b) *Smarter Food Procurement in the Public Sector*. Report by the Comptroller and Auditor General. HC 963–1 Session 2005–2006. 30 March 2006. London: TSO.

National Offender Management Service (2007). Sample pre-select menu. Received via email September 2007.

Northern Ireland Prison Service & Health Promotion Agency. *Promoting Healthy Prisons*. Report of a conference held on 12 September 2006 in Lisburn, Northern Ireland. www.niprisonservice.gov.uk/

Northern Ireland Prison Service (NIPS). *Catering*. www.niprisonservice.gov.uk. Accessed April 2007. NIPS website page.

Northern Ireland Prison Service (NIPS) (1995) Statutory Rules of Northern Ireland. 1995, no. 8. Prisons and Young Offenders Centres.

Northern Ireland Prison Service (NIPS) (2006a). *NIPS Food Safety & Catering Manual*.

Northern Ireland Prison Service (NIPS) (2006b) *Press release issued by the Butler trust*. www.niprisonservice.gov.uk. 31 March 2006.

Northern Ireland Prison Service (NIPS) (2007) Sample pre-select menu. Received via email September 2007.

Pratt, J. (1999) Norbert Elias and the civilised prison. *British Journal of Sociology*, 50(2):271–296.

Priestly, P. (1999) *Victorian Prison Lives*. London: Pimlico.

Prison Commission (1925) Report of Departmental Committee on Diets.

Prison Department (1990s – full date unknown) Manual V. Supply and Transport Branch. Vol. 4: supply.

Prison Reform Trust (1991) *The Woolf report. A Summary of the Main Findings and Recommendations of the Inquiry into Prison Disturbances*. London: Prison Reform Trust.

Prison Reform Trust (2008). *Bromley Briefings: Prison Fact File June 2008*. London: Prison Reform Trust.

Prison Reform Trust and National AIDS Trust (2005) HIV and hepatitis in UK prisons: Addressing prisoners' healthcare needs. In: Prison Reform Trust (2006). *Prison Fact File November 2006: Bromley Briefings*. London: Prison Reform Trust.

Prison Rules (1933) *Concordance with Rules of 1898* (1933) London: HMSO.

Private email correspondence with NIPS catering adviser 2000–05, 23/08/07.

Private email correspondence with HMPS head of catering, 29/08/07.

Private email correspondence with the SPS, 23/10/07.

Private email correspondence with the SPS, 21/11/07.

Private email correspondence with the DH, 13/07/07.

Raine, R., Mellingen, K., Liu, J. *et al.* (2003) Effects of environmental enrichment at ages 3–5 years on schizotypal personality and antisocial behaviour at ages 17 and 23 years. *American Journal of Psychiatry*, **160**:1627–1635.

Schauss, A.G. (1984) Nutrition and antisocial behaviour. *International Clinical Nutrition Review*, 4(4):172–177.

Schauss, A.G. & Simonsen, C.E. (1979) A critical analysis of the diets of chronic juvenile offenders. *Orthomolecular Psychiatry*, 8(3):149–157.

Schoenthaler, S., Amos, S., Doraz, W. *et al.* (1997) The effect of randomised vitamin-mineral supplementation on violent and non-violent behaviour among incarcerated juveniles. *Journal of Nutritional and Environmental Medicine*, 7(4):343–352.

Schoenthaler, S.J. & Bier, I.D. (2000) The effect of vitamin-mineral supplementation on juvenile delinquency among American schoolchildren: A randomized, double-blind placebo-controlled trial. *Journal of Alternative & Complementary Medicine*, 6(1):7–17.

Scottish Government (2004) *Integrating Sustainable Development into Procurement of Food and Catering Services*. Published May 2004. Edinburgh.

Scottish Government (2005) *Public Sector Food Procurement in Scotland: Incentives and Constraints for Buyers and Producers*. Published 29 April, 2005. www.scotland.gov.uk.

Scottish Office (1996) *Eating for health: a diet action plan for Scotland*. http://www.scotland.gov

Scottish Prison Service. *Prison Rules*. www.sps.gov.uk. Accessed March 2007.

Scottish Prison Service (2002) *The Health Promoting Prison: A Framework for Promoting Health in the Scottish Prison Service*. Edinburgh: The Health Education Board for Scotland.

Scottish Prison Service (2006) *9th Prisoner Survey 2006*. www.sps.gov.uk

Scraton, P. & Moore, L. (2007) The prison within. The imprisonment of women at Hydebank Wood 2004–06. *Northern Ireland Human Rights Commission*.

Smith, C. (2002) Punishment and pleasure: Women, food and the imprisoned body. *The Sociological Review*, 50(2):197–214.

Smith, W. (1776) *The state of the gaols in London, Westminister*. In Drummond, J.C. & Wilbraham, A. (1957) *The Englishman's Food*. Oxford: Alden.

Solomon, E. (2004) *A measure of success: An analysis of the Prison Service's performance against its Key Performance Indicators 2003–4*. London: The Prison Reform Trust.

Tomlinson, M.H. (1978) Not an instrument of punishment: Prison diet in the mid nineteenth century. *Journal of Consumer Studies and Home Economics*, 2:15–26.

United Nations (1955) *Standard Minimum Rules for the Treatment of Prisoners*. Geneva: UN.

Wheatley, P. (2006) (Director General of the Prison Service). Oral evidence taken before the Committee of Public Accounts on Wednesday 19 April 2006. Fifty-sixth Report of Session 2005–06.

Wilde, O. (1978) *The Ballad of Reading Gaol*. London: Journeyman Press.

World Health Organization Europe (2003a) *Prison health as part of public health*. Declaration, Moscow, 24 October 2003.

World Health Organization Europe (2003b) Health in Prisons Update. *Newsletter*, 1 (2003) WHO Regional Office for Europe. Web download.

WHO/UNAIDS (1998) HIV/AIDS, sexually transmitted diseases and tuberculosis in prisons. Joint Consensus Statement. Geneva: World Health Organization. In Gatherer, A., Moller, L. & Hayton, P. *et al.* (2005) The World Health Organization European Health in Prisons Project after 10 years: Persistent barriers and achievements. *American Journal of Public Health*, 95(10):1696–1700.

World Health Organization (2003) *Diet, Nutrition and the Prevention of Chronic Diseases*. WHO Technical Report Series, No. 916. Geneva: WHO.

5 Armed forces

Maria Cross

5.1 Introduction

'If the soldier is to be kept fit on active service he must depend chiefly upon Doctor Diet'. (Cope, 1959)

The importance of adequately feeding members of the armed forces has long been recognised as being crucial to the smooth functioning of the military machine, and to successful campaigns. Whereas there has, from time to time, been considerable public outrage at the quality of food served up to those in other institutions, such as schools, hospitals and care homes, no such outrage has been required when it comes to feeding military personnel. Napoleon was not the first to observe the role of food in maintaining a fighting force when he famously remarked that 'an army marches on its stomach'. Before him, Frederick the Great (1712–1786) is credited with the remark that 'An army, like a serpent, goes on its belly'.

The armed forces is an organisation comprised of three services: the Army, the Royal Navy (RN) and the Royal Air Force (RAF). The inter-service nature of military operations is highly sophisticated, requiring ultra-efficient coordination. There were around 190 400 members of the armed forces in 2007, not including reserves, cadets and civilian Ministry of Defence (MoD) staff.

The armed forces constitute an institution comprised of mainly adult individuals, the majority of whom are men, who are presumed to be both fit and healthy, and frequently engaged in strenuous physical activity. Intense physical activity demands additional energy input. The MoD recruits up to 18 000 people every year – and the physical fitness of these recruits, as well as of serving personnel, is an important part of preparing for military operations.

As well as meeting the additional energy requirements of military personnel, those involved with armed forces catering must meet a broad spectrum of criteria. The logistics of feeding soldiers engaged in operations, or on the move, at sea and so on are highly complex. Food is often prepared and eaten in challenging or hazardous environments, or in extreme climates. Personnel are deployed all over the world and may be based in diverse environments where extreme climate conditions can impact on nutritional requirements. Food supplied during operations has to be nutritious and calorific but at the same time weigh little and occupy minimal space. The diversity of personnel is as important a consideration as the diversity of the environment in which they are deployed. A large number of recruits are from the Commonwealth, so cultural dietary habits are wide-ranging, and the provision of food needs to accommodate religious as well as cultural requirements.

Food can also be deeply meaningful for those serving in the armed forces. For those engaged in campaigns far from home, the role of food extends beyond supplying energy and sustenance to providing comfort and building morale. Eating together under extremely difficult circumstances can be a comforting, bonding experience. The MoD is well aware of the importance of providing food to its overseas members which is as similar as possible to the food served at 'home'. It also knows the value of regularly surveying personnel about what they want to see on the menu. For those not engaged in overseas operations, the unit and mess are to all intents and purposes home, where they can choose to eat most if not all their meals.

5.2   History of feeding the armed forces – the Army

5.2.1   Seventeenth century

The present British Army was founded following the English Civil War (1642–1649) and the restoration of the monarchy in 1660. During the Civil War provisions were basic: the Commissariat provided the men with bread and cheese, and those who could afford to do so bought meat and vegetables at market (Fortescue, 1928). Following the war and the establishment of the army, soldiers were billeted in inns or with private citizens, whose responsibilities included feeding the men (Cole, 1984).

5.2.2   Eighteenth century

When Britain became involved in military undertakings on the continent, such as the War of Spanish Succession (1701–1714), the only rationed food the men received was bread. To supplement their diet, they had to rely on sutlers who accompanied armies in the field (Cole, 1984). These private adventurers followed armies on their campaigns and offered foodstuffs for sale. So essential did sutlers become to the army in the field that they were eventually placed under military regulation (Fortescue, 1928). Each regiment had one grand sutler, and each troop or company one petty sutler. It was later ordered that the men were to receive meat twice a week, with the cost deducted from their pay. The soldier's diet was further supplemented by food growing wild: parties of troops were sent out ahead to forage for vegetables and leafy greens. Butchers were encouraged to follow regiments with a stock of butchered meat as well as cattle on the hoof (Cole, 1984).

By the end of the eighteenth century, it was evident that the British Army was becoming larger and more sophisticated and could no longer survive by relying on the gains of foraging parties. The need to provide regular supplies was first met by the Royal Wagonners, set up in 1794 and which became the Royal Wagon Train in 1802, serving the army during the Napoleonic Wars.

5.2.3   Nineteenth and twentieth centuries

By the early nineteenth century it had become clear that feeding the soldier well was crucial to a successful campaign, even if the science to back up this certainty was scarce. It was believed that meat in particular promoted fighting qualities (Crowdy, 1980). To provide the men with meat there would be cattle – up to 500 heads – following behind the troops. Tea and coffee were issued to the troops when available, as these beverages were considered revitalising, especially coffee (Cole, 1984).

In the series of wars and battles leading up to the Battle of Waterloo in 1815, Wellington's army had to supply vast amounts of food for thousands of troops, not to mention horses, and this was the job of the Commissariat Department. The Commissariat was far from proficient and there was still no effective central control over feeding, with supplies being provided in a haphazard manner, and often failing to arrive. Part of the problem was fatigue of transport animals (Cole, 1984).

The first basic form of food ration was provided in 1816 when a decree was ordained for a common ration scale for the whole British army. The daily allowance per man was:

Bread	1 lb
Meat (fresh or salted)	1 lb
Wine	1 pint
(or spirits in lieu	1/3 pint)

For this, 6d a day was deducted from the soldier's pay.

Over the course of the Napoleonic Wars, the life of the soldier at home underwent enormous changes. Barracks were built on a large scale, and the old system of billeting in ale-houses came to an end. The first rudimentary canteens were set up in barracks, with the aim not so much to feed the men, but to provide them with liquor, to prevent smuggling. The original canteens sold rather rough spirits only (Fortescue, 1928). More goods were added to the canteen provision, but they were of poor quality and at high prices. Canteens were let out to contractors, and the state made a healthy profit from these contracts.

Cooking facilities were basic, and the staple diet was meat and potatoes (Cole, 1984). The meat was always boiled beef, for there were no means of roasting or baking it. The soldier had two meals a day – breakfast and lunch.

As a result of having no food in the evening, he would frequently take to drink. In 1840 a third daily meal was made obligatory, in an effort to limit excessive alcohol consumption, which was a serious problem among soldiers. In 1847 Parliament reluctantly prohibited the sale of spirits in canteens, following pressure from concerned commanding officers.

5.2.3.1   Crimean War (1854–1856) and Alexis Benoît Soyer (1810–1858)

When engaged in military campaigns abroad, soldiers routinely experienced hunger, due to poor logistical organisation. The Crimean War was to prove a turning point for military feeding, when it became clear just how poorly the men who were expected to fight were provided for. A breakdown in logistics meant that there was insufficient transport to move rations from harbour to the soldiers in the field, who were frequently virtually starving. Although each man was supplied with a camp kettle, few had any idea how to cook and they had no fuel allowance. Men who returned exhausted to camp had to grub up roots for fuel, a necessity made all the harsher by winter snow and frost (Cole, 1984). They were issued with coffee beans, but no means of grinding or roasting them. Nor were there facilities to bake bread. By November 1854 severe malnutrition had set in, and scurvy had begun to appear. The story of the provision of food at the time was effectively a saga of mismanagement – for example, nearly one ton of lime juice, which would have eliminated scurvy, was held in Balaclava, having been ordered by the Medical Department but with no authority given to issue it. Not that the men would have been satisfied had they had access to all their rations: in 1856 a report into the soldier's ration declared it to be inadequate, even if supplied in full (Crowdy, 1980).

The Crimean War was not by any means the first campaign where men starved and died in their thousands. But in 1854 war correspondents were present for the first time on the battlefield, making the public at home aware of the many horrors of war. The consequence of this early media presence was a strong urge back home to help the suffering soldiers in whatever way possible. The appalling conditions faced by the men in the Crimea led to the formation of the Land Transport Corps in 1855 which delivered supplies to the British Army during the remainder of the war. Also in 1855 a letter appeared in *The Times*, appealing to famous London chef and catering reformer Alexis Soyer to help out. Soyer, a Frenchman, responded by offering to go to the Crimea (and Scutari), at his own expense, in order to improve the diet of the military. The Government accepted his offer.

Much is owed to the work and influence of Alexis Soyer, who changed the nature of military catering forever. He revolutionised mass catering for the army during the Crimea War, during which time he became friends with Florence Nightingale. After his death Nightingale wrote: '*His death is a great disaster. Others have studied cooking for the purposes of gormandising, some for show, but none but he for the purpose of cooking large quantities of food in the most nutritious manner for great numbers of men'* (Le Gros Clark, 1959). Soyer was the celebrity chef of his day, combining an interest in the nutritional aspect of feeding with a philanthropic impetus – before heading off to the Crimea in 1855, he went to Ireland to superintend soup kitchens for famine relief.

In Scutari, Soyer found that the hospital catering was poorly organised and lacked trained cooks. Within a month he had set up new kitchens and greatly improved the hitherto miserable diet of the hospitalised. He also reorganised the system of issuing rations and created recipes to make them more palatable. He designed menus for soups, stews and seasoned meat, and supplemented the regular diet of soldiers with local purchases. He introduced tinned, dried vegetables to prevent scurvy and set about designing his portable cooking stove, which was to become a basic component of camp equipment. The stove was smokeless, making its use invisible to the enemy, and with modifications was still being used by the British Army during the first Gulf War. He left Scutari and sailed, with Florence Nightingale, to the Crimea, where he introduced his new stove into army cooking. The efficiency of the system of catering he instigated brought about considerable savings in fuel and labour. Soyer returned from the Crimea in 1857 to London, where, on behalf of the new Barracks and Hospitals Sub-Commission, he organised schools of regimental and hospital cookery. He wrote his *Instructions to Military Hospital Cooks*, which was adopted by all military hospitals (Le Gros Clark, 1959). He lectured on military dietetics at the United Services Institute and designed a cooking wagon for armies on the march. Today, Alexis Soyer is still toasted at an annual Soyer dinner held for serving army caterers.

The Commission that Soyer helped to organise was tasked with reviewing the living conditions and diet of soldiers. These conditions were found to be poor, and as a result immediate steps were taken to improve accommodation and catering. Barrack kitchens were equipped with ovens for roasting and baking and cooks were given basic instructions in catering (Cole, 1984). The Commissariat set up its own butcheries and bakeries, and started buying groceries in bulk. The introduction of recreational rooms and sports grounds and gymnasia was also part of the steady progress towards improving the soldier's lot.

In 1858 a Royal Commission stated that the soldier should be supplied with food '*sufficient both in quantity and quality to provide him with three meals and to keep him in health and efficiency*'. In 1869 the Army Service Corps was established as the organisation tasked with supplying and transporting provisions. There were reforms to the canteens, which put an end to the old contract system and established the canteen as a regimental affair. The steward, waiters and barmen (selling liquor never completely ceased, despite legislative efforts to ban it from canteens) were generally drawn from the regiment and the retail profits went back to the regiment. The system was still by no means perfect and corruption and abuses sprang up quickly, whilst complaints of bad quality food and high prices continued.

After 1870 the army slowly underwent complete transformation, which included the abolition of long service. The Army School of Cookery was established at

Aldershot in 1883, where men were sent from different regiments to learn culinary skills before returning to their regiments. The second Army Service Corps was formed in 1888, when the whole supply service finally came under the control of the central military authority. At that time, the daily diet of most men consisted of:

Breakfast	bowl of tea
Lunch	beef and potatoes
Evening	tea and bread (Cole, 1984)

The diet was not exactly excessive, nor appetising, but it did continue to improve following the establishment of the ASC, with more variety. In 1894, in a further effort to improve the canteen system for soldiers at home, the Canteen and Mess Co-operative Society was formed by a handful of army captains and others. Members held shares but the amount held and interest gained was limited, with excess profits returned to the canteens (Fortescue, 1928). The Canteen and Mess Society was very successful, and when it came to war (in South Africa) the Society placed canteen-stores upon every troopship and supplemented these supplies with regular shipments to South Africa.

5.2.3.2   Boer War 1899–1902

Concerns were raised again about the nutritional status of soldiers during the Boer War of 1899–1902. In 1899 the military in Aldershot were reminded, in a series of lectures, that 'If we are going to get the best value out of our troops, we must feed them well' (Clayton, 1899). The regimental supply wagon would carry two days' groceries and one day's preserved meat and biscuit, together with one day's grain for the horses. The groceries consisted of salt, sugar, tea, cocoa and pepper. Each man also carried in his haversack the emergency ration: a small tin cylinder containing about 4 oz of cocoa paste and 4 oz of pemmican;[1] the latter could be used as a semi-solid or made into soup. Army rations were frugal and the men supplemented their diet either through thieving or bargaining with locals (Cole, 1984).

Despite poor supplies, the British army in South Africa during the period of the Boer War was competent in field cookery. Field ovens were constructed and bread was supplied regularly. Each army corps had a bakery company which was supplied with Aldershot Ovens which were able to supply sufficient bread for the whole corps, when given the opportunity – that is, when the army was halted for a period of 24 hours or more (Clayton, 1899). The Aldershot Oven was introduced generally in the 1860s and remained in service until the 1950s. Constructed of wrought iron, it could bake 108 rations of bread and dinner for about 220 men in each batch (Cole, 1984).

At the beginning of the twentieth century, attempts were made to estimate the energy requirements of the soldier at war. In 1909 and 1910 two experimental marches of two weeks' duration were carried out. After the first march the average daily intake of each soldier was estimated to be about 3500 kcal. Each soldier had lost weight and was judged to have been underfed. For the second march, each man was given about 1000 kcal extra per day. This was judged to be about right, to prevent weight loss. It was from this that the 1913 field scale was produced, designed to provide between 4500 and 5000 kcal daily (Crowdy, 1980).

In the five years leading up to World War I, training in field cookery had become part of training generally. Officers were instructed in cooking and kitchen management (Cole, 1984). The first *Manual of Military Cooking and Dietary* was published, giving advice on improvised methods of field cooking, such as how to make best use of mess tins as cooking utensils. The manual contained a number of recipes, including s*oup with preserved meat, curried stew, preserved meat fritters* and *toad-in-the-hole* (Cole, 1984).

5.2.3.3 World War I

When the British Expeditionary Force of 1914 went to war, it was on the ration scale laid down in the revised edition of the Field Service Pocket Book published earlier that year (Cole, 1984). The field ration consisted of:

- 1¾ lb preserved or salted meat
- 1¼ lb bread or 1lb biscuits or flour
- 4 oz bacon
- tea
- sugar
- jam
- salt & pepper
- cheese
- mustard

Fresh vegetables were only issued by the Army Service Corps when available. By 1916 the ration had been reduced, due to the difficulty of maintaining a large army during the German blockade. Soldiers on the Western Front were living on canned corned beef (bully beef), bread and biscuits. Soldiers experienced many hardships, not least of all food shortages, especially when advancing into enemy territory. Kitchen staff foraged for wild leaves to supplement the meagre diet. By the winter of 1916 bread was being made from dried ground turnips.

In addition to the standard field ration, each man carried an iron ration, which was an emergency pack consisting of tinned corned beef, tea, sugar, biscuit and 2 cubes of meat extract. The iron ration could only be opened with the permission of an officer.

Never before had the army had to provide food on such an enormous scale, and it frequently failed to do so. Men complained regularly of not receiving the full ration. At the start of the war, there was still no provision made by the military authorities for any canteen organisation in the field. In France and Flanders local tradesmen saw their opportunity and raised prices accordingly. The Canteen and

Mess Society acted to remedy the situation, and the Expeditionary Force Canteen (EFC) was created in 1915. The EFC was controlled by the Canteen and Mess Society and became the universal provider for all the wants of the army and of its auxiliary services at the Western Front. Because operations there were static, it was possible to establish permanent kitchens that were able to provide a regular catering service (Cole, 1984). Horse-drawn travelling field kitchens were used to prepare hot meals to sustain the men in the front line. Field kitchens moved with the men as they marched, cooking food as they went along. This meal usually consisted of a stew with potatoes, peas or carrots. A cold pudding – usually custard – was also provided.

More and more base-depots were established and these pushed forward almost to the firing line. The EFC supplied everything 'from a button to a bottle of champagne' (Fortescue, 1928). It even took over the Valroy Springs at Etaples in 1915 to supply the army with mineral water. It brewed its own beer for the men, and sought out wine for the officers.

Of course canteens could not have operated in the field, and rations could not have been provided, without the logistics of transporting goods there. This was carried out by the Army Service Corps which transported prodigious amounts of food, equipment and ammunition from England, using horses, motor vehicles, railways and waterways. At the end of WWI, the Army Service Corps was awarded the Royal prefix in recognition of the role it played during the conflict.

After the war, in 1917, the Army Canteen Committee was formed, charged with the task of supervising the administration of canteens and maintaining standards. This committee recommended that all canteens should be conducted by a central organisation owned and controlled by the army itself. This move was intended to rid the system of corruption, high prices and bad food. The committee began to take over all business from the civil contractors and to establish itself as a central organisation not only for general control but for the provision of supplies. The Canteen and Mess Society was then subsumed into the Army Canteen Committee. By April 1917 over two thousand canteens were being controlled by the Committee. In June 1917 the Navy asked that the British sailor might enjoy the same benefits as the British soldier. As a result the Committee assumed the new title of the Navy and Army Canteen Board. By the end of the War the RAF had also joined up.

Following a review of canteen facilities, on the orders of Winston Churchill, it was then decided that the canteens, or institutes as they were by then called, should be administered by a joint organisation styled the Navy, Army and Air Force Institute (NAAFI), which came into being on 1 January 1921 as a cooperative, with profits returned to the Forces. NAAFI provided a restaurant service in barracks, with food such as meat pies, eggs and chips served at reasonable prices. By the end of WWII, it was operating 10 000 outlets, including 800 ships' canteens. It is still in operation today, as the 'official trading organisation of HM Forces'. However it is currently being withdrawn from all UK non-operational establishments.

5.2.3.4   *World War II and the Army Catering Corps*

The British Army went to war in 1939 equipped with the Field Service Pocket Book, with instructions and guide to camp cooking, little changed since the First World War edition (Cole, 1984).

Improvements were made to the provision of food when, in 1941, the Army Catering Corps (ACC) (1941–1993) was founded. Its purpose was to improve military catering and cookery skills. A new Army School of Cookery had been opened just a fortnight before, in St. Omer Barracks in Aldershot. During the Second World War the ACC played a central role not just in providing food but also in maintaining morale amongst the troops. ACC soldiers were attached to regiments and corps of the British Army and were present at every battle and on every front throughout the world.

The Second World War was the first war to be fought on a truly global scale, meaning that food and other supplies had to be transported in vast quantities across vast distances. Previous ration packs were deemed too heavy, so experts set about devising a more compact, lightweight solution. The result was the 24-hour, individual composite ('compo') ration. This 90-cubic inch pack weighed just over a kilo and provided around 4000 calories. Much of the food, including meat, was dehydrated, in the shape of square blocks. Typical components of the composite ration included bully beef, sausages and beans as well as cigarettes. Rations were supplemented with any food units were able to source locally. Mobile bakeries and field butchery units were set up as soon as it was possible to do so (Wickham Smith, 2006).

5.2.3.5   *Post-war years*

After the War, it was decided to retain the Army Catering Corps as an integral part of the Army. The ACC became increasingly professional as it became more evident that army catering required properly trained staff. The ACC developed a well-defined career structure which allowed for progress through the ranks. By the 1980s the Corps was made up of well-trained caterers who were also fit, professional soldiers. But it was to have a short history. In the early 1990s, it was decided to amalgamate several service-providing corps, including the ACC, into the Royal Logistic Corps, which had its inception in April 1993.

The RLC has various responsibilities, including the movement of personnel throughout the world, transport and provision of supplies and the training and provision of cooks to almost all Army units. The RLC is under the authority of the Defence Logistic Support Training Group.

5.3   History of feeding the armed forces – the Navy

5.3.1   The Tudor era (1485–1603) and Stuart era (1603–1714)

During the Tudor era the seaman's diet was generally poor and putrid. The staple diet consisted of salt beef, salt fish, biscuit and cheese. Disease was rife and death from disease and malnutrition common. Sailors during the Stuart period fared no better, with the food 'as bad as ever it had been' (Kemp, 1970). A ration scale was laid down which consisted of biscuit, beer, salt beef, salted pork, peas, butter, fish and cheese. Complaints were not so much about quantity as quality: 'stinking beer', 'salt beef which causes sickness' and 'mouldy bread from Hull' and 'the butter very bad' were among the sailors' grievances (Kemp, 1970). Food preservation methods were limited to pickling in brine.

Conditions for the seaman did not improve much under Cromwell. It is Samuel Pepys (1633–1703) who, through his reforms, is credited with contributing towards the improvement of the seaman's diet. Pepys was a naval administrator and was Britain's first secretary of the Admiralty. In 1677 he drew up a contract which set the ration for each seaman: one pound of biscuit and one gallon of beer a day (Macdonald, 2004). This was in addition to the weekly ration of eight pounds of beef, or four pounds of beef with pork and pease. Fish was served three days a week with butter and cheese. Fish was later dropped from the seaman's diet, but other than that the basic ration did not change until after 1847 (Macdonald, 2004). Meals were consumed in messes of six men, at a table with a wooden bench to sit on. By the beginning of the eighteenth century conditions all round for the seaman had considerably improved all round, with better living and working conditions.

5.3.2 The Georgian era (1714–1837)

During the Georgian era feeding men on ships with no refrigeration system and limited preservation methods (salting, pickling and drying) was not so difficult in peacetime, when ships operated in home waters, but considerably tricky when the navy was engaged in war. Ships could be away from land for many months at a time. The solution was to base rations on foodstuffs with a long shelf-life: salted meat, salted or dried fish, dried pease and beans and items made from cereal grains such as biscuits. It had been observed that eating salted food was a prime cause of sickness, and from the early eighteenth century onwards fresh provisions were issued to ships returning from long expeditions, and the crews of ships in harbour were issued with fresh provisions two days each week (Kemp, 1970).

What the standard ration lacked in freshness and appeal was made up for by calories – almost 5000 per day (Kemp, 1970). The diet of the Georgian seaman was probably nowhere near as bad, frugal or revolting as history often suggests, even if it did lack palatability and freshness. According to Janet Macdonald in her book *Feeding Nelson's Navy: The True Story of Food at Sea in the Georgian Era* (Chatham) stories of malnourished seamen, fed on rotten meat and weevilly biscuits may have been true of merchant seamen, but almost certainly not of Navy seamen. The Navy would have been aware that in order to work and fight, its men needed energy; they worked extremely hard, with few luxuries such as heating to keep warm, or waterproof clothing.

By the mid-1790s, the Admiralty had systems in place which ensured that naval seamen were supplied with good and plentiful food. The job of supplying ships with food was the responsibility of the Victualling Board, under the command of the Board of Admiralty. Alcohol was a normal part of the daily diet – officially, the daily allowance for seamen was a gallon of beer, though in reality the men had unlimited access to it (Hill, 2002). Beer in those days was however considerably weaker than today's – around 2–3 per cent proof. A gallon then would have been the equivalent of five-sixths of a modern gallon. Beer kept well in casks so was more practical than holding water for long periods of time. When beer ran out, wine was provided. In certain areas such as the West Indies, rum was provided when the wine ran out (Hill, 2002). Fresh vegetables were served when the ship was in port. Onions and cabbages get particular mention in log entries, and carrots and turnips are sometimes mentioned. Nelson (1758–1805) believed that fresh meat and vegetables were essential for the health of his men, and had his pursers obtain these whenever possible.

Livestock also was brought on board – bullocks, sheep and pigs. These would have been slaughtered on board. A goat may have been kept for its milk, and poultry was kept on most ships for eggs and meat (Macdonald, 2004). Food was prepared by the ship's cook (a man who did not necessarily have any culinary credentials and whose sole qualification was that he was a pensioner of the Chest at Greenwich, which meant that he often had a limb missing) and at least one assistant, plus the services of a boy. Virtually all food was boiled, as there were at that time no facilities for any other form of cooking.

Scurvy was the scourge of the Navy, and for a long time its cause was unknown. When ships were at sea for long periods of time they would have had no access to fresh fruits and vegetables. The cause of the disease however eluded medics. There were many theories and most of these were wildly inaccurate. The symptoms were however clear: bleeding gums and loose teeth, bruising and ulceration, hair loss, hallucinations, depression, blindness and, eventually, death. In 1600 the surgeon John Wooddall had recommended citrus fruit as an antiscorbutic, but it was not until the Scottish naval surgeon James Lind conducted an experiment in 1747 on twelve sailors with the disease that the link was made between scurvy and citrus fruits, or rather something that they contained. He divided the 12 men into pairs, each pair receiving the same diet plus something extra – either citrus fruit, vinegar, seawater, cider, garlic paste or elixir of vitriol. It was the group receiving citrus fruit every day which recovered. However Lind did not publish his *Treatise of the Scurvy* until 1753, when it was all but ignored. In this paper, Lind claimed that citrus fruit contained a substance which could cure scurvy. In 1757 he recommended that seamen arriving home from a long voyage should be given fresh provisions, including lots of green vegetables. Continual uncertainty as to the cause of scurvy meant that these recommendations were not met. It was not until more than forty years later, in 1795, that the order was issued to supply bottled lemon juice to ships. The results were immediate: scurvy vanished. Lemons were then added to the regular diet on board ship.

The seaman's lot continued to improve throughout the Napoleonic Wars (1803–1815). The quality and quantity of food was better, with more captains ensuring that their ships bought fresh meat and vegetables at every port (Kemp, 1970). The weekly allowance by this time consisted of: 7 lb bread/biscuit; 7 gallons of beer; 4 lb beef; 2 lb pork; 2 pints of pease; 3 pints of oatmeal; 6 oz butter; 12 oz cheese and 6 oz sugar. In addition each man received a daily ration of half a pint of rum, though this was later reduced by half because of the enduring problem of drunkenness. Fresh meat replaced salt meat when in port (Kemp, 1970).

5.3.3   Nineteenth and twentieth centuries

The introduction of canned foods in 1813 was a turning point in navy feeding, even though they did not become a standard part of a ship's provisions until 1847 – the Victualling Board thought them too expensive (Macdonald, 2004). By the middle of the nineteenth century a Royal Commission led to further improvements in the seaman's diet. The daily ration was increased so that it compared favourably with the diet of the working classes in towns. The daily entitlement was 1½ lb biscuit, 1 lb fresh meat and ½ lb of vegetables. Sugar, chocolate and tea were in generous supply. When at sea, the fresh meat was substitute by an equivalent amount of preserved meat. Even though the daily ration really only provided enough for one proper meal a day, it still left the seaman better off than his land-based peer (Wells, 1994).

Canteens were introduced on board ships, selling fresh foods, eggs and bacon for those who could afford them. In 1892 these canteens were taken over by the Royal Naval Canteen Board to prevent excess profiteering. Persistent grumblings below deck led to an investigation into the poor standard of naval cooking. The result was the introduction of a messing allowance which enabled the sailor to supplement his rations and vary his diet (Wells, 1994). Three daily meals were introduced and proper menus devised.

During the 1930s the Royal Naval Canteen Board was integrated into NAAFI and canteens expanded to provide a wider range of foods. There were by now bakeries on board all large ships. Centralised messing was introduced in the first half of the twentieth century, meaning that the whole ship's company could be fed meals during a continuous sitting in a cafeteria-style dining hall (Wells, 1994). Well-trained chefs (the Central School of Naval Cookery had been established in Chatham) offering a choice of hot and cold food was a further improvement to feeding the navy in the twentieth century. The traditional ration of rum, so long a staple of the Navy diet, was abolished in 1970.

5.4   Current provision

'Catering is tremendously important to our Armed Forces' morale, especially of course in Afghanistan and Iraq where chefs go to great efforts to feed our troops, constantly improving and varying their menus'. (Lord Drayson, MoD website).

5.4.1 Organisation

There are three main areas of food provision within the armed forces: non-operational (UK bases), operational (ration packs, overseas bases and active theatres) and civilian. Each unit of all three services has a catering manager in charge of all aspects of the catering operation, from standards of food production to accounts and stock.

Until March 2006 the supply of food to the armed forces was managed by the Defence Catering Group (DCG), which, as part of the Defence Logistics Organisation (DLO), was launched in 2000 as an amalgamation of the three single service catering directorates. In March 2006 the role of the DCG was taken over by the newly formed Defence Food Services Integrated Project Team (DFS IPT), which provides catering support to the armed forces worldwide, whether on operations, exercises or in barracks. It manages the Ministry of Defence food supply contract (now with the company Purple Foodservice Solutions) and oversees training of catering personnel, as well as providing catering policy, guidance and technical support.

The DFS IPT is responsible for the quality and types of meals prepared for the UK's armed forces worldwide, including Royal Navy ships and submarines. It is also involved in researching and developing the operational ration pack (ORP). The term 'military precision' lends itself well to the management of the feeding of the armed forces, whether in barracks or on global operations. The DFS IPT is organised into various departments with clearly defined responsibilities. These departments include:

DFS IPT Support for Operations. The DFS IPT has to provide food to exercises worldwide and support current operations, which include Iraq, Afghanistan, the Falklands, and the Balkans. The operations team manages the procurement, production and quality control of operational ration packs and provides guidance on their distribution and storage. The team also conducts research and development of ORPs.

DFS IPT Catering, Retail and Leisure Contracts. This department manages services contracts such as cleaning, catering, shops and leisure clubs such as the servicemen's club. It is also involved in the delivery of the new *Pay-as-You-Dine* (PAYD) contracts (see page 374).

DFS IPT Food Supply Management. This team oversees the procurement and distribution of food through the MoD supply company which in October 2006 switched from *3663 First for Foodservice* to *Purple Foodservice Solutions*. The team also manages and approves the monthly core range (page 392) and organises the monthly *Food Selection Panels* (page 384) which '*ensure that the Core Range remains dynamic, meets the customers' needs and provides value for money*'. The panel consists of members of each armed service who blind-taste new products. Members of the Food Supply Management team also form part of the Expert Panel for Armed Forces Feeding (see page 384).

DFS IPT Policy Concepts & Information Strategy. This team is responsible for catering accounting and the management of the JSP 456 range of catering manuals (see page 375). It also ensures that national and EU food safety policies are adhered to. Members sit on the *Expert Panel for Armed Forces Feeding* and contribute to the development of the core menu.

DFS IPT Equipment and Infrastructure. This team is commonly known as the MoD Kitchen Design & Equipment Authority and is involved in the improvement of MoD kitchens worldwide. It gives advice on the design and equipping of catering facilities and ensures that equipment meets current legislation and specifications.

DFS IPT Quality Assurance. This team is charged with monitoring the quality of food supplied to ensure that it meets the standards required to feed the armed forces. Key areas of the team's work include inspection of food premises, monitoring of manufacturing processes and the assessment of quality management systems, with particular regard to operational ration packs and their components.

In addition to the above, there are other teams which provide supporting functions, involved in such issues as personnel and training, budget management and technical advice. The logistical organisation is managed by a software system called Tricat, a *'bespoke catering management system'* which manages all three services and covers stock management, supply chain procurement, financial control, recipe and menu planning and other kitchen activities, as well as full financial reporting (Fretwell downing). According to the producers of Tricat, out-of-barracks catering has been significantly improved as a result of the employment of the system – previously, problems such as over-ordering were common, leading to inefficiencies and extra costs. The Policy Concepts & Information Strategy department was responsible for rolling out the Tricat software catering system across all three services (previously employed only by the Royal Navy).

5.4.2   Pay-As-You-Dine and the core menu

Food is free to personnel on exercises and operations. Personnel based at units pay for their food. A new system, known as Pay-As-You-Dine (PAYD) has been introduced which will put an end to the old system which was (and still is, in some establishments) based on the 'daily food charge'. This is the amount of money automatically deducted from the salary of a live-in serviceman or woman's pay, regardless of whether or not meals are taken. The PAYD scheme was piloted at 11 sites starting in 2002 and is in place in many but not all establishments. It is expected to be in place across all three services by 2009.

PAYD means that personnel only pay for food taken. The decision to use this new system came about as a result of a 1999 survey which identified an 'overwhelming desire for change' amongst service personnel. PAYD is considered to be a fairer system: many recruits are away at weekends and resent paying for meals which are not taken. The survey found that approximately only half of armed forces personnel were taking meal entitlement (National Audit Office (NAO), 2006). With PAYD, armed forces members can choose to purchase food from catering facilities on military bases or from any other outlet. The system has been found to reduce wastage, with meals more often cooked to order. However it has also been found to increase queuing and waiting times at the counter (NAO, 2006).

When PAYD is introduced at a base, an approved core menu must continue to be offered which costs the same, when all three meals are aggregated over the day, as the daily food charge and has a similar nutritional value. At the time of writing the daily food charge was £3.76. The three meals provided by the core menu should provide a minimum of 3300 kcals. The *Defence Catering Manual*, which governs every aspect of food provision in the armed forces, provides a 'shopping basket', or list of example ingredients needed to make up the core menu. These are basic ingredients which include dairy products, flour, sauces, cooking oils, jams and so on. The manual also produces a sample core menu, an extract of which is provided in Table 5.1. This sample gives a good indication of the variety and appeal of the menu.

All personnel are entitled to receive the core menu at the daily food charge. They are also entitled to have access to *nutritionally balanced and healthy food at each establishment* (MoD, 2007a). The core menu must offer, as a minimum, a six-item breakfast, lunch, and a 3-course dinner. Furthermore, there must always be a vegetarian option available, on demand, in addition to the number of core choices. Provision must also be made for religious, medical and lifestyle requirements. These must be planned in advance, to avoid repetition.

The menu may be restricted at weekends or other times when there may be a reduced number of personnel eating from the servery. The level of restriction must be agreed by unit authorities.

5.4.3 JSP 456 *Defence Catering Manual*

JSP 456, *Defence Catering Manual* (MoD, 2007a) is an extensive set of regulations, instructions and advice, to be used as a point of reference for caterers and managers to assist them in the delivery of the catering service across the armed forces.

The manual is comprised of four volumes:

Volume 1: Catering Management
Volume 2: Catering Accounting Regulations
Volume 3: Food Safety Management
Volume 4: Catering, Retail and Leisure.

The contents of each volume were agreed through consultation between the DFS IPT and lead commands of each of the three services. Volume 1 alone covers issues which include management and administration, inspections, deliveries, receipts

Table 5.1 Sample of core menu dinner choices over one week.

Monday	Tuesday	Wednesday	Thursday	Friday	Saturday	Sunday
Lentil soup	Scotch broth	Mushroom soup	Cream of tomato soup	Cream of celery soup	Vegetable soup	Cauliflower soup
Pork with beans sprouts	Noisettes of lamb & garlic sauce	Stir fried beef with green beans	Sweet & sour chicken	Pork cutlets with mushroom sauce	Beef bourguignonne	Roast leg of lamb with mint sauce
Steak & kidney pie	Cod d'orly	Pork stroganoff	Fish & potato pie	Curried beef & boiled rice	Salmon steak	Pork escalope cordon bleu
Mixed grill	Roast turkey & stuffing	Gammon steak hawaiian	Lasagne and garlic bread	Turkey stroganoff & braised rise	Breast of duck a l'orange	Deep-fried chicken in lemon sauce
Vegetable lasagne	Vegetable pudding (suet mix) flavoured with basil & tomato	Chinese stir fry vegetables with egg fried rice	Vegetable stroganoff	Vegetable croquettes	Mushroom & pepper bake	Button mushrooms & spaghetti in a cream sauce
Anna potatoes &/or lorette potatoes	Roast potatoes &/or croquette potatoes	Savoury potatoes &/or parisienne potatoes	Byron potatoes &/or delmonico potatoes	New/boiled potatoes &/or potato rissoles	Marquise potatoes &/or chateau potatoes	Creamed potatoes &/or savoyard potatoes
Boiled french beans &/or fried aubergine or side salad	Boiled swede &/or corn on the cob or side salad	Courgette provençal &/or creamed carrots or side salad	Mixed vegetables &/or grilled mushrooms or side salad	Green peas &/or roast parsnips or side salad	Sauté brussel sprouts &/or stuffed peppers or side salad	Curried mixed vegetables &/or braised cabbage or side salad
Boiled rice or pasta	Fried rice or pasta	Braised rice or pasta	Savoury rice or pasty	Boiled rice or pasta	Fried rice or pasta	Braised rice or pasta
Gravy	Gravy	Gravy	Gravy	Gravy	Gravy	Gravy

Chicken salad	Beef salad	Ham & egg roll	Salmon salad	Gala pie salad	Corned beef salad	Ham salad
Minimum choice of 4 simple salads & 3 compound salads & dressings	Minimum choice of 4 simple salads & 3 compound salads & dressings	Minimum choice of 4 simple salads & 3 compound salads & dressings	Minimum choice of 4 simple salads & 3 compound salads & dressings	Minimum choice of 4 simple salads & 3 compound salads & dressings	Minimum choice of 4 simple salads & 3 compound salads & dressings	Minimum choice of 4 simple salads & 3 compound salads & dressings
Steamed lemon sponge	Rhubarb crumble	Baked jam roll	Break & butter pudding	Baked rice pudding	Apple & blackcurrant pie	Apple crumble
Pineapple fritters	Jam puffs	Lemon sponge pudding	Devonshire roll	Gooseberry crumble	Cherry crumble	Break & butter pudding
Custard sauce	Custard sauce	Custard sauce	Custard sauce	Custard sauce	Custard sauce	Custard sauce
Fresh fruit	Fresh fruit	Fresh fruit	Fresh fruit	Fresh fruit	Fresh fruit	Fresh fruit
Yoghurt	Yoghurt	Yoghurt	Yoghurt	Yoghurt	Yoghurt	Yoghurt
Treacle tart	Peach melba	Meringue buns	Apple strudel	Devonshire splits	Fruit scone	Chocolate gateau

Source: Ministry of Defence (2007c). © Crown copyright/MOD 2007.

and storage, mess management, operational catering, equipment, contracts, information systems (Tricat) and catering competitions.

5.5   Food and nutrient guidelines

Box 5.1 gives the MoD nutrition policy statement. This statement '*commits all catering staff to provide a catering service based on sound nutritional principles reflecting current UK Government advice and initiatives and to support the rigorous physical fitness requirements of an expeditionary Armed Forces Policy*' (MoD, 2007a).

There are currently no nutrient specifications for food provided for the armed forces, but the MoD plans to develop evidence-based UK Military Reference Dietary Intakes (MRDI) for a range of macro- and micro-nutrients. These guidelines are to be informed by the American College of Sports Medicine recommendations for macronutrients in combination with US Nutritional Standards for Operational and Restricted Rations recommendations for overall energy and micronutrient intakes.

Box 5.1   UK MoD nutrition policy statement.

1   The UK Ministry of Defence (MOD) undertakes to provide military personnel with a basic knowledge of nutrition, with the aim of optimising physical and mental function, long-term health, and morale. Educators will use effective education techniques, and programmes developed by, or in consultation with, registered dieticians and other qualified personnel. Programmes will reflect current nutrition knowledge and scientific research findings, and may contain other appropriate information, such as that provided by the UK Department of Health. Advice on the nutritional needs of pregnant or lactating female military personnel, or individuals requiring nutrition therapy for conditions such as illness, injury, infection, chronic disease, or trauma, will be available from qualified personnel on request.

2   The UK MOD undertakes to provide a variety of healthy and palatable food and beverage choices to military personnel to enable them to adopt healthy eating habits, a balanced diet, and to ensure optimal fitness and performance. Contract caterers will be required to provide food at the point of service that meets these requirements.

3   UK Operational Ration Pack/s (ORP) will continue to be provided to sustain troops on operations and during field exercises, with the aim of preserving life, preserving both physical and mental function, maintaining mood and motivation, preventing fatigue, and speeding up recovery. ORP will be designed to meet the energy and nutrient requirements of military personnel operating for periods of at least 30 days in both temperate and extreme environments. The exception to this will be any form of nutritionally incomplete survival ration, or restricted ration, e.g. Assault ORP.

From: Ministry of Defence (2007a). Crown copyright /MOD 2007.

5.5.1   Healthy catering

The DFS IPT policy on healthy catering is:

'To educate and inform personnel of the benefits of maintaining a healthy and balanced diet. To provide and market an adequate variety of foods from which our consumers can select meals to meet individual dietary needs within nutritional guidelines'.   (MoD, 2007a)

The *Defence Catering Manual* provides general information on the role of nutrition in maintaining and promoting health, based on the Government's *Balance of Good Health* (now the *eatwell plate*) (see page 18). Generally, catering managers are advised to:

* *ensure that there is always a choice of food. Do not force healthy choices on people.*
* *Change menus to support sound nutrition and healthy eating and identify the healthier options.*
* *Effect recipe changes to improve the 'healthiness' of popular dishes, for example, measure and gradually reduce salt used in standards recipes.*
* *Highlight the fact that healthier ingredients are being used – for example 'We only fry in polyunsaturated oil' or 'All our recipes use less salt and sugar than before and every opportunity is taken to increase the amount of dietary fibre available'.*
* *Not allow your healthy eating initiative to rely solely upon gimmicky promotional material on the servery. The initiative should be deeper and more comprehensive through menu planning and the cookery processes adopted in the mess.*
* *Change promotional displays frequently to catch the eye and maintain interest.*

The manual wisely, perhaps, advises catering managers that in order to implement healthy catering practices, customers need to be prepared for change. Caterers are advised to achieve this through education and promotional material such as posters and information leaflets which explain the benefits of a healthy diet. It is advised that food should be displayed attractively, with healthy dishes displayed prominently. The manual gives more specific guidance on presentation of food. These include:

* placing healthier choices within the customer's eye and reach;
* presenting vegetables without fat or cream sauces, reducing mayonnaise on dressed salads;
* avoiding using cream in desserts;
* providing a variety of homemade breads and rolls, including wholemeal varieties;

- keeping salt at the servery rather than on the table;
- keeping sugar sachets at beverage dispensers rather than on the table;
- offering a choice of skimmed, semi-skimmed and full-fat milk.

Specific advice is given on how to reduce the amount of fat in the diet, increasing the amount of fibre-rich starchy foods, reducing the amount of sugar and salt. Caterers are advised that they should:

- Reduce the amount of fat, particularly saturated fat, in recipes, by grilling, providing more chicken and fish than red meat, trimming red meat, avoiding frying and using alternative cooking methods such as baking, boiling or steam roasting. Suggestions such as low fat cheeses and yoghurt instead of cream are made.
- Increase fibre-rich foods, by offering wholemeal bread, jacket potatoes, wholegrain cereals, beans, pulses. Other suggestions include the use of raw vegetables in salads and leaving skins on vegetables.
- Reduce the amount of sugar in recipes by, for example, offering fruit as a pudding, unsweetened fruit juice as an alternative to soft drinks, artificial sweeteners.
- Reduce salt in recipes by, for example, using herbs and spices to enhance flavour, or substitute with a low fat product; avoid tinned vegetables with added salt; avoid using processed food and make homemade soup rather than use tinned or dried. Further suggestions include not adding salt to food before serving, but leaving the choice to the customer.

5.5.2   Menu planning

'In accordance with current UK legislation and Government guidelines it is incumbent on HM Forces to cater for all personnel irrespective of gender, race, religious belief, medical requirements and committed lifestyle choices. It is fundamental to menu planning to know your consumer base'.   (MoD, 2007a)

The *Defence Catering Manual* provides advice on the dietary requirements of the main religions including Judaism, Islam and Hinduism. Advice is also given on common medical requirements such as weight loss diets, diabetic and gluten-free diets and lifestyle diets, such as the various forms of vegetarianism.

The menu is to be drawn from the five food groups of the Balance of Good Health: meat, poultry and fish; grains; dairy; fruits and vegetables; fats and oils. The menu must provide compatibility, variety, availability, nutrition and seasonality (to reduce menu boredom and 'reflect tradition'). Convenience foods should be avoided as much as possible. Although it is acknowledged that these may occasionally be appropriate, *the principle of military catering is to provide fresh food, which is freshly prepared* (MoD, 2007a).

The number of choices to be made available depends on the number of people being catered for. Table 5.2 specifies the number of choices which are to be offered

Table 5.2 The number of choices to be offered at both the main meal of the day and the third meal.

Matrix of number of menu choices according to feeding strength

Number to be fed	Main course	Potato	Vegetables	Main meal only	
				Hot sweets	Cold sweets
1–30	2	2	2	1	2
30–60	3	2	2	1	2
60–100	4	2	2	1	1
100–200	5	2	3	2	3
200+	6	2	3	2	3

Source: Ministry of Defence, 2007a. © Crown copyright/MOD 2007.

Table 5.3 Breakfast choices.

First-course options	Second-course options	Third-course options
Cereals and accompaniments	A choice of at least three high quality proteins (eggs, bacon, cheese, ham etc.)	Bread (toast) and bread rolls, pastries, croissants
Fruit (fresh and dried); juice	A choice of at least two portions of vegetables and fruit (tomatoes, mushrooms, beans, potatoes, etc.)	Marmalades, honey, jam and other spreads
		Butter and non-butter spreads
		Tea, coffee, milk and accompaniments including sweeteners

Source: Ministry of Defence, 2007a.

at both the main meal of the day and the third meal. Caterers are advised to avoid repetition.

5.5.2.1 Breakfast

Breakfast must be varied, to avoid 'menu fatigue'. An alternative to the traditional cooked breakfast should always be available, and the choices reviewed regularly. There must be a minimum of three courses plus drinks. Suggestions given for breakfast ideas are presented in Table 5.3.

5.5.2.2 Third meal (usually lunch)

The third meal of the day is similar to the main meal, the exception being that starters are only provided 'where funds permit'. Hot/cold sweets are optional, but fresh fruit and yoghurts should be provided, again where funds permit. Where feasible, cakes can also be offered. Bread and spreads should also be available.

Box 5.2   Guidelines for the main meal of the day.

The starter should consist of a choice from a fresh homemade soup or a simple dish

The main course menu should include a choice of freshly cooked hot main meat, fish and egg dishes.

A non-meat dish and a salad should always be on offer.

In larger messes the salad should take the form of a cold buffet. Where practical, salads should be provided without dressings, but with a choice of dressing available to the diner.

Two choices of potato should be available throughout the meal period. At least one choice should not be fried. Pasta or rice can also be offered either in replacement of, or in addition to a potato choice.

Two or three choices of vegetables should be available throughout the meal period. At least one should be fresh, but ideally both.

Freshly made hot and cold sweets should be available. In addition, fresh fruit and yoghurts should be available to be offered in lieu of a cold sweet choice.

Drinks should include tea, coffee and cold water. Squash may also be provided.

Source: Ministry of Defence, 2007a. © Crown copyright/MOD 2007.

5.5.2.3   Main meal (usually dinner)

The main meal of the day should consist of three courses: starter, hot or cold main course and hot or cold sweet. Box 5.2 provides the guidelines stipulated for planning the main meal.

5.5.2.4   Packed meal

Packed meals must be provided for those on duty away from their unit or unable to attend the mess. They must be prepared fresh on the day of consumption and kept refrigerated until collected. A vegetarian option must be available. A packed meal must contain a minimum of five items:

- Two rounds of sandwiches or similar (such as a tortilla wrap) with a variety of fillings. A pie or pasty may be offered in lieu of one round of sandwiches.
- Two snack/confectionery items
- At least one piece of fruit (more fruit should be offered in exchange for a confectionery item, if requested).

5.6   The provision of food during operations

'UK Operational Ration Packs (ORPs) are designed to sustain troops on operations and during field exercises, with the aim of preserving life,

preserving both physical and mental function, maintaining mood and motivation, preventing fatigue and speeding up recovery'.   (Expert Panel on Armed Forces Feeding (EPAFF), 2006)

'Cooking in a tent, outside in winter with basic equipment and basic, mostly dried, ingredients really tests your ingenuity and skill'. Andrew Preston, Combined Services Culinary Competition winner.   (MoD website)

Food is of particular importance to personnel in the field, especially when far from home. There are few diversions from the normal routine, so food assumes a greater role than it might usually. Operating in the field can be arduous, and the ration pack has to sustain a soldier experiencing physical stressors such as climatic extremes, sleep deprivation and intense physical activity. The food provided is considered fundamental to the physical and mental wellbeing of military personnel, and to play a role in maintaining morale among troops often living and working in difficult and hazardous conditions (DCG, 2005).

The DFS IPT provides food to operations worldwide, including Iraq and Afghanistan. There are currently (May 2008) over 8000 personnel deployed in Afghanistan and 4000 in Iraq. In Iraq, the most shipped product is water – about six litres of bottled water per person per day. Fruit and vegetables can be sent by air freight by the RAF, but dry goods have to be sent by sea from Hampshire to Kabul, a process which takes about 8 weeks. This can be dangerous, as escorted military conveys come under attack from enemy fire. Food supplies are often stolen en route, or supply vehicles even blown up. Suppliers have to negotiate poor roads and hostile terrain. Despite the obstacles they face, catering personnel manage to serve up a surprisingly varied and appetising menu. Breakfast may include cooked foods, porridge, cereals, fruit, yoghurts, toast and jams, and there may be between five and seven hot choices at lunchtime. These choices include meatballs, pasta, chips, omelettes, hot baguettes, baked potato and soup. Also available are filled rolls, salads, fresh fruits and yoghurts. Similar choices are available in the evening, as well as puddings and pastries. There are often themed events, such as curry, chip shop or kebab nights (MoD, 2007d).

Military personnel are issued with ORPs but when troops are engaged in operations, the aim is to provide fresh feeding as soon as possible. The MoD strives to provide a diet to troops serving overseas as close as possible to that served in home establishments. Fresh feeding can take place once centralised cooking facilities have been established. A mobile field bakery system is usually set up, capable of producing in excess of 4000 kilos of bread in a 20-hour working period, supporting 13 000 service personnel a day. Centralised cooking depends on the availability of refrigeration and power generation, and it may be necessary to establish a food distribution centre or create a purpose-built facility (MoD, 2007d). In Afghanistan, food is provided by a distribution centre in Kabul, an ex-Russian food warehouse refurbished by the MoD at the outset of operations in January 2002. A distribution centre in Kuwait provides food to troops in Iraq. A full core range is offered with units receiving three multi-temperature deliveries per week.

When operations become prolonged, it is likely that catering may be transferred to contract support – Contractors on Deployed Operations (CONDO). This depends on the friendliness of the environment and the availability of a local workforce. This is advantageous in that it frees up military manpower, although the decision to use CONDO depends on a risk assessment of the individual situation.

At the beginning of operations, it is inevitable that military personnel will depend exclusively on ORPs. The ORP is designed to meet specific operational requirements which demand quick efficient feeding of troops in the field. Personnel from all three services receive the same ORP. When operations begin, the order of feeding plan is:

(1)   the issue of 24-hour ORPs
(2)   the transition to central feeding, once field kitchens are established. This is based around the 10-man ORP.
(3)   The 10-man ORP is supplemented with fresh foods
(4)   Fresh foods supplemented with ORPs, as required.

ORP meals are either in dehydrated, boil-in-the-bag or tinned format. The ORP is based around a 24-hour cycle, and is normally limited to the first 44 days of an operation. The aim is to move from ORP to fresh feeding as fast as logistics permit, and to ensure that personnel are not feed exclusively on ORPs for more than 14 consecutive days. However, in combat situations it is inevitable that troops will remain on the ORP as the main, if not sole, source of food for prolonged periods (EPAFF, 2006). For small scale operations, it may be appropriate to purchase rations locally, using *cash in lieu of rations* (CILOR).

The Defence Food Services Integrated Project Team (DFS IPT) is responsible for researching, developing, field-testing, evaluating, procuring and packing UK military rations. Meals are packed in 'retort pouches' made of aluminium foil laminate, which can be submerged in boiling water. The components are then packed into a light-weight cardboard carton. The distribution of food to the armed forces in operations is overseen by the Food Supply Management team which also ensures that the ORP is 'fit for purpose' (DCG, 2005). The components of the 24-hour ORP are subject to constant review and assessed by professional *Food Selection Panels* for taste and conformity to MoD specifications on safety, shelf-life, macronutrient composition and packaging. These panels are made up of service personnel of all ranks.

In early 2004 the Expert Panel on Armed Forces Feeding (EPAFF) was set up to examine all aspects of defence catering. One of the first things the EPAFF looked at was the 24-hour ORP. It was felt that the ORP was outdated and did not reflect contemporary, multicultural tastes. In 2004 the EPAFF devised new menus designed to be both tasty and nutritious. These menus included dishes such as chicken balti curry and Italian meatballs with pasta.

Table 5.4   Core items in each ration pack.

Snacks	Drinks	Sundries
Oatmeal block	Instant coffee	Tabasco sauce
Fruit biscuits	Black tea	Chewing gum
Brown biscuits	Whitener	Weatherproof
Chocolate	Sugar	matches
Boiled sweets		Water purification
Vegemite		tablets
Fruit grains		Paper tissues

Source: Ministry of Defence, 2007a. © Crown copyright/MOD 2007.

The ORP range is designed to cater for the specialist needs of ethnic and religious groups and vegetarians. The components of the ORP allow it to be used in both hot and cold conditions and are packed into 10-man and single-man variants, with a shelf life of three years. Inside the box is a menu sheet and cooking instructions. In addition to the meal, the pack is supplied with core items, as listed in Table 5.4: Matches are included for lighting the hexiburner cooker which each soldier carries. This is a small, light cooker designed for burning hexamine fuel tablets. Each soldier is issued with sufficient tablets to last 24 hours, as well as two mess tins, knife, fork, spoon and water bottle.

5.6.1   Types of ORP

'You can often tell the temperature from what's not used in a 10 man ration pack'.   (Little, 2004)

There are two main types of ration packs: those suitable for group feeding and those intended for individual feeding. These ORPs are regularly reviewed and are currently as described below.

5.6.1.1   Group feeding

The 10-man ORP. This pack is designed for feeding 10 men for 24 hours, and requires a chef to prepare the components, so its use depends upon access to a field kitchen (EPAFF, 2006). Basic catering equipment and utensils are required. Chefs – who double up as drivers, stretcher-bearers and soldiers – have to be creative and be able to combine fresh ingredients with standard ORP components. A balance must be struck between preserving food stocks and providing nutritious food. The 10-man ORP box contains commercial tinned and packet foods, plus sauces, herbs and spices for flavouring. There are four menu variants, but no ethnic or religious variants as the components can meet all dietary requirements. The pack may be supplemented with fresh fruit and/or vegetables and other produce such as bread and potatoes.

5.6.1.2   *Individual feeding*

The *24-hour general purpose ORP* is described as the 'backbone' of UK operational feeding (EPAFF, 2006). Each box – which has a shelf life of at least three years in temperate conditions – feeds one man per day. There are seven 'general purpose' menu variants (A to G, Table 5.5). The food it contains can be prepared and consumed in the field, however extreme the conditions, requiring only additional water. The main components are packed in retort pouches designed

Table 5.5   Operational ration packs menu variants.

Menu	Breakfast	Main meal
A (GP)	Hamburger & beans	Soup Chicken mushroom & pasta Treacle pudding
B (GP)	Corned beef hash	Soup Beef stew & dumplings Chocolate pudding in chocolate sauce
C (GP)	Sausage & beans	Soup Lamb stew with potatoes Fruit dumplings & custard sauce
D (GP)	Corned beef hash	Soup Pork casserole Treacle pudding`
E (GP)	Bacon & beans	Soup Lancashire hotpot Fruit dumplings & custard sauce
F (GP)	Beefburger & beans	Soup Steak & vegetables with potatoes Rice pudding
G (GP)	Meatballs and pasta in tomato sauce	Soup Chicken stew and dumplings Chocolate pudding in chocolate sauce
S1 (Sikh/Hindu)	Meat-free sausage & beans	Soup Vegetable tikka masala Treacle pudding
S2 (Sikh/Hindu)	Meat-free mini burger & beans	Soup Vegetable chilli Chocolate pudding in chocolate sauce
S3 (Sikh/Hindu)	Meat-free sausage & beans	Soup Vegetable casserole Rice pudding
H1 (Halal)	Meat-free sausage & beans	Soup Chicken casserole with dumplings Treacle pudding
H2 (Halal)	Meat-free mini burger & beans	Soup Steak & vegetables Chocolate pudding in chocolate sauce
H3 (Halal)	Meat-free sausage & beans	Soup Lamb stew with potatoes Rice pudding

Table 5.5   (Continued)

Menu	Breakfast	Main meal
V1 (veg)	Non-meat sausage & beans	Soup Vegetable tikka masala Treacle pudding
V2 (veg)	Meat-free burger & beans	Soup Pasta with mushrooms & sweetcorn Chocolate pudding in chocolate sauce
V3 (veg)	Potato & beans	Soup Spicy vegetable rigatoni Rice pudding
P1 (patrol)	Hot cereal start	Soup Potato & beef with herbs Rice pudding with apple & cinnamon
P2 (patrol)	Instant oats & apple flakes	Soup Pasta carbonara Chocolate chip pudding
P3 (patrol)	Hot cereal start	Soup Chicken balti Apple with custard
P4 (patrol)	Instant oats & apple flakes	Soup Chicken with noodles Peach & pineapple pudding

Source: Ministry of Defence, 2007a. © Crown copyright/MOD 2007.

to be carried by the soldier in the absence of field kitchens, requiring minimal preparation – they are designed for re-heating by boiling in the bag using the hexamine stove, or eating cold from the pack. The pack may be supplemented with long-life milk and cereal; it contains core ingredients common to all individual ORPs, as shown in Table 5.4. The pack, which weighs on average 1.8 kg, is primarily for use in temperate climatic conditions but is also suitable for both tropical and Arctic conditions.

The 24-hour hot climate ORP. This pack also has seven menu variants (A–G) and is the same as the general purpose ORP but contains additional beverages to make it suitable for use in tropical and humid climatic conditions.

The 24-hour vegetarian ORP is based on the general purpose pack but has contents suitable for lacto-ovo-vegetarian diets. It contains components which have all been approved by the Vegetarian Society. There are three menu variants (V1–V3).

The 24-hour halal ORP is based on the general purpose pack but with contents which meet the dietary requirements of Muslims. The components have all been approved by Islam authorities. There are three menu variants (H1–H3).

The 24-hour Sikh/Hindu pack is based on the general purpose pack but with contents suitable for personnel of both the Sikh and Hindu faiths. It also meets the requirements of a lacto-ovo-vegetarian diet. There are three menu variants (S1–S3).

The 24-hour patrol ORP is a high-calorie pack used mainly by the Royal Marines and Special Forces. Its lightweight, dehydrated formula is designed for training exercises and operations above the snow line, such as Arctic warfare training. The little water that is required to reconstitute a meal can be obtained from snow. Its low moisture content means it can be used in very cold climates without freezing (EPAFF, 2006). There are four menu variants (P1–P4).

In addition to the 24-hour ration packs are the survival rations. These are intended strictly for short-term use in cases of sea and air survival situations. There are three varieties: Emergency Flying Ration (EFR), Submarine Survival Ration (SSR) and Life Raft Survival Ration. There are two types of EFR: mark 4 and mark 9. Mark 4 is designed to sustain fast-jet aircrew disaster survivors and is built into the ejection seat. It consists of a flattened tin, two spring handles, plastic bag and 100 g of fruit-flavoured sweets. Nine sweets are to be eaten each day, at intervals of about an hour. The tin can is intended to hold drinking water and can be used for boiling water to dissolve sweets to make a hot drink.

The mark 9 EFR is used to sustain the crew of multi-engined aircraft disasters. It consists of:

- Two-piece aluminium alloy container.
- Four wire spring handles
- Two emergency foods packs (8 portions per pack)
- One packet of beef stock drinking cubes (6 cubes)
- Two packets of sugar cubes (12 cubes per pack)
- One packet containing beverages and creamer (7 sachets instant coffee, 4 sachets instant tea, 7 sachets of vegetable creamer)
- Two spatulas
- One polythene bag
- Instruction leaflet (with advice on using the survival pack) (EPAFF, 2006).

The Submarine Survival Ration (SSR) takes the form of a bar wrapped in foil, to be consumed in submarine disaster situations. The bar is made of maltodextrine, glucose, sugar, malt extract and vegetable fat (EPAFF, 2006).

5.6.2   Nutritional value of the ORP

The UK ORP currently provides between approximately 3788 and 4996 kcal. The approximate percentage contribution of each macronutrient is: carbohydrate 57%, fat 33%, protein 10% (EPAFF, 2006).

5.6.3   The ORP in maritime operations

Food is either stored on board ship or in what is called solid support ships (SSSs) operated by the Royal Fleet Auxilliary (RFA). Each SSS acts as a food warehouse which distributes food into operations areas. A range of food items is stored, in quantities known as thousands of man months. Storage space is extremely limited and provisions compete with other resources within the hull space available on board. Limited storage space for dried, chilled and frozen foodstuffs means that there is a greater requirement for trained catering specialists within naval vessels. A careful balance must be struck between conserving food stocks and producing attractive menus.

There are two basic types of catering on ships: *defence watch messing* and *action stations*. RN chefs work in 2–4 watches, according to the size of the ship. Three watches are the norm. During tension or war, chefs are allocated to galleys and work in two watches, providing meals, snacks and drinks. During action stations, food and drink must be available at short notice when ordered by the command. Hot food is served to the ship's company at designated points, within the quickest possible time. The galley may only be used once clearance has been given, during a lull in the action. Only 25% of the ship's company may be fed at any one time, in order to maintain 75% fighting efficiency. Simple dishes, requiring minimum preparation are provided to personnel who eat standing up, using disposable utensils wherever possible. Suggested meals are meat stews, Cornish pasties, meat pies, pasta or curry dishes. Energy-boosting snacks (chocolate bars and biscuits are recommended) provided at action messes during a lull in the action may be consumed when authorised by the command.

5.6.4   The ORP in air operations

Because air operations now cover much wider areas but are thought less likely to be conducted in areas with extensive host nation support, there is an increased need for stand-alone support units. Catering support systems for air units are the same as those used in land operations, and are dependent upon the operational environment and prevailing level of activity. There is a need to ensure that aircrew receive a balanced diet at appropriate intervals, and catering personnel must also be able to undertake the full range of military duties, including armed guarding.

5.6.5   Water supplies

During operations, all water in the field is regarded as unsafe unless it comes from an approved source, or has undergone purification. The Army (Royal Engineers) is responsible for ensuring that potable water is provided to all services in all theatres, during both war and peace time. Calculations for the provision of domestic water supplies are based on a requirement of 22.5 litres of person per day (MoD, 2007a).

5.7   Monitoring of standards

Internal inspections are carried out by mess managers or catering managers who then compile inspection reports. Each of the three services has its own system of inspections in place. There is no formal standardised inspection report, but unit inspections must:

- ensure compliance with legislation, regulations and the contract
- ensure economy efficiency and value for money
- identify any necessary changes required to reflect new developments
- provide the foundation for any risk analysis-based inspections (MoD, 2007c).

A performance review is carried out 'on a regular basis' which must consider, among other issues:

- purchasing and food supply
- recipe development and costing
- calculating selling prices
- menu planning
- production planning and control
- food service
- marketing and merchandising
- consumer satisfaction   (MoD, 2007c)

The unit Commanding Officer is ultimately responsible for ensuring that a satisfactory standard of messing is maintained. It is the responsibility of the orderly officer in each unit to check that what is stated on the menu is the same as what is provided on the hot plate, and to listen to feedback from personnel. In 2006, the National Audit Office published the results of commissioned research into in-house catering at a 'typical' armed forces base and found that:

- food displays and presentation were very good
- menus were balanced nutritionally
- food was stored and labelled appropriately
- monitoring systems were in place
- cleaning schedules were in place (NAO, 2006)

The catering manager of each unit is expected to monitor changes in sales and consumption patterns of foods high in fats, salt and sugar and record customer comments and feedback. Customer feedback on food standards is monitored regularly. The software system Tricat (page 374) which is used to manage every aspect of armed forces catering, can also be used to provide a full nutritional analysis of a meal or full menu cycle. However, although menus are based on recommendations and recipes from the *Defence Catering Manual* there are currently no mandated nutritional standards to which the daily menu must comply.

Overall, the DFS IPT Quality Assurance team ensures that the quality of food supplied under contract meets standards, whether in messes or on operations. The team is responsible for inspecting food premises, monitoring manufacturing processes and assessing the effectiveness of the quality management systems used by suppliers, particularly in the production of operational ration packs.

5.8   Catering costs

The catering department of each of the three services within the armed forces is responsible for ensuring that expenditure on food is kept within the budget. It is estimated by the MoD that 127 million meals were served in 2004–05 at a procurement cost of approximately £135 million. Around £100 million was spent on non-operational feeding, which covers UK bases and £35 million spent on operational feeding (Casey & Wood, 2006). The amount spent per day per person on food (three meals) is known as the daily messing rate (DMR). The DMR is based on a 'shopping basket' of around 100 staple foodstuffs (bread, milk, fruit and vegetables, etc.) costed at current food source prices, calculated on a monthly basis. The DMR is the same for all three services, but may be set higher if local prices are more expensive. In early 2007 the DMR was approximately £1.51 per day per person in the UK. The DMR for personnel serving in both Iraq and Afghanistan was £3.11 per day in early 2007.

The cost of producing an operational pack is much higher. In July 2008 it was reported that the Ministry of Defence had purchased 9.8 million 24-hour ORPs since 2003 (Hansard, 2008a) and the average cost of producing a general purpose ORP was £8.75 (Hansard, 2008b). It is not surprising that the military aims to move from ORPs to fresh feeding as soon as possible.

5.9   Catering contracts and procurement

The Defence Food Services Integrated Project Team (DFS IPT) oversees the Ministry of Defence food supply contract, which was granted, in October 2006, to Purple Foodservice Solutions (PFS) in a deal worth up to £300 million over five years. From 1997 to 2006 the contract was with the UK's largest food service distributor, 3663 First for Foodservice.

Known as the 'publicly funded messing (PFM) contractor', Purple Food Service is the main supplier to the armed services and is a consortium of three shareholding partners: DBC Foodservice Limited, which supplies food to the armed forces in the UK; Supreme Foodservice Solutions A.G., which manages all overseas deliveries and Vestey Foods UK Limited, which is a major supplier of meat and poultry products. According to Purple Food Service, *The contract seeks a value for money approach in procuring an efficient, effective and economical food supply to troops throughout the globe'* (Purple website). Because the contract is aggregated and managed across the whole of the armed forces, it is considered to be more economically efficient – the MoD expects to generate savings of £19.4 million by 2010 (NAO, 2006).

The contractor supplies an extensive approved list of food items known as the 'core list' consisting of over 1400 products. It is also responsible for security and any administration involved. An updated core range price list is distributed to units once a month. In order to feature on the core list, a food product must meet seven criteria:

(1) it must have a long shelf life wherever possible
(2) packaging must be strong enough to survive transit and meet shelf life
(3) it must provide value for money by offering the best quality at the optimum price
(4) it must have security of supply: each item requires year-round availability and suitability for export
(5) it must meet government guidelines for reduced salt, fat and sugar levels
(6) it must meet surge capacity – that is, be available in larger amounts at short notice
(7) it must meet the mandate to buy British wherever possible (NAO, 2006).

Every month a Food Selection Panel meets to confirm existing core range products or select new products to be added to the range. The decisions of the panel are discussed by a standing committee comprised of a representative of each of three services, together with a dietitian and any other interested parties and then a final decision is made on the selection of items for the core list.

The Food Selection Panel ensures that members of the armed forces retain some control over the quality of the food provided. Although value for money is considered of paramount importance, the panel can help ensure that other issues are taken into consideration, such as healthy options and quality. Members of the panel can also ensure that no products containing genetically modified ingredients make it onto the core list, thus relieving chefs of their obligation to declare their presence on their menus (Defra, 2007).

Other contracts, known as *Local Service Contracts* are in place in theatres throughout the world where there is no permanent contract in place. The range tends to be less comprehensive than the core list and purchases must be kept to a minimum (MoD, 2007a).

Procurement of food not on the core list is the responsibility of the Defence Logistics Organisation (DLO). The armed forces are subject, like other public sector procurers, to the EU Treaty of Rome which protects the free movement of goods and service and prohibits discrimination on the grounds of nationality. Therefore, public sector buyers cannot restrict their purchases to specific locations or buyers. However, in 2004 the European Parliament endorsed two new directives on public procurement which were enshrined in law in early 2006. These introduced a change in the European regulatory context of public procurement by stating that:

'Contracting authorities may lay down special conditions relating to the performance of a contract ... The conditions governing the performance of a contract

may, in particular, concern social and environmental considerations' (European Parliament and Council, 2004).

This means that the public sector can be more environment-minded in its procurement of food. Currently the proportion of UK produced food procured by the MoD is 43%. There is no figure available for schools, but the MoD figure is similar to that of the NHS – 40% – but compares poorly to the Prison Service, which procures 67% of its food from the UK (Psfpi, 2008). The MoD has acknowledged that '*... There has been increasing interest in using public sector procurement to make the transition to a more sustainable economy*' (DFS IPT, 2007). In 2007 the DFS IPT published its *Sustainable procurement action plan* (DFS IPT, 2007). Among the 'guiding principles' laid down in the action plan, the DFS IPT says it will, in future:

- *Consider, and include reference to, the achievement of environmental and sustainable development objectives in our business plan*
- *Ensure non-discrimination against local and UK suppliers and, where suppliers are located in overseas countries, ensure that 'fair trade' terms are applied.*
- *Promote food with health benefits including those organically produced. Promote menu planning which encourages the use of seasonal and, where possible, locally grown products (currently the armed forces do not source any organic foods or ingredients (PSFPI proportion).*
- *Where practicable, reduce air and road mileage of products.*
- *Improve waste management, in particular the removal of unnecessary packaging and use of biodegradable materials.*

Because MoD contracts have always, in the past, been awarded on the basis of best value for money, it would have been difficult, before the introduction of the new European directives in 2004, to apply these new guiding principles. The DFS IPS in its *action plan* states that in future, contracts will also take into account environmental and social criteria. Food Selection Panels will also assess the core range on its sustainability credentials. Box 5.3 outlines the decision-making criteria that the DFS IPS has defined for future procurement of food, services and catering equipment.

On a practical level, the DFS IPS has organised a sustainable procurement pilot with its key suppliers to improve their awareness of the subject and all commercial staff are expected to have completed sustainable awareness training. The results of the pilot were due to be assessed by April 2008.

5.10   Catering training

Uniquely among institutions, armed forces chefs and caterers are drawn from the forces themselves. Furthermore, the armed forces have a long history of ensuring that their chefs and caterers are well trained. Until 2004, each service had its own

---

Box 5.3   Criteria for integrating sustainable procurement into goods, works and service procurement.

Identify requirement	Is the product really necessary? Am I replacing an existing product? Can I include environmental criteria within the specification? Is there an eco-label or equivalent for this product? Will its purchase require subsequent items? Will I be able to return it to the manufacturer at the end of its life for responsible disposal? What alternative disposal routes are available?
Select product	Is there a more sustainable equivalent? Can I buy locally? Are any associated items sustainable, e.g. batteries/consumables? Have I recorded my decision in the audit trail for future information?
Disposal	How can I dispose of the item? Re-use/re-cycle or return to the manufacturer?

Source: DFS IPT, 2007. © Crown copyright/MOD 2007.

---

separate catering school: the Army, RAF and RN Schools of Catering. The three services are now in the process of being brought together under the Defence Food Services School (DFSS) established at St Omer Barracks in Aldershot in 2004 and where TV chef Jamie Oliver famously sent his school dinner ladies to learn to cook. The DFSS is part of the Defence Logistic Support Training Group, and it trains students in all aspects of military feeding, including sourcing and supply of food, accounting, healthy eating and serving the finished product. The school trains up to 1200 students a year on 40 different courses.

The main components of the DFSS are:

- Cookery Training Squadron (CTS (Army)) which trains recruits as military chefs, bakers, butchers and victuallers.
- Cookery Training Squadron (CTS RAF) which trains personnel in chef and steward craft and management at RAF Halton.
- Royal Naval Logistic School, based at HMS Raleigh in Cornwall, which provides all RN and most Royal Marine catering-related training alongside other logistic training.
- Operations Food Services Squadron which trains personnel in catering and stewarding management in operational (field) cookery.
- The Catering Support Regiment – a regular unit based in Grantham which trains and provides around 400 reservist chefs to territorial army and regular units in support of operations and training.

All new recruits to the armed forces must first undergo basic military training regardless of their ultimate specialisation. This is known as phase one training. Only then can they opt to enrol at the DFSS, as part of their 16-week phase two training. During phase two training, recruits learn basic craft chef training and field cookery – catering for groups of soldiers under difficult circumstances and with limited facilities. They also gain certificates in food hygiene and health and safety.

The DFSS is a City & Guilds awarding body, and its personnel are trained initially to NVQ Level 2 standard. Recruits are trained in food preparation and cooking; food and drink service and customer service. Of the recruits who attend the school, 96% receive their NVQ qualification at the first attempt (personal communication, 08/05/06). For those who wish to pursue a food service career in the armed forces, phase three training allows personnel to graduate as military chefs or catering managers. Non-chef courses lead to qualifications in victualling, butchering and baking. Officers can study for a diploma in logistics and nutrition (awarded by Swansea University) and take modules towards a masters degree in logistics (personal communication, 08/05/06).

5.11 Nutritional requirements of armed forces personnel

'Military personnel who establish a strong nutritional status will better endure the harsh environments encountered in today's battlefield'. (Thomas *et al.*, 1993)

Strenuous physical activity places extra demands on the body for nutrients and water. A 2004 US study estimated the mean total energy requirement of male military personnel to be 4610 kcal/day, and 2850 kcal/day for female personnel (Tharion *et al.*, 2004). Requirements for the average male civilian are estimated to be 2500 kcal/day and 2000 kcal/day for the average female civilian.

The physical demands of performing military duties are generally thought to be similar to those of endurance athletes. However there are occasions when those demands are even greater for military personnel. Combat training, for example, has been found to produce higher energy requirements than non-combat training, and cold weather and high-altitude conditions to result in higher energy expenditure than hot weather conditions, which do not appear to influence total energy expenditure (Tharion *et al.*, 2004).

In an extremely cold environment, personnel are at risk of physical exhaustion and hypothermia. Energy expenditure increases in the cold and it is estimated that work in the cold may require 4000–5000 calories a day (Thomas *et al.*, 1993). This is especially true in conditions of high altitude, where reliance on carbohydrates is considered even greater. Energy requirements for high-altitude operations are estimated to increase 15–50% above sea-level requirements (Thomas *et al.*, 1993). It is harder to work at high altitude, so more energy is required. However, reduced oxygen suppresses the appetite. Weight loss is considered inevitable for those involved in high-altitude operations.

Weight loss is also fairly common in the field and is a serious concern for the armed forces. Soldiers can reduce their food intake by up to 40%, and this weight loss can quickly result in impaired physical and mental performance (Thomas *et al.*, 1993). The cause of this weight loss is due partly to ration pack boredom and failure to consume all components of the pack. This one of the many reasons why it is important to establish fresh feeding in the field as soon as possible. Even so, soldiers often endure periods of limited food intake (Montain & Young, 2003). Some of the earliest US military research into diet and performance, focussed on health and the consequences of under-feeding in soldiers and examined methods of producing the optimal survival rations to mitigate the adverse effects of fasting (Montain & Young, 2003). A review of studies into the effects of fasting and performance among military personnel found that, in the long term, underfeeding had detrimental effects on soldier physical performance capability. However, in the short term, underfeeding was found to have limited impact on muscle strength and aerobic endurance. Nutritional supplementation was not found to have any advantage over a well-balanced diet (Montain & Young, 2003).

5.11.1   Expert Panel on Armed Forces Feeding (EPAFF)

In early 2004 the MoD established the *Expert Panel on Armed Forces Feeding* (EPAFF), a joint venture of the Defence Catering Group (now the Defence Food Services Integrated Project Team (DFS IPT), the defence technology company QinetiQ and food research company CCFRA (Chipping Campden Food Research Association). The panel is made up of catering and medical staff, plus external experts. When it was established, the EPAFF's remit was to examine all aspects of defence catering and 'provide a world-class military feeding capability' (EPAFF, 2006). EPAFF reviews and examines development in food and nutrition *to meet the challenges of feeding service personnel under demanding operations as well as in barracks* (MoD, 2007a). EPAFF was responsible for overhauling the operational ration pack in 2004 in order to produce more appealing, as well as more nutritious packs for personnel in the field (see page 384).

5.12   Nutrition education

The new Pay-as-You-Dine system, which is expected to be rolled out across all three services of the armed forces by 2009, means that personnel are not penalised for choosing to eat outside the mess canteen. What this financial freedom means is that it has become harder to monitor the nutritional value of foods selected. Personnel are under no obligation to choose healthy, nutritious foods – they can only be encouraged to do so. To this end, the EPAFF produced a series of educational literature aimed at both new recruits and commanders, whom, it is hoped, would influence the dietary choices of those under their command.

5.12.1   The UK Armed Forces Personal Guide to Nutrition

This guide (Casey & Wood, 2006) was published in October 2006 'to ensure that all new entry trainees passing through training establishments have at least a basic understanding of the principles of nutrition and healthy eating' (MoD, 2007a). It replaced an earlier version, *Recruits Guide to Nutriition* (Casey *et al.*, 2005), published in 2005. This updated, simpler and more reader-friendly colour brochure is written in a plain, easy to understand format and is intended for all recruits.

The guide is divided into five sections:

(1) *Eating a balanced diet.* This section provides basic dietary advice on the main food groups, based on the *Balance of Good Health* (see page 18). There is a heavy emphasis on loading up on carbohydrates, with the recommendation that at least half of the total energy intake should be in the form of carbohydrate. The five-a-day message is emphasised and recruits are advised to avoid sugary food and decrease saturated fat. Recruits are also advised on how to cut down on salt and alcohol.

(2) *Your energy requirements.* Recruits are advised that energy input must be equal to energy output in order to be able to sustain training. A table is provided showing how much energy male and female recruits require, depending on the amount of physical activity they are engaged in (Table 5.6).

(3) *Your fluid requirements.* This section offers advice on recognising and preventing dehydration.

(4) *Operational ration packs (ORPs).* This brief section emphasises the need to ensure that the ration pack is consumed so that energy requirements may be met and physical and mental functions maintained.

Table 5.6   Energy input requirements for average-size personnel.

Amount of energy needed from food and drink each day	Megajoules (MJ)	Kilocalories (kcal)
Men		
UK Phase 1 Recruit Training (Army)	15.0	3570
UK Officer Cadet Training (RMA Sandhurst) (average of training in RMAS and on Exercise)	20.1	4780
UK SAS Selection, Brecon Beacons, Weeks 1–4. Includes 64 km march with 25 kg bergen and weapon.	27.5	6550
British Infantry, Collective Training, Kenya (hot, dry)	16.1	3833
Training once per day (e.g. 30 minute run)	12.8	3050
Mainly sedentary (no physical training)	10.6	2550
Bedrest (no walking about at all)	7.3	1740
Women		
UK Phase 1 Recruit Training (Army)	12.4	2960
UK Officer Cadet Training (RMA Sandhurst) (average of training in RMAS and on Exercise)	15.9	3780
Training once per day (e.g. 30 minute run)	9.2	2200
Mainly sedentary (no physical training)	8.1	1940
Bedrest (no walking about at all)	6.0	1400

From: Casey & Wood, 2006. Reproduced with kind permission from QiniteQ.

(5)   *Sports drinks and food supplements.* Sports drinks are recommended because they replace fluid and carbohydrates. Vitamin and mineral supplements are not considered necessary if a balanced diet is being consumed.

5.12.2   Commanders' Guide to Nutrition

The Commander's Guide (Messer *et al.*, 2005) was launched at the same time as the original Recruit's Guide, and constitutes a much more detailed resource package for use by senior members of the armed forces. It is designed to teach commanders 'the basics of good nutrition' and to help them 'improve both the physical and mental performance' of their troops and themselves. Indeed, the guide states that improving diet can increase performance, reduce the chance of being injured, help an individual stay healthy and fit and recover more quickly from training sessions. The guide is in four sections:

(1)   *Good nutrition.* The section is fundamentally a short course in the basics of nutrition and provides detailed advice on macronutrients, micronutrients, fibre and fluids. It describes dietary reference values, guidance on how to calculate individual energy requirements using a basal metabolic rate table and physical activity level table as well as precise information on how to read food labels.

(2)   *Nutrition and physical performance.* Athletes and those undertaking regular physical exercise have different dietary requirements than the general population. Emphasis is very much on carbohydrates and maintaining glycogen stores in muscle through eating and drinking extra carbohydrates. 'Sports' drinks are recommended to sustain both glycogen and fluid levels. This is considered to be especially important in the first few hours after exercise to ensure recovery and prepare for future performance. Immediately following heavy, prolonged exercise, military personnel are advised to consume approximately 1 g/kg body mass of carbohydrate and to continue to do so every 2 hours until the next mealtime. The meal itself should be carbohydrate-dense. The guide advises that this level of carbohydrate loading, a common strategy employed by athletes to increase glycogen stores before prolonged exercise, is only likely to confer benefits when the exercise carried out lasts more than 60 minutes. Exercise lasting less than that time requires a normal diet.

Advice is also provided concerning nutritional requirements for military operations in extreme environments. Not only can exposure to extreme environments impair military performance, it can also be life-threatening. One concern is that soldiers in the field tend to reduce their food intake. It is advised that, in a hot environment, soldiers should be encouraged to eat adequately in order to ensure that sufficient sodium is being consumed. Sodium is lost in sweat, and deficiency causes dehydration, nausea and cramp. It is advised that in high temperatures stimulants such as caffeine and alcohol should be avoided.

(3) *Nutrition and health.* This section provides information on disease prevention, including obesity and diabetes; food allergies and intolerances; malnutrition; the needs of adolescents and vegetarians and cultural minorities; eating disorders; common dietary deficiencies (calcium, iron folate) and nutrition and injury. The latter is particularly important to the military because there is a high incidence of musculoskeletal injuries during military training, especially among new recruits, females in particular. Good nutrition can reduce the risk of injury by delaying the onset of muscle fatigue. To avoid injury, the guide advises commanders to:

- encourage personnel to eat meals
- encourage the consumption of carbohydrate and fluids
- encourage consumption of high calcium foods, particularly by females

(4) *Military operational ration packs – nutrition in the field.* Commanders are told that military personnel should be encouraged to consume as much of their ORP as possible, and to educate their personnel to *'believe that adequate nutrition and hydration are essential for maintaining their "fitness to fight"'*. Personnel are discouraged from eating local foods, which should be considered unsafe to eat, because of the risk of debilitating gastrointestinal complaints.

5.12.3 *Commanders' Guide to Fluid Intake During Military Operations in the Heat*

Dehydration can have a significant impact on performance: even a 2% decrease in body weight, due to water loss, can significantly decrease performance (Thomas *et al.*, 1993). Electrolytes are lost in sweat, which can result in deficiency. Soldiers need to drink even when they do not feel thirsty; the thirst mechanism is poor and awareness of thirst only occurs once dehydration has begun. Recognising that dehydration could become a serious problem, the Defence Logistics Organisation (DLO) produced *Commanders' Guide to Fluid Intake During Military Operations in the Heat* (Nevola *et al.*, 2005). The guide outlines the causes and dangers of dehydration and offers advice on how to avoid dehydration whilst carrying out military activities in the heat. The DLO and defence technology company QinetiQ have also produced a factsheet based on the guide, called *10 Top Tips on Hydration* (Box 5.4). This factsheet provides information on recognising dehydration by the colour of urine and ensuring that troops are aware of the importance of remaining in a hydrated state during training or operational activity.

5.12.4 Armed Forces Nutritional Advisory Service (AFNAS)

In January 2006, the DFS IPT launched AFNAS to provide advice and information on diet, nutrition and military feeding to UK military personnel and military civil servants. This is a free, confidential email service. Personnel may enquire about

Box 5.4   Ten Top Tips on Hydration.

1 Check your urine – this is the best test. If you are well hydrated your urine will be light in colour and there will be plenty of it. If you are dehydrated your urine will be darker and there will be less of it. Use the urine colour chart in the Commanders' Guide to Fluid Intake to help you.

2 Ensure you begin training or operational activity in a hydrated state. A small degree of dehydration will not affect you, but severe dehydration harms both performance and health.

3 Take responsibility for finding out how much fluid you require. Sweat losses vary a great deal between individuals and some soldiers will need to drink more than others. Do the urine test above to establish your personal fluid requirement. It doesn't take long to do this, but remember that your needs will change depending upon the amount of exercise you do, the type and amount of clothing you are required to wear, and the weather. If you can, try to weigh yourself before and after exercise to help you gauge how much fluid you need (see below).

4 If you can, weigh yourself, either nude or in the same dry clothing, before and after exercise. Weight loss during a single period of exercise equates largely to fluid loss (1 kg body weight lost = 1 litre of water lost). This is a simple and accurate way to find out how much fluid you need to drink after exercise. If you can, drink up to one and a half times the amount lost (e.g. if you have lost 2 kg in weight, aim to drink 3 litres of fluid during the recovery period). Scientific studies have shown that this strategy restores hydration status more effectively than simply matching weight loss because it takes account of the urine you will continue to pass in the hours after exercise.

5 Where possible, drink cool fluids before, during, and after training and operational activity. If you have access to them, sports-type drinks (usually isotonic) are best. The small amounts of carbohydrate and sodium they contain increase the rate of fluid uptake by the body, improve taste, and maintain the desire to drink, thereby helping to ensure the replacement of body fluids (and salts) lost in sweat. Plain water is fine, but you may stop feeling thirsty, and therefore stop drinking, before you are properly rehydrated. Scientific studies have shown that consumption of water alone is unlikely to restore and maintain hydration status after exercise as effectively as a sports-type drink.

6 Carry drinks when you can, or try to ensure you will have access to safe drinking water.

7 Pay attention to drinking during and after exercise in all weather conditions. We all know that, in the heat, body water is lost as sweat and must be replaced. Fewer soldiers are aware that there is a real risk of dehydration during cold weather training and operations. In the cold, soldiers still sweat during exercise, and breathing in cold, dry air draws water out of the airways. Indeed, some soldiers on cold weather deployments may actually lose more fluid than those operating in temperate or warm environments because the insulation provided by their clothing can reduce heat loss and promote sweating. If clothing is inadequate and the body cools, they will lose water by urinating more often. Despite this, the cold will make them feel less thirsty. The effort of producing potable water from snow, difficulties in preparing and serving food in cold conditions, and the dehydrated nature of cold climate meals, which are sometimes eaten without being reconstituted, also increase the risk of dehydration.

8 Avoid fizzy drinks and alcohol. Fizzy drinks tend to fill you up before you are hydrated, and alcohol can lead to further dehydration.

9 Don't drink too much! Continually having to stop to go to the toilet won't help you or your Unit, and the extra body weight won't help you either. Do the urine test on a regular basis, and find out how much you need to remain properly hydrated, but, again, remember that it will change depending upon the amount of exercise you do, the clothing you are required to wear, and the weather.

10 Look out for 'salty sweaters'. Some individuals lose a lot of salt in their sweat during exercise, and this can sometimes be seen as white crumbly patches dried on the skin and clothing after exercise. These individuals may be at greater risk of muscle cramps during exercise, and may benefit from drinks containing salts such as sodium. They should try to eat a meal after exercise as foods (particularly foods in operational ration packs) are also a good source of salt.

From: Nevola *et al.*, 2005. Reproduced with kind permission from QinetiQ.

general nutrition, meal ideas, how to follow specific diets, how to eat to improve training and performance, read labels, lose weight and so on.

5.13 Competitions

'Participation in catering competitions leads ultimately to an improvement in an individual's craft skill which in turn, enhances the quality of catering provided to the Armed Forces'.   (MoD, 2007a)

Within the armed forces a number of catering competitions have long been established. Indeed, army cookery competitions were held as early as 1896 (Cole, 1984). It may be argued that the armed forces are by their very nature competitive, but there is a real need to maintain the impetus to provide quality food. The Armed Forces Catering Manager of the Year award was introduced in recognition that 'the feeding of military personnel is a unique skill', deserving of particular recognition (MoD, 2007a).

The most important competition today is the Combined Services Culinary Challenge (CSCC), an annual, inter-service competition. The main aim of this competition is *'to provide chefs and stewards of the Armed Forces with a competition which will further develop their culinary skills, nurture pride in their professional achievement and build team spirit for the ultimate benefit of the Armed Forces as a whole'* (MoD website). All types of armed forces catering are featured and the judging panel includes Michelin-starred chefs. According to Royal Navy Captain Paul Cunningham, head of the Defence Food Services project team at Defence Equipment and Support and organiser of the Combined Services Culinary Challenge, *'The Combined Services Culinary Challenge really does bring out the best from chefs in all three Services and civilians; there is fierce inter-Service rivalry, creating a unique atmosphere throughout the event. Service chefs take enormous pride in their work and in ensuring they maintain their very high professional standards. This competition ensures that those high standards are maintained and keeps everyone on their toes'* (MoD, 2007e).

The CSCC includes cookery skill classes and exhibitions and a field cookery competition. It also provides the opportunity to select personnel for the Combined Services Culinary Arts Team (CSCAT), which represents the UK armed forces at national and international culinary events. CSCAT enters two competitions a year, usually one of which is national and the other international.

In addition to the combined services competitions, each individual service also has its own award events. The Royal Navy has a number of annual awards for proficiency and catering. The army has awards for field cookery and catering, among others, and the RAF, which makes a number of awards including RAF Catering Student of the Year, believes that the competitions it holds *'did a great deal to improve cheerless RAF dining halls throughout the UK'* (MoD website).

5.14   Discussion and conclusion

The provision of food in the armed forces is considered a matter of paramount importance, which is why catering is an integral part of the forces, rather than an out-sourced service. Food is valued not only as a source of fuel but also for its role in building morale. It has powerful symbolic meaning, which is why food provided in overseas operations is designed to resemble food provided at 'home'.

It is the military's grasp of food's many functions which is the key to its success. For this reason, the armed forces are able to serve up more than passable meals in places such as Afghanistan and Iraq, and overcome numerous obstacles to do so, whilst other institutions struggle to provide a decent meal in the UK. The success of armed forces catering is not ascribable to one particular factor, but a combination of factors, driven by will and commitment. These include:

Central control. The entire catering system of the armed forces, whether in the UK or on operations abroad, is under the direction of the Defence Food Services Integrated Project Team (DFS IPT). As a result, the armed forces are able to make 'smart' procurements. With one central organisation aggregating and managing the contract, the service is highly efficient, both practically and financially.

Centralised software management. The work of the DFS IPT is facilitated by a computer software system – Tricat, which manages all aspects of catering, from supply chain procurement to full financial reporting.

Catering is a valued and integral part of the armed forces. The various culinary competitions within the forces ensure that creativity and standards are constantly driven upwards.

Food Selection Panels ensure that standards are upheld and that the views of personnel from all three services are represented.

Despite the achievements of armed forces catering, there are still challenges to be met. The MoD ensures that members of the armed forces are educated on the need to make healthy dietary choices, and produces good, clear literature to this effect. The email service provided by the Armed Forces Nutritional Advisory Service offers individualised advice to anyone requiring specific dietary advice. In short, there is no lack of information available to members wishing to better educate themselves on the subject of dietetics.

However, there is no guarantee that important messages will assimilated, or even read. Each new recruit receives a raft of literature offering advice on military life and there is no obligation to read any of it. Furthermore, members of the armed forces, when not on exercises or operations, are free to eat whatever they choose. In fact, over 50% of personnel live outside units, usually because they are married.

Despite the efforts of the armed forces to encourage healthy catering and healthy eating practices, there is concern that recruits continue to shun healthy options in favour of less healthy ones. Chips remain a universal favourite, and vegetable dishes, which are always provided, frequently end up in the bin at the end of the meal service (personal communication, 26/04/06). The head chef in each unit has to develop strategies to persuade recruits to eat more vegetables – by disguising them in sauces, for example. Vegetables are not popular, though salads generally are and fruit is frequently taken away for later consumption (personal communication, 26/04/06).

Paradoxically, personnel are at risk of both under-nutrition and obesity, depending on the stage of training they have arrived at. It is generally assumed that military personnel undergo intense physical training throughout their career. However, this is really only true of new recruits, during phase 1 training. Although there are no studies on the nutritional status of armed forces personnel undergoing phase 1 training, surveys in the US have found that a large proportion of female soldiers have sub-optimal levels of energy and protein intake, as well as calcium and iron (King *et al.*, 1993). It is believed that this could present health problems during extended periods of action.

The level of activity experienced during phase 1 training may be greatly reduced by the time recruits begin phase 2 training. This has given rise to concerns regarding overweight and obesity within the armed forces (personal communication, 08/05/06). A phase 2 soldier may spend a great deal of time behind a desk, but still be consuming as much food as during phase 1.

Perhaps the greatest challenge to armed forces catering lies in the outcome of the PAYD scheme. The mess canteens need to keep their customers, and they can only do this if prices remain competitive and the food remains appetising. Three daily meals at a total cost of £3.76 is certainly good value for money, but caterers cannot afford to maintain these prices and throw away unpopular food, such as vegetables. Providing meals which are both popular and nutritious remains an ongoing challenge. Weaning personnel off staples such as chips and other, less nutritious foods may prove a challenge too far.

Finally, it remains to be seen how the forces will rise to the challenges outlined in the DFS IPT document on sustainability – *Sustainable procurement action plan* (DFS IPT, 2007). As the document states, *Sustainable Procurement involves a change in mindset rather than simply the implementation of a varied range of policies.* However, the armed forces appear to enjoy a challenge and it will be interesting to observe how a new mindset, which values not only the individual but the environment, is created.

Note

1   A small cake of compressed, shredded dried meat, made into a paste with fat and berries, or dried fruit. '*Of the cocoa I have nothing but good to say, it is excellent, but I don't think that much can be said of the pemmican; it is no doubt theoretically very nourishing, but at the same time I think it very nasty; it may be my bad taste, but I think that if any of you like to taste it you will agree with me that it is not the sort of food the British soldier would like to make a hearty meal from*'. (Clayton, 1899)

References

Casey, A., Messer, P. & Owen, G. (2005) *Recruits Guide to Nutrition.* QinetiQ Report no. QINETIQ/KI/CHS/CRO21121.

Casey, A. & Wood, P. (2006) *UK Armed Forces Personal Guide to Nutrition. Expert Panel on Armed Forces Feeding.* Farnborough: QinetiQ.

Clayton, F.T. (1899) *Supply of an army in the field.* Aldershot Military Lectures 64–90 (355.4) (Tuesday, 28 March).

Cole, H.N. (1984) *The Story of the Army Catering Corps and its Predecessors.* Army Catering Corps Association.

Cope, Z. (1959) The human factor in group feeding. Alexis Soyer and the Crimean War. *Proceedings of the Nutrition Society*, 18(1):6–8.

Crowdy, J.P. (1980) The science of the soldier's food. *The Army Quarterly and Defence Journal*, 110(3):266–279.

Defence Catering Group (2005) *Customer Information Pack. Feeding the Forces.* Bath: Defence Catering Group.

Defence Food Services Integrated Project Team (2007) *Sustainable procurement action plan.* 800/15. 2 November 2007, version 1.1. MoD.

Defra (2007) *MoD's central food supply.* www.defra.gov.uk. Accessed February 2008.

Expert Panel on Armed Forces Feeding (EPAFF) UK (2006) Operation Ration Packs of the British Armed Forces. Bath: DCG.

European Parliament and Council (2004) Directive 2004/18/EC of 31 March 2004 on the coordination of procedures for the award of public works contracts, public supply contracts and public service contracts. *Official Journal of the European Union*, 47:1–127.

Fortescue, J. (1928) *A Short Account of Canteens in the British Army.* Cambridge: Cambridge University Press.

Fretwell Downing Hospitality. Tricat – Feeding the forces with technology. www.fdhospitality. com. Accessed February 2008.

Hansard (2008a) House of Commons written answers, 16 July 2008. www.parliament.co.uk. Bob Ainsworth responding to Bob Spink.

Hansard (2008b) House of Commons written answers, 15 July 2008. www.parliament.co.uk. Bob Ainsworth responding to Bob Spink.

Hill, J.R. (ed.) (2002) *The Oxford Illustrated History of the Royal Navy.* Oxford: Oxford University Press.

Hussain, H. (2007) Active service. *Hotelkeeper*, 29 November 2007.

Kemp, P. (1970) *The British Sailor: A Social History of the Lower Deck*. London: Dent.

King, N., Fridlund, K.E. & Askew, E.W. (1993) Nutrition issues of military women. *Journal of the American College of Nutrition*, **40**(4):344–348.

Le Gros Clark, F. (1959) Alex Soyer (1809–1858) – an historical note on his contributions in applied nutrition. *Proceedings of the Nutrition Society*, **18**(1):1–6.

Little, J. (2004) Feeding the forces. *Defence Management Journal*, 17 June 2004.

Macdonald, J. (2004) *Feeding Nelson's Navy. The True Story of Food at Sea in the Georgian Era*. London: Chatham Publishing.

Messer, P., Owen, G. & Casey, A. (2005) *Commander's Guide. Nutrition for Health and Performance – A Reference Guide for Commanders*. QinetiQ Report no. QINETIQ/KI/CHS/CR021120.

Ministry of Defence (2007a) *JSP 456 Defence Catering Manual*, Vol. 1. MoD.

Ministry of Defence (2007b) *JSP 456 Defence Catering Manual*, Vol. 2. MoD.

Ministry of Defence (2007c) *JSP 456 Defence Catering Manual*, Vol. 4. MoD.

Ministry of Defence (2007d) Feeding the forces on food's front line. www.mod.uk. Accessed February 2008.

Ministry of Defence (2007e) *Forces' chefs in challenge to serve up feast fit for front line*. www.mod.uk. Accessed January 2008.

Ministry of Defence. MoD website. Accessed February 2008.

Montain, S.J. & Young, A.J. (2003) Diet and physical performance. *Appetite*, **40**:255–267.

National Audit Office (NAO) (2006) *Smarter Food Procurement in the Public Sector: Case Studies*. Report by the Comptroller and Auditor General HC963-II session 2005–2006, 30 March 2006. London: The Stationery Office.

Nevola, V.R., Staerck, J. & Harrison, M. (2005) *Commanders' Guide to Fluid Intake During Military Operations in the Heat*. DLO & QinetiQ Defence Science and Technology Laboratory.

Private communication with Col. E. Budd, Commandant, Defence Food Services School, St Omer Barracks, Aldershot. 08 May 2006.

Private communication with head of catering Defence Food Services School & St Omer Barracks, 26/04/06.

Public Sector Food Procurement Initiative (2008) *Proportion of domestically produced food used by Goverment departments and also supplied to hospitals and prisons under contracts negotiated by NHS Supply Chain and HM Prison Service*. www.defra.gov.uk. Accessed February 2008.

Purple Foodservice Solutions. www.purplefoodservicesolutions.com. Accessed February 2008.

Tharion, W.J., Lieberman, H.R., Montain, S.J., Young, A.J., Baker-Fulco, C.J., Delany, J.P. & Hoyt, R.W. (2004) Energy requirements of military personnel. *Appetite*, **44**(1):47–65.

Thomas, C.D., Baker-Fulco, C.J., Jones, T.E. *et al.* (1993) *Nutritional Guidance for Military Field Operations in Temperate and Extreme Environment*. Natick: US Army Research Institute of Environmental Medicine.

Wells, J. (1994) *The Royal Navy. An Illustrated Social History 1870–1982*. Stroud: Alan Sutton.

Wickham Smith, C. (2006) Looking back at logistics. *DLO News – The Newsletter for the Defence Logistics Organisation*, **42**:38–41.

Index